GROUPS IN CONTEXT

Leadership and Participation in Small Groups

GERALD L. WILSON & MICHAEL S. HANNA
University of South Alabama

SECOND EDITION

McGRAW-HILL PUBLISHING COMPANY

New York   St. Louis   San Francisco   Auckland   Bogotá   Caracas   Hamburg   Lisbon   London
Madrid   Mexico   Milan   Montreal   New Delhi   Oklahoma City   Paris   San Juan   São Paulo
Singapore   Sydney   Tokyo   Toronto

GROUPS IN CONTEXT: LEADERSHIP AND PARTICIPATION IN SMALL GROUPS

3 4 5 6 7 8 9 0 **DOH DOH** 9 4 3 2 1

ISBN 0-07-557314-8

This book was set in Serif by Monotype Composition Company.
The editors were Hilary Jackson and Sheila H. Gillams;
the designer was Leon Bolognese;
the production supervisor was Laura Lamorte.
Arcata Graphics/Halliday was printer and binder.

Cover Photos: Top left, Rae Russel;
top right, Jim Pickerell / Stock, Boston;
bottom left, David M. Grossman;
bottom right, Richard Kalvar / Magnum.

Library of Congress Cataloging-in-Publication Data

Wilson, Gerald L., (date).
    Groups in context: leadership and participation in small groups /
    Gerald L. Wilson and Michael S. Hanna.
        p.   cm.
    Includes bibliographical references.
    ISBN 0-07-557314-8
    1. Small groups.   2. Decision-making, Group.   3. Leadership.
I. Hanna, Michael S., (date).   II. Title.
HM133.W52   1990
302.3′4—dc20
                                                89-13456

ABOUT THE AUTHORS

Gerald L. Wilson is Associate Professor of Communication at the University of South Alabama where he teaches courses in organizational communication. He received his B.S. from Bowling Green State University, his M.A. from Miami University, and his Ph.D. from the University of Wisconsin–Madison. Professor Wilson is a consultant to business and industry, working over the past ten years with such organizations as RCA Corporation, Jefferson National Life Insurance Company, Scott Paper Company, and International Paper Company.

Michael S. Hanna is Professor of Communication at the University of South Alabama. He has been a college-level teacher for some twenty-five years, teaching courses in interpersonal and organizational communication. Professor Hanna received his A.B. and M.A. from Central Missouri State College and his Ph.D. from the University of Missouri–Columbia. Over the past five years, Professor Hanna has trained more than 2500 working adults to improve their communication skills in such companies as International Paper, Monsanto, Ciba-Geigy, Del Monte, A. O. Smith Harvestore, and Teledyne Continental Motors.

Professors Hanna and Wilson have authored numerous articles for journals as well as papers for professional meetings. In addition, they have co-authored *Communicating in Business and Professional Settings*, 2nd Edition, and *Interpersonal Growth Through Communication*, 2nd Edition. Professor Hanna is also co-author of *Public Speaking for Personal Success*, 2nd Edition. Professor Wilson is co-author of *Organizational Communication*.

We dedicate this book to Robert Maurice Wilson and Kathryn Fahndrich Wilson, and to the memory of Russell Talbot Hanna and Marguerite Esser Hanna— our parents. Each of these four people valued achievement through disciplined effort and tried to teach it to us. We are very grateful.

CONTENTS

Preface xiii

PART I

Approaching Communication in Group Contexts   1

Chapter 1   **Introduction to Groups and Group Processes   2**

WHY STUDY GROUP COMMUNICATION?   5

GROUPS DEFINED   6

KINDS OF GROUP MEETINGS   7
  Information-Sharing Meetings   7
  Decision-Making Meetings   8
  Special-Events Meetings   8

COMMUNICATION: THE BASIC IDEA   9
  Source/Encoder   9
  Messages   10
  Channels   11
  Receiver/Decoder   11
  Feedback   12
  Noise   12
  Situation   14

UNDERSTANDING SOME BASIC DYNAMICS OF GROUPS   15
  Group Culture   15
  Group Norms   17
  Tasks and Relationships   19

THE SMALL GROUP AS AN INFORMATION PROCESSING-SYSTEM   22

ETHICAL RESPONSIBILITIES IN SMALL GROUP DISCUSSION   23
  Determine To Do Your Best   23
  Determine To Behave Rationally and with the Group's Good in Mind   23
  Make a Commitment To Fair Play   24
  Determine To Listen Carefully and To Participate Fully   24
  Take On a Participant-Analyst Role   25

Summary   25

Exercises   26

Notes   27

Recommended Readings   28

PART II
Preparing for Group Meetings   29

Chapter 2   **Preparing for Group Discussion**   30

SELECTING THE PARTICIPANTS   32

CONSIDERING DISCUSSION ISSUES   34
  Kinds of Discussion Issues   34
  Focusing the Discussion Issue   35

DECIDING ABOUT STRUCTURE   36
  Need for Order   36
  Time Considerations   37
  Group Size Considerations   37
  Group Members' Emotional Involvement   37
  Nature of the Task   38

SECURING INFORMATION   39
  Conducting an Inventory and Analysis of What You Know   40
  Gathering Additional Information   40
  Evaluating the Information   43
  Preparing the Material for Use   44

Summary   45

Exercises   46

Notes   46

Recommended Readings   47

Chapter 3   **Decision Making in Small Group Meetings**   48

INDIVIDUAL OR GROUP DECISION MAKING?   50

AGENDAS FOR SMALL GROUP DECISION MAKING   51
  Agendas Based On Reflective Thinking   51
  Brilhart-Jochem Ideation Criteria   55
  Ideal Solution Sequence   57
  Single Question Sequence   58
  Adapting the Agenda to the Group's Needs   60
  Using the Agenda Effectively   61

DISCUSSION TECHNIQUES   62
  Brainstorming   62
  Nominal Group Technique (NGT)   63

Buzz Groups 65
Quality Circles 66

METHODS OF DECIDING 68
Consensus 68
Compromise 68
Majority Vote 69
Decision by the Leader 69
Arbitration 70

Summary 70

Exercises 72

Notes 73

Recommended Readings 74

Chapter 4 **Understanding Verbal and Nonverbal Messages** 76

UNDERSTANDING VERBAL MESSAGES 79
The Concept of Meaning 79
Frame of Reference 81
Overlap of Experience 81
Denotative and Connotative Meaning 82

PROBLEMS WITH VERBAL COMMUNICATION 82
Perceptual Difficulties 83
Abstraction in Language Use 84
Labels and Language 85
Too Much Information 86
Too Little Information 87

INCREASING VERBAL EFFECTIVENESS 90

UNDERSTANDING NONVERBAL MESSAGES 92
The Functions of Nonverbal Messages 94

USING NONVERBAL CODES 96
Physical Environments 96
Appearance 98
Gesture, Posture, and Movement 99
Face and Eye Behavior 99
Vocalics 100
Use of Time 100
Problems in Using Nonverbal Messages 101

INCREASING NONVERBAL EFFECTIVENESS 102

LISTENING 104
The Components of the Listening Process 104

Listening Problems   105
Developing Listening Skills   108

Summary   112

Exercises   113

Notes   114

Recommended Readings   116

PART III
Participating in Group Meetings   117

Chapter 5   Encouraging Group Development and Evolution   118

MOTIVATIONS FOR MEMBER PARTICIPATION IN GROUPS   120
Attraction to Others in the Group   121
Attraction to Group Activities   122
Attraction to Group Goal   122
Attraction to Being Affiliated with the Group   123
Attraction to Needs Outside the Group   123
Encouraging Group Development: Motivation through Meeting Needs   124

PHASES IN GROUP DEVELOPMENT   124
Group Development   125
Fitting Together the Models of Group Development   129
*Encouraging Group Development: Application of Task-Group Development
    Theory*   130
Social Tension   133
Encouraging Group Development: Application of Social Tension Theory   135
Idea Development   137
*Encouraging Group Development: Application of the Spiral Model of Idea
    Development*   140

Summary   141

Exercises   142

Notes   143

Recommended Readings   144

Chapter 6   Roles and Role Emergence   146

THE CONCEPT OF ROLE   149

ROLE EMERGENCE IN SMALL GROUPS   150

ROLE CONFLICT   153

FUNCTIONAL ROLES IN SMALL GROUPS   154
Group Task Roles   154

Group Building and Maintenance Roles   157
Self-Centered Roles   160

Summary   162

Exercises   163

Notes   163

Recommended Readings   164

Chapter 7   **Leading Group Meetings**   166

LEADERSHIP AND LEADERS   169

PERSPECTIVES ON LEADER BEHAVIOR   171
Trait Perspective   171
Style Perspective   175
Functional Perspective   177
Situational Perspective   178
Contingency Perspective   179

CHARACTERISTICS OF THE EFFECTIVE LEADER   182

IMPROVING YOUR LEADERSHIP SKILL   184
Preparing for Leading a Meeting   185
Structuring and Guiding the Group Activity   187
Stimulating Creative and Critical Thinking   190

Summary   191

Exercises   192

Notes   193

Recommended Readings   195

Chapter 8   **Promoting Group Cohesiveness**   196

THE RELATIONSHIP BETWEEN COHESIVENESS
AND PRODUCTIVITY   198
Determinants of Cohesiveness   200

SOURCES OF MEMBER SATISFACTION IN GROUPS   202
Perceived Freedom to Participate   202
Perceived Progress Toward Group Goals   203
Status Consensus   203

PROMOTING COHESIVENESS   204
Leadership Style   204
Group Size   204
Effective Participation   206
Commitment to Group Goals   209

GROUPTHINK   212
Conditions That Promote Groupthink   214
Symptoms of the Groupthink Syndrome   214
Consequences of the Groupthink Syndrome   215

Summary   216

Exercises   218

Notes   219

Recommended Readings   220

Chapter 9   **Managing Relationships in Groups   222**

MEETING INTERPERSONAL NEEDS   225
Perception   227
Cognition   228
Motivation   228
The Ideas of William Schutz   229

SELF-DISCLOSURE, EMPATHY, AND TRUST   232
Self-Disclosure   232
Empathy   235
Trust   236

CREATING AN EFFECTIVE COMMUNICATION CLIMATE   237
Defensive Climates   238
Supportive Climates   240

COMMUNICATION NETWORKS   244

Summary   247

Exercises   248

Notes   249

Recommended Readings   250

Chapter 10   **Managing Conflict in the Group   252**

**EVOLUTION OF CONFLICT IN A SMALL GROUP:
A MEMBER'S REPORT   254**
First Meeting   254
Second Meeting   254
Third Meeting   254
Fourth Meeting   255

THE NATURE OF CONFLICT   255

THE EFFECT OF CONFLICT IN GROUPS   256
Functional and Dysfunctional Conflict   257

INTRAPERSONAL, INTERPERSONAL, AND INTERGROUP
CONFLICT 257
    Intrapersonal Conflict 258
    Interpersonal Conflict 258

SUBSTANTIVE AND AFFECTIVE CONFLICT 259

FUNCTIONS OF CONFLICT 260
    Conflict Increases Involvement 260
    Conflict Provides an Outlet for Hostility 260
    Conflict Promotes Cohesiveness 261
    Conflict Increases Group Productivity 261
    Conflict Increases the Chance of Genuine Commitment 261

SOURCES OF CONFLICT 262
    Ideational Conflict 262
    Status and Power Conflict 262
    Goal Conflict 263

MANAGING CONFLICT EFFECTIVELY 264
    Dysfunctional Conflict-Management Strategies 264
    Strategies for Managing Conflict 266

MANAGING INTERPERSONAL CONFLICT 268
    Preliminary Considerations 268
    Effective Confrontation in Groups 270
    Managing Ideational Conflict 274
    A Parting Plea 279

Summary 279

Exercises 281

Notes 282

Recommended Readings 284

PART IV
Analyzing Small Group Decision Making 285

Chapter 11 **Observing and Evaluating Groups 286**

OBSERVING SMALL GROUP INTERACTION 288
    Ground Rules for Observing Groups 289

INSTRUMENTS FOR COLLECTING DATA 289
    Interaction Observation Forms 290
    Role Analysis in Discussion 291
    Leadership Rating Form 293

OBSERVING GROUP PROCESSES 293

SELF-REPORT RATING SHEETS 294

Summary 300

Exercises 302

Recommended Readings 304

PART V
Preparing for and Participating in Public Group Meetings 307

Chapter 12 Groups in Public Settings 308

FORMATS FOR PUBLIC DISCUSSION 310
  Forum 310
  Panel 311
  Symposium 312
  Colloquium 312
  Selecting a Public Discussion Format 313

LEADING THE PUBLIC DISCUSSION 314

PLANNING THE CONFERENCE 315
  Decide Your Purpose 315
  Plan the Agenda 316
  Identify the Other Participants 316
  Select the Setting 316
  Plan for Mechanical Details 317
  Publish the Agenda with the Invitation 322
  Plan the Arrangement of Participants 323
  Arrange to Meet, Greet, Identify, and Introduce Participants 323
  Begin and End on Time 324
  Follow Through after the Meeting 324
  A Conference-Planning Checklist 325

Summary 325

Exercises 328

Notes 328

Recommended Readings 328

Glossary 329

Troubleshooting the Small Group 343

Permissions/Acknowledgments 353

Name Index 355

Subject Index 357

PREFACE

Our aim in writing *Groups in Context* was to provide a book that would meet the needs of discussion and small group communication courses that prepare students for decision-making groups in private and professional settings. What was needed, we thought, was a lively textbook that presented a balanced approach—a blend of current theory and research with practical skills and applications. Clearly, there is a relationship between theory and practice. A book that is only theoretical does not help the student. A book that is only a list of prescribed behaviors cannot help the student, either. Understanding and skill go hand in hand. To this end, we have carefully documented this book with both classic and current research. We have worked diligently to provide clear explanations of theoretical ideas. We have also richly illustrated the concepts with real-life examples from a broad range of contexts. We have become convinced, on the basis of our teaching, research, consulting experience, and use of the first edition, that such a book is much needed.

The title *Groups in Context* was selected to reflect our belief that the study of small group communication is best understood when the concepts are presented within specific contexts. We meet with others to make decisions in the workplace, in neighborhoods, in churches, in social groups, and in civic organizations. We illustrate the concepts we present with examples from these contexts.

Our use of context flows out of another concern. We want our students to communicate better in groups and to diagnose and act on decisions made about their group's process. To achieve this goal we believe it is necessary for the student to be able to make the connection between what he or she is studying and real-world groups. Our use of contexts to provide illustrations and examples of important principles shows students how to make that transfer.

Groups in Context focuses primarily on decision-making groups. We selected this focus for two reasons. First, the decision-making process is one of the most difficult tasks a group might undertake. It requires systematic analysis of the particular group situation, vigilance in the decision-making process, and well-developed communication and leadership skills. Second, decision making is one of the most prevalent of group activities. We *deliberate to plan and set policies* for groups in both our private and professional lives. The ability to carry out well the group decision-making activity is vital to the life of an educated person. It is an activity that most adults cannot avoid.

Our coverage of material and our sequencing of chapters creates a model of small groups as an information processing system. This model is presented in Chapter 1 so that students can see the layout of the book. We believe that this sequence fits many of the courses in small group communication. Since individual teachers vary in their approach to this course, we have written the chapters to be self-contained and thoroughly cross-referenced. Instructors can present them in any sequence that meets their particular course requirements.

We also carefully reviewed our experiences as teachers and consultants to discover what has helped our students function more effectively in groups. The features of this book are designed to respond to student needs on the basis of this careful review.

SPECIAL FEATURES

We think that certain features of this book will make it stand out in small group communication courses. We have made every effort to achieve an appropriate blend of *current theory and research* with practical explanations, skills, and applications.

We firmly believe that examples can make the difference between books that are useful in a classroom and books that are not. So we have filled our book with *examples from group contexts* to show how concepts work in actual group meetings.

Each chapter encourages students to analyze their own communication behavior, and place that *behavior in a group context*. For example, our book includes exceptionally *thorough coverage of leadership and conflict*, and not merely from the view of a designated leader but from all potential group participants.

We have been especially sensitive to the need to provide comprehensive coverage of the *current hot topics* in group communication, such as group culture, conflict management, and group development.

We pioneered the *Troubleshooting Guide* when it appeared in the first edition of our business and professional communication book. Such a guide is included at the end of this book, set off for readers by the bar at the trimmed edge. This guide is organized around the questions most commonly asked by our students and clients. We think students ought to be able to find answers to questions that are couched in language they use to talk about group problems. To use it, a reader need only identify a general category that a question falls into, turn to the questions in that category to find one close to their own question, then identify the page or pages on which the answer to it may be found. The positive feedback we have received about the Troubleshooting Guide suggests that students find it helpful.

FEATURES IN THE SECOND EDITION

We have updated our coverage of theory, research, and practice in this second edition. We have added new or greatly expanded sections on evaluating and preparing information by using questions to encourage research, fostering group development and lead-ins for public discussion. Beyond this, we have given added emphasis to ethical responsibilities of group members, the participant-analyst approach to studying groups, and the need for groups to evaluate their decisions critically. In all of this, we have tried to keep the student reader in mind, repeatedly asking ourselves: What does the student need to know about this concept? Can we provide a real example of that idea? Will the student reader be able to relate to this explanation?

ORGANIZATION OF THE BOOK

Part I: Approaching Communication in Group Contexts

This book is organized in deductive fashion. Part I, *Approaching Communication in Group Contexts*, clarifies what we mean by small group communication and provides a conceptual foundation for the rest of the book.

Chapter 1: Introduction to Groups and Group Processes In this first chapter we explain what is meant by groups and describe the communication process. We focus on how groups develop culture and norms as they seek to manage task and relationship concerns. Ethical responsibilities are important, too, if the group is to be effective.

Part II: Preparing for Group Meetings

The chapters that comprise Part II help the reader understand what is involved in and how to prepare for group meetings.

Chapter 2: Preparing for Group Discussion Chapter 2 examines concerns about the need for structure, selecting participants, and securing and preparing information for use.

Chapter 3: Decision Making in Small Group Meetings Chapter 3 highlights the importance of making choices about and planning for decision making. Should an individual or a group make the decision? How should the group organize its decision-making process? What special group techniques might facilitate the group's effort?

Chapter 4: Understanding Verbal and Nonverbal Messages Chapter 4 examines the nature of verbal and nonverbal messages. Recurring problems with these kinds of messages are explored, along with suggestions for handling them. Issues of message reception are presented, with suggestions for improving the receiving process.

Part III: Participating in Group Meetings

The six chapters in Part III work together to form a thorough treatment of the theories, applications, and skills that help a member participate more effectively in group meetings.

Chapter 5: Encouraging Group Development and Evolution Chapter 5 focuses on the evolutionary processes of groups. It begins with a discussion of the motivations for joining a group. This is followed by an explanation of the development of phases, social tension, and ideas.

Chapter 6: Roles and Role Emergence Chapter 6 presents the concept of roles and how they emerge in small decision-making groups. Group task roles, maintenance roles, and self-centered roles are explained. Conclusions are drawn about critical role functions for groups.

Chapter 7:   Leading Group Meetings   Chapter 7 focuses specifically on the leadership function in groups. Perspectives on leader behavior are examined and conclusions drawn from these regarding effective leadership. Concrete suggestions are provided for improving leadership to meet specific group needs.

Chapter 8:   Promoting Group Cohesiveness   Chapter 8 addresses cohesiveness as a central concern of group effectiveness. What can be done to enhance the cohesiveness of a group? How can cohesiveness be promoted? These two central issues are addressed in this chapter. Then, too, participants need to be aware of and guard against the effects of too much cohesiveness.

Chapter 9:   Managing Relationships in Groups   Chapter 9 takes up relational concerns of groups. Members have needs that must be understood and addressed. Beyond this a group must foster a relationship-building process. Members will want to understand and be able to facilitate appropriate relationships and climate.

Chapter 10:   Managing Conflict in the Group   Chapter 10 takes the perspective that conflict in groups can be managed so that it is functional. Whether the conflict is substantive or affective, understanding the source of the conflict and how to manage it effectively allows for a potential beneficial outcome.

Part IV: Analyzing Small Group Decision Making

Members can make greater contributions to their understanding of groups if they are able to analyze the process carefully. Part IV provides the understanding and tools to carry out analysis.

Chapter 11:   Observing and Evaluating Groups   Chapter 11 provides instruction in the process of observing and analyzing groups. Data-collecting instruments are provided to study interaction, roles, leadership, and the decision-making process.

Part V: Preparing for and Participating in Public Group Meetings

Chapter 12:   Groups in Public Settings   Chapter 12 rounds out our presentation of groups by addressing public discussion settings. Formats for public discussion are presented, along with specific suggestions for leading groups in this unique setting. A special public setting is the conference, for which a step-by-step guide is provided to aid in planning.

The Troubleshooting Guide

This guide is a reference tool designed for quick use by the reader. It covers a wide range of group communication problems discussed in the book and provides page numbers for easy location of solutions presented in the book.

LEARNING AIDS

Our effort has been to make the intent of our book, chapter by chapter, as clear as possible to our readers. Each chapter begins with a list of *objectives* that highlight the most important themes in the chapter. *Chapter summaries* at the end of each chapter recast the important ideas of the chapters into overview statements that should leave no doubt in the reader's mind about which are key ideas and which are not.

Over the years we have found that understanding of the material is facilitated by experiences and *exercises*. The first of these for each chapter can be used in an ongoing *journal assignment*. Others may be selected to emphasize particular concepts.

Recommended readings, a new feature in this edition, are found at the end of each chapter. These have been carefully selected with the aim of identifying the best, and in some cases most influential, works available in our literature. We think students should be made aware of the benchmarks in a discipline. We also think less well-known works, when they are especially relevant, should be brought to the reader's attention, and so we have mentioned some of them, too. We have also included a *glossary* of terms of small-group communication at the end of the book.

Resources for Instructors

An Instructor's Manual has been prepared to aid instructors in their teaching. It provides sample syllabi and assignments, and cases for problem solving, as well as other teaching materials.

ACKNOWLEDGMENTS

The following individuals have provided excellent suggestions as we revised this book. We are grateful, and we take this opportunity to express our sincere thanks.

Elizabeth S. Bishop, College of Lake County

Randall L. Bytwerk, Calvin College

Joann Keyton, University of South Alabama

Paul Reid, Syracuse University

William J. Schenck-Hamlin, Kansas State University

We do not want to overlook our obligation to the many colleagues who helped us as we prepared the first edition for publication. We remain indebted to these people:

Delindus R. Brown, University of Florida

Ronald K. Burke, Syracuse University

RoLayne S. DeStephen, Sinclair Community College

William E. Holdridge, Southern Illinois University

Virginia Kidd, California State University, Sacramento

Margaret L. McLaughlin, University of Southern California

John T. Morello, Simpson College

Marjorie K. Nadler, Miami University

James E. Norwig, Louisiana Technical University

Patricia J. Palm, Mankato State University

Gerry Philipsen, University of Washington

Richard Quianthy, Broward Community College

David W. Shepard, Ball State University

Charles H. Tardy, The University of Southern Mississippi

David E. Walker, Jr., Middle Tennessee State University

Mary O. Wiemann, Santa Barbara City College

Authors write manuscripts, which are then turned into books by extraordinarily able, dedicated people employed by the publishing company. We especially want to thank our editors, Kathleen Domenig, Hilary Jackson, Peter Labella, Sheila Gillams, and Roth Wilkofsky, who contributed their exceptional expertise and knowledge to this project.

Finally, we thank our wives, Lin and Nancy, and our children for their patience, understanding, and encouragement during the revision of this book.

GERALD L. WILSON
MICHAEL S. HANNA

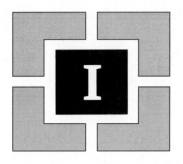

Approaching Communication in Group Contexts

CHAPTER 1

Introduction to Groups and Group Processes

OBJECTIVES

After reading this chapter you should be able to:

Specify in your own words the personal and professional advantages that accrue from the study of group communication.

Specify and explain the defining characteristics of decision-making groups: size, goal orientation, and mutual influence.

Identify and describe three different categories of group meetings, and explain the differentiating characteristics of each: information-sharing meetings, decision-making meetings, and special-events meetings.

Recall and explain a basic model of the communication process, including these components: source/encoder, messages, channels, receiver/decoder, feedback, noise, and situation.

Explain and provide examples of three different categories of noise: physical, semantic, and systemic.

Explain the concept of group culture.

State in your own words what is meant by norm; suggest how an unproductive norm might be changed.

Distinguish between the task and relationship dimensions of group communication.

Specify and explain a personal code of ethics for group discussion.

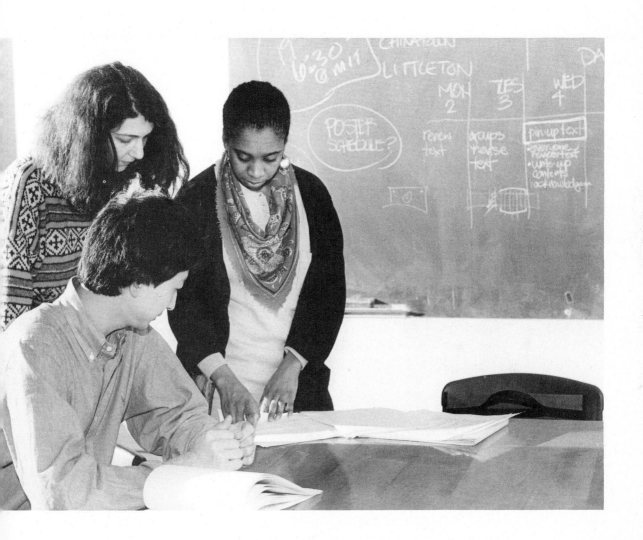

What a useful thing you are doing for yourself when you study small group communication! Learning to be an effective contributor in group meetings is certainly among the really important skills you will need in your professional and personal life.

In *Working Smart '87* John J. Franco, the president of Learning International (formerly Xerox Learning Systems), argued that, today, business is increasingly done in the team mode, and that the higher a person rises in an organization, the more work he or she will do in meetings. Franco's argument is borne out by the fact that the average chief executive officer in the United States spends about six hours of every day working on or participating in meetings.

We know, too, that the best way to enhance upward mobility in a working organization is to become an effective group participant, someone who is skillful at giving the group leadership when the situation warrants.[1] That stands to reason. Groups, whether they be a business meeting, conference, or quality circle, are the best place to meet and work with (and impress) individuals from other parts of your organization. Groups provide you with the best opportunity to shine as a decision maker. Groups give you the best organizational setting to demonstrate your political skill, your analytical ability, and your emotional stability.

Of course, the business community is only a part of your total life. Your study of group communication will also be of benefit in your personal and social life. You will be a member of many groups across the course of your life; you are already a member of many groups. You may be a member of a church-related group. You certainly are a member of more than one informal, social group. You are undoubtedly a member of a family group. And undoubtedly both the social groups and the family group meet to make decisions. Each of these groups provides you with opportunities to make some productive contribution, enhance the quality of others' lives, and cement your relationships with the other group members.[2] Your study of group communication is designed to help you perfect the task-related and social skills that will be most useful to you in these pursuits.

Groups are everywhere. Groups are at school, at church, at work, in your social life, in your avocational and recreational life, and in your private life. If you think about it, you will discover that you are a member in good standing of many more groups than you might have realized. You even have cards to prove your membership in some groups. And for every group that issues a card, you may belong to a dozen groups that do not.

Yet there is also evidence that not all the people who participate in groups have the required skill and knowledge to make group meetings productive. Many executives complain about the number of meetings they have to attend. They wish they knew how to get more out of those meetings, and how to make them less of a waste of time. Some executives will admit that they actually duck out of meetings, even though they know that the meetings are important. Others delegate leadership of the meetings to their subordinates.

Clearly, with so much involvement in group behavior, you cannot afford not to be a skillful member. You want what that skill will bring, and every one of the groups to which you belong will benefit because you have it. What a useful thing you have done to decide to study small group communication!

WHY STUDY GROUP COMMUNICATION?

Definite advantages come to those who learn to be successful and skillful group participants. At the personal level, if you develop your skills in groups you stand to gain enormous benefits, which range from monetary and position-enhancement rewards to your own self-actualization.[3] The better you are in group contexts, the more likely you are to accomplish your own goals and projects. The more of your goals and projects you accomplish, the better you feel about yourself. Thus, even at the personal level, group communication skills are valuable.

At a second level, you can make a very important contribution to the success of any group you join. Not everyone understands the complex nature of group processes, and fewer still have the understanding to be able to intervene in behalf of better group decision making and more successful participation by individual members. These are the conditions (at least, two of the conditions) that are extremely important to group success. If, because of your study of small group communication, you can help a group member to participate, and if you can intervene to help the group make decisions more effectively, your contribution will have been significant. If the group's success is important to you (why would you be a member if it weren't?), your ability to help the group achieve success is certainly going to be rewarding personally, too.

At a third level, you can make a better contribution to the world you live in if you have better group communication skills. Does that statement sound idealistic or altruistic? Then consider that the decision-making processes that run our society take place every day in small groups, and that those groups do not always include highly placed government or business officials.

Consider the ongoing problem that most communities face in striving to maintain high-quality education for their children. Often groups of ordinary citizens organize— as they did in one Alabama community—to do something about the situation. To some, the schools seemed too small, in poor repair, badly lighted, not air-conditioned. Private citizens met in small groups to propose solutions to meet this growing concern, and their effort had a significant influence upon the community. A referendum was proposed to increase tax revenue for the schools. The point is that betterment of the community is part of the responsibility of its citizens, and small group commuication is a major tool for groups of citizens to achieve their ends.

Groups and group behaviors are fundamental to your world and culture. Groups meet for personal growth, for study and learning, for cooperative activity, for public discussion, for problem solving, and for countless other tasks. The list of groups that meet to solve problems is equally extensive.

Yet most of us take groups and group behaviors for granted in that we fail to perceive and understand what is happening in them. Perhaps even more important, we fail to perceive and understand how what we are personally doing affects what does or does not happen in a group. Rarely do we consider our performance in group settings and how to make it more effective. This kind of neglect is unfortunate. The better you perform in group contexts, the more likely you are to be successful in terms of personal satisfaction and achievement of your goals.

GROUPS DEFINED

The communication process in groups is so pervasive in our society that we need to focus and limit our consideration if this book is to be of reasonable length. After all, communication takes place in all kinds of groups. And it happens all the time, in an amazingly complex process of variables that can have an effect on accuracy and efficacy. So some terms need to be defined at this point. The purpose of doing so is to limit the arena in which you will be working in this course and to develop a basic understanding of the common characteristics of groups.

Group

We will understand the terms *group* and *decision-making group* to be nearly synonymous. These terms will mean a collection of three or more individuals who interact about some common problem or goal so that they exert mutual influence over one another. A small decision-making group—the kind that is of most interest to us—is one in which members communicate with one another face to face, aware of one another's roles. The three key elements in this definition are size, goal orientation, and mutual influence.

Size   By this definition, two people cannot be a group. When three people join together they create a unique environment because of the ability of two of the members to unite to exert pressure on the other. That is not possible with only two people. Almost everything that may be said about two persons interacting can apply to groups, but this book focuses upon those variables that influence group processes. (Along the way, ideas about interpersonal communication are integrated, of course. This book could not be written without doing so.)

Goal Orientation   A group usually shares some problem or wishes to deal with a commonly shared need or to achieve some commonly shared goal. By this requirement, a collection of people who do not experience a need to work jointly on some project does not constitute a group. As you will see shortly, this simple idea can be pretty important. If you want a word to describe a gathering of individuals who are not a group, you could call them a collection. You may be amused that some authors refer to such a collection of people as a heap.

Mutual Influence   The interactions and behaviors of individual group members influence all the members of the group. This means that the members of a group exert mutual influence. They listen to one another. They talk with one another. They attempt to affect one another's attitudes, thinking, and behavior. They influence the collective mentality and the collective behavior of the group. They respond to each other in a variety of ways. The members of a group are interdependent. They are related by talk and intention and they interact from a shared motive.

It is because of this mutual influence and the uniqueness of each group member that the group itself is a "new experience" each time it meets. Countless examples of collections that *are* groups and countless examples of others that are not could be offered. But perhaps these comparisons will help to clarify the kinds of groups this book will focus upon. By our definition, five students who meet by prior agreement to study for an examination would qualify as a decision-making group. Five students who bump into one another outside a classroom building, and who pause to chat for a moment between classes, would not be a decision-making group. In the first example, people share a common goal or problem, and probably have an awareness of one another's roles. An ad hoc committee appointed by the president of the student government association to make a recommendation about dates for the upcoming freshman mixer would also be a decision-making group.

On the other hand, when several old friends agree to go fishing and then do so, they are not a decision-making group. They may have some personal goals, but it is not clear that they share them. (If they actually met to plan the trip, they would qualify as a decision-making group for that meeting.)

To provide another example of the differences between groups that are not decision making and groups that are, suppose four faculty members and two students meet to plan the fall semester of the coming year. They would be a decision-making group. But if four faculty members and twenty students gather to celebrate the end of a rigorous semester by holding a picnic in the park, they would not be a decision-making group.

With this idea of what we mean by group in mind, it is possible to identify some common kinds of group meetings that occur across a variety of contexts.

KINDS OF GROUP MEETINGS

Information-Sharing Meetings

One kind of group meeting, found in families, learning groups, work groups, and groups generally, is the *information-sharing meeting*. This type of meeting occurs on a regular basis, with a predictable agenda format and a clear set of procedural traditions.

To illustrate the information-sharing meeting, consider the regular Monday morning conference of department heads at a local hospital. In that meeting they follow a predictable agenda—announcements, ongoing concerns, assignments for the week, and adjournment. Such a meeting allows members of the group to express themselves, to be informed of the activities and events of the other members of the group, to get and give assistance, to clarify the group's goals, to clarify their own short-term goals, and to establish and maintain their working relationships with one another. Routine meetings happen in corporations, churches, schools, service clubs, social fraternities and sororities, and any other organization or agency in which people do business together over a long period of time.

Decision-Making Meetings

A second very important group experience you will almost certainly encounter is the *decision-making meeting*. This experience can occur in ad hoc (one meeting only, or limited numbers of meetings) and ongoing groups. Task groups meet to focus upon some particular concern. They typically follow a loose agenda, and they are very free to deviate from that agenda. It should be noted here that effective leadership will monitor the progress of a decision-making group through the various stages in the evolution of an agenda designed to get the task accomplished in the allowed time. But the leadership will almost certainly not hold the group members to a lock-step commitment to some prearranged agenda. To do so would be a disastrous hampering of the group's decision-making creativity.

Decision-making group experiences are the most interesting and most common of all group meetings. They are found in families, therapeutic groups, and work groups. In fact, routine information-sharing meetings may evolve into decision-making meetings. For example, the regular Monday meeting group of hospital department heads may identify that it has to confront some particular task. The group may realize that it has to generate a holiday schedule, or make a decision about the problem of sudden higher-than-normal power and heat consumption, or generate some creative means to reduce hospital spending by 3 percent in the next quarter. In these examples, the routine meeting group becomes a decision-making group with a particular problem to consider. Its behaviors will be governed by the new context it has imposed upon itself.

Special-Events Meetings

A third, and somewhat less frequent, kind of group experience you are likely to encounter is the *special-events meeting*. A group that calls itself into conference once each spring, for example, is having an annual meeting. This is a special event. A group of employees being entertained by a sales representative from one of the company's suppliers—typically called a sales meeting—is involved in a special-event meeting. Individuals who gather at a resort hotel to attend a seminar on fund-raising methods for nonprofit organizations are involved in a special-event meeting. The special-event experience is different from the other two in some very particular ways, but it is also sufficiently like the others—it may involve information sharing and/or decision making—to allow you to find some overlap in the impact that the context can have on group behaviors and performance.

Thus groups work within three very different yet very predictable contexts; these contexts tend to overlap in some ways; and it is useful to identify the experiences that are common. Groups abound in private and professional life. Groups are so important to our culture that they are fundamental to the culture's pursuits and to our own pursuits as well.

COMMUNICATION: THE BASIC IDEA

When many people think about communication, they get a mental image of something as simple as water flowing through a pipe. They have the basic idea that—assuming there are no blockages in the pipe—once the water is put into one end of the pipe and sent on its way, it will get to the other end essentially intact.

If your own private model of communication is something like this, then it is very seriously limited. For communication is far more complex than can be exemplified by such a model.

In every communication event, such as one-to-one talk, or a small task-group meeting, or even a public speaking situation, everyone involved in the event is both sending and receiving messages—a variety of messages, and through a variety of channels—at the same moment. Communication is not a static thing; it is ongoing and continuous.

To illustrate this idea, consider a business meeting of a local service club. A particular member is speaking to the group about upgrading the facilities of a inner-city youth center. She is intent on the task of getting members to consider her ideas seriously. So she has taken on a slightly impersonal and formal style. Even in such a situation, this group member is at once both a source and receiver of ideas. Although she is doing all the talking, and although she is primarily in control of the timing and pacing of the talk, she is still receiving a number of messages from her fellow club members.

Perhaps you can imagine the group sitting around a table. The responses of members are easily noticed. Group members fidget, they squirm, they whisper, they take notes, they listen attentively, they plan the evening's entertainment, they read over their notes, they yawn—they live. In doing so, they communicate something to the speaking member. Hence she is both a source and a receiver.

So a contemporary communication model is something quite different from a model that shows a straight-line relationship between speaker and listener. It is patterned after some of the more contemporary ideas about what happens in dyads (that is, two people) and groups. This model is displayed in Figure 1.1. It includes the key elements source/encoder, messages, channels, receiver/decoder, feedback, noise, and situation. Each of these is important enough to need a working definition. This basic communication model applies in nearly all group contexts, and describes every communication situation.

Source/Encoder

The communication process begins with the source/encoder. The *source* is the location of an idea. In group communication this is a person, obviously, generating ideas at a fantastic rate. Each of those ideas must be encoded—that is, translated into words and behavior. That is why we identify this first part of the process as the source/encoder. The source has to put ideas into codes. A *code* is a set of symbols used to express an idea. One form of code, for example, is a series of dots and dashes—Morse code. In our group communication situation, the codes are the English language and such nonverbal

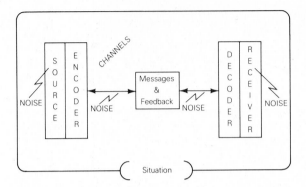

FIGURE 1.1
A Transactional Model of Communication

messages as facial expression, body position, vocal characteristics, and clothing. Each of these nonverbal elements utilizes symbols to encode ideas as surely as does English.

Messages

Messages are arrangements of symbols that have meaning for the source. That is, the source selects and arranges symbols in such a way that they create information. The source hopes the receiver will understand, too.

An interesting thing about messages—one that is extremely important to you and a fundamental assumption to this book—is that messages in themselves do not have meaning. Put another way, meaning does not obtain in the messages we send and receive. Meaning obtains in the people who send and receive the messages. Understanding is a function of assigning meaning, and of the message exchange itself. Thus communication has an inherently transactional nature. Meaning is attached to symbols through a process in which one person initiates a message, the other person or persons take in the message and respond, and the initiator notes the response. Meaning is what *you* make of the messages throughout the communication transaction with the other person. As you will see, losing sight of this idea gets people into a great deal of trouble in their day-to-day communication. It is certainly one of the principal sources of trouble for groups.

Consider that the meanings one group member might have for the codes used to transmit an idea may be different from those of other group members. For example, when one group began talking about male-female relationships, a female member seemed to become particularly angry and emotionally involved. Later the group discovered that she was processing the information through the memory of an intensely unpleasant experience with a male. A person's understanding of the meaning of a code he or she uses lies not in the word itself, but in the head of the user. In other words, when someone uses a word, that person's translation is based on what he or she takes the word to mean. This idea is illustrated in situations where you and another person use a word differently. Who is "correct"? Both of you are correct from your own perspectives. The meaning is in the person and not in the word itself.

Channels

In order for the source/encoder to communicate, the ideas that are encoded must be transmitted as message*s* through channel*s*. A *message* is the idea or combination of ideas expressed to a receiver. It is created by the arrangement of symbols that are meaningful to the source/encoder. *Channels* are the medium through which the message is sent. Thus the channels may be aural channels (such as speech sounds, music, pausing, and phrasing) or they may be visual channels (such as gestures and facial expressions). The channels may be any combination of phenomena that impinge upon your perceptual mechanisms. You see, you hear, you touch, you smell things, and you taste them. These five senses allow you to establish some kind of relationship with the world outside you. They suggest the communication channels at issue in the model in Figure 1.1.

Notice that up to this point, the letter *s* in the words *channels* and *messages* has been consistently italicized. This is to emphasize that you rarely communicate through only one channel, and that you rarely communicate only one message. Consider a group leader, who is trying to motivate sales managers to strive harder. He might be especially careful to pick the right words. But he would also try to maintain direct eye contact, raise the volume of his voice slightly above normal, use more emphasis than normal, and so forth. He is using multiple channels to enhance the reception of his message by the group.

Use of multiple channels sometimes complicates the effort to create clear messages. What you communicate through multiple channels are multiple messages. Just as you rarely use only one channel, you rarely send only one message. What you *say* has message value, of course. But so does what you wear, how you use space, the gender cues you provide, and so forth. These messages are the substance of any communication event. Understanding this fact about messages alerts us to a benefit and a problem. When multiple messages convey the same idea, they reinforce one another, adding impact to the message. On the other hand, when they contradict one another, they send mixed messages, creating confusion. Suppose a group member uses words to say that her idea is important, but her tone of voice and other nonverbal symbols suggest the opposite. What will the impact of these mixed messages be? Which message will be believed?

Receiver/Decoder

Just as a source has to encode ideas into messages in order to send them through channels, the *receiver* of the messages must decode them in order to process the ideas. Thus we include in our model of the communication event language that appears to be opposite from that of the source/encoder. There is a sense, of course, in which this approach is correct. When you are sending, you want the other person to receive. You will certainly be better able to decode a message from a group member if it is encoded into English.

In a larger sense, however, the use of opposites—source/encoder and receiver/decoder—creates a false impression that the transactional model is very much like the linear model. This is not true. Each person in the communication event is at once source and receiver. The arrowheads on both ends of the line between source/encoder and receiver/decoder in Figure 1.1 serve to make this point—they symbolize a simultaneous, two-way flow of messages.

Feedback

Feedback is information that is the receiver's response to the source's message. The arrowheads, identified earlier in discussing the simultaneous exchange of messages between source and receiver, make possible the notion of feedback. *Feedback* is the idea that, so far as communication systems are concerned, one participant's response helps to correct and control another's message by an ongoing feedback process. For example, consider, Susan, a member of a program committee at her church. Imagine that as she speaks to the group she becomes too distant and verbally flat. She may soon notice the other members of the group shifting in their chairs, yawning, gazing out the window, and looking glassy-eyed. She has lost them and the feedback is telling her that. Susan has a choice if she is being sensitive to her colleagues. So the feedback has served the purpose of correcting and controlling her behavior. Although the response of group members may differ in kind, feedback is an important part of the communication transaction. Without it the success and morale of the group would surely suffer.

Noise

You could say that the communication event is a pretty noisy one. If anything in the situation tends to damage the fidelity of message exchange between group members, whatever it is, it may be called noise. Thus there are at least two, and possibly three, separate and distinct categories of noise.

Physical noise is that which exists in a situation, but outside the participants. The clattering and humming of the air-conditioning system produces noise. The unnecessary chill in the room temperature that distracts you is a form of noise. The glaring light that causes you to "take cover" while someone is trying to make a point is a form of noise by our definition. If something is outside group participants, and if it gets in the way of the fidelity of message exchange, call it physical noise.

A second category of noise can be called *semantic noise.* This kind of noise is inside the individuals involved in a communication event. It includes all the distortions of reality that occur as a result of being human, including such things as imposing one's own reality on the talk of others.

You can call this kind of semantic noise to mind by imagining these events. A paper-manufacturing firm was in deep financial trouble. One of the reasons for their difficulty was a very high-paid labor force. Another factor was a depressed economy that resulted in fewer orders. A group of top managers met to decide on a strategy for coping with the problem. As soon as one manager uttered the words "union" and "strike," productive decision making was impossible. With the possibility of the firm folding if the union chose to strike, the words "union" and "strike" introduced a great deal of semantic noise.

Semantic noise can be created in a variety of ways. One of the typical ways is through the use of emotionally charged words. When a member uses a racial slur, semantic noise may be created. If a member attaches highly judgmental labels to ideas, semantic noise may be created. The potential for semantic noise is great in groups, and it is something you must be prepared to deal with. This noise can sometimes be reduced by merely avoiding the emotionally charged words. Yet in the case of "union" and "strike," some of the tension-reducing strategies discussed in Chapter 10 might be employed.

Similarly, group members always bring to each communication event such things as their own feelings, wants or expectations, and intentions. They bring with them their attitudes and beliefs. They bring with them a constantly shifting latitude of acceptance for other people and their ideas. They bring with them images of themselves and images of the people with whom they communicate. These are always there, and they often generate semantic noise.

We want to add what may seem obvious. Not all semantic noise is equally damaging to communication fidelity. For example, a group member may bring to a group meeting some noise that has little or nothing to do with the other group members. The person may be preoccupied with personal thoughts, such as a pending exam or a car, and therefore attend in a different way. His or her noise may not be at all damaging.

Every group communication event includes two dimensions: a *content dimension*—the behavior and ideas related to the task—and a *relationship dimension*—the behavior and ideas related to how people are connected socially. Each of these dimensions has potential as a source of noise. Semantic noise related to content—topics and ideas—generally involves words. This is the kind of noise illustrated by the example of the words "union" and "strike." But another kind of noise among group members is more often expressed nonverbally—the message exchange is left to such nonverbal cues as body posture, facial expression, tone of voice, and eye contact—but that is always present and very frequently noisy. This noise is generated through cues about the relationship—a relational definition that, perhaps, one or more of the group members believes to be inappropriate.

To illustrate this second kind of semantic noise, suppose that you are attending a hastily called meeting of your work group. Your boss says to the group, "I have noticed a lot of complaining around here lately. I want to talk with you about what is going on!" How she says this may communicate a number of things about how she is defining her relationship to you. Perhaps she wants to remind you that she is the boss, and that her job is to give orders and yours is to take them. Perhaps she is concerned about the problems that her employees are experiencing and would like to help. Thus the relationship dimension of the communication event allows you to know how to understand the content dimension. It is simultaneous with the content dimension, and it is one kind of metacommunication (that is, communication about communication). As you will see, in group communication events, the relationship between the task, or content, dimension and the relationship dimension, is very important indeed. And the point is that the relationship between the two can be a source of semantic noise.

A third category of noise that often produces trouble for a group is called *systemic noise*. Systemic noise occurs as a product of the communication system in which any particular communication event might occur. It is a noise that affects a group but is generated by forces outside the group. For example, many decision-making groups meet as part of the expectations of some larger organization of which they are part. A sales and marketing department might meet as a group, for example, to hammer out its quota schedule for the next two quarters. Suppose it does that, and after a lengthy process, agrees on a tentative quota system, only to discover that the production group cannot accommodate that plan. Such a situation might create frustration and error in the message exchange. An even better example is the loss, by an inexperienced worker in the interoffice mail system, of a communiqué from the sales department to the production group manager, whose office is in an adjoining building. Inexperience allows for good examples of systemic noise. As you will see, systemic noise can be very perplexing to groups.

Situation

Finally, in order for the communication event to make sense, it has to occur within some situation. The box around the model in Figure 1.1 is marked *situation*. It is important for you to understand what is implied by that word. First, of course, all the marked elements of the communication process happen in the situation. But the situation includes much, much more. It includes all the information available to a group at that point in their communication event. It includes such outside data as the temperature, lighting conditions, and noise in the environment; the texture and color of the walls; and the acoustics in the room. Perhaps more important, it also includes everything that the parties in the event brought to the event. This means their motives, their fears and hopes, their self-confidence, their skill with language, their images of one another, and the like.

The situation also has to have a beginning and an ending. Interaction sequences, like word sequences, must be grouped if they are to make sense. They never occur in isolation. To illustrate how this idea works, imagine two members of a management team reporting their experience of a fight they witnessed in the Monday morning meeting. Nancy says, "I couldn't believe Linda this morning. She was really riding Phil about those sales figures." John replies, "I didn't see it that way at all. I thought she was being quite reasonable. Phil was the person who was being unreasonable. He ought to have those figures and be able to explain them." Nancy continues, "I agree that he ought to have those figures, but Linda was really being testy today! I don't think that kind of behavior is called for in a team meeting." John replies, "I think Linda calls them like she sees them. She is a good team player. Remember that just last week . . . ."

Each event exists in relation to what came before it. What is happening in a group meeting at any given time is related to the events that surround it. In our illustration, Nancy observed the event, began to understand it from its place in the sequence of events, and drew conclusions about what was happening. Her conclusions were that Linda was being testy and that the situation did not warrant this behavior. John, on the other hand, selected a different sequence of events as relevant. When he made sense out of what was going on he came to a different conclusion—that Linda's behavior was necessary, perhaps even justified.

Who was correct, Nancy or John? The matter of correctness in this case depends on perspective. How the incident is understood will depend on *where* you start to understand it. This idea is called *punctuation,* and it is a very important idea for you to understand. A group member who understands that he or she may be punctuating the sequence differently from other members may check out his or her perception. A member who does not understand punctuation may not think that it is possible for others to see the situation differently.

A model of communication that shows a frozen moment in time and space, and that includes all the elements in a single communicative moment—source/encoder, messages, channels, feedback, receiver/decoder, noise, situation—must be understood to be always in a state of flux, changing to meet the whims or caprices of the individuals involved, as well as to accommodate the constantly changing world in which it exists. It seems useful to look at the communicative moment from a different perspective—what happens inside an individual communicator. This perspective is very important to group members, for it makes clear that merely because one person defines something in a particular way does not mean the others will understand! (More will be said about this issue in Chapter 4, when verbal and nonverbal messages are discussed.)

UNDERSTANDING SOME BASIC DYNAMICS OF GROUPS

If you want to prepare for a small group discussion, either as a participant or as a group leader, you must understand some of the basic dynamics of groups. How a group evolves the rules by which its members play bears directly on participation in that group at every level. These two categories (group culture and group norms) are very closely interrelated. Beyond these, you will want to understand the two basic dimensions of group communication that are evolving: task and relationship.

Group Culture

Just as societies evolve cultures, so do the subgroups within those societies. Your dictionary will define the term *culture* in a way that is similar to ours: "The sum total of ways of living built up by a group of human beings and transmitted from one generation to another."[4] That definition bears closer examination, for it implies the components in a group's dynamics.

A culture, including a group's culture, generates from the values or ideals of a group, as agreed upon over time by its members, and from the customs or ways of doing things that the members have traditionally followed. These may be helpful to a culture, or they may be harmful. To illustrate at the grossest level, American culture values personal independence. You can find evidence of this value in such language as "self-made man" and "rugged individualist." Our cultural mythology and fantasy are full of the value system that surrounds personal independence.

At the same time, Americans drive their cars everywhere. They don't pay much attention to city advertising campaigns that aim at getting them to use mass transportation facilities, or at least to share in car pools for their daily trips into town and back home. On any given morning in any city in America, you can see many more individuals using their cars than you can see groups. These observations provide an example of a cultural ideal (personal independence) coupled with a behavioral custom (one person driving a personal automobile to work). This is the traditional way of doing things. It was probably the most useful way of doing things during the early stages of development of the American nation, when neighbors were many miles apart and connected only by horse cart and dirt roads. An individual under those circumstances had to be rugged and self-sufficient.

But in our time such independence may be counterproductive. For the society as a whole, thousands of individual drivers honking their way to the center of the city are damaging because of such effects as traffic jams, air and noise pollution, and energy inefficiency. For the individuals involved, the symbol of rugged individualism probably costs more in time and convenience, and certainly more in actual operating costs, than would using mass transit. Notwithstanding these arguments, Americans cling tenaciously to the custom of driving to work alone.

Notice that this custom (to preserve personal independence by driving a personal automobile to work) enjoys the collective support of the society. Indeed, all cultural artifacts of value or custom evolve out of the collective support of the members.[5] You can say that they evolve as the result of trial and error through the functioning of human interaction.

At a much more focused level, these same ideas hold for the lives of small groups. That is, small groups evolve ideals and traditional ways of doing things, and those ideals and traditions become their culture.

For example, six engineers who work for a large papermaking company in Oregon were all appointed to their positions within a six-month period. They were hired to help run an automated plant that makes pasteboard for boxes. The plant was described by one of the six as "state of the art," meaning that all the equipment and all the processes used to make paper from pulpwood at that location were technologically sophisticated and advanced. Naturally, the individual engineers identified with one another immediately. They were all relatively new. They were all relatively young. They were all highly trained, but they were all relatively inexperienced. They had all been hired by the company to meet the same company goals to make paper as well, as fast, and as efficiently as possible. As these six worked together to make decisions, they began to evolve a group ideal. Their performance became as sophisticated and efficient as they perceived their plant to be.

To accomplish this informal group goal, the six engineers began to meet regularly after hours to discuss ways of ensuring excellent on-the-job performance. Their thinking was that they might be able to help one another do their jobs better. They decided that group performance would improve if they planned to cover one another's assignments. Each member learned not only his or her own job but one of the other group members' jobs as well. In this way they were able to minimize the effect if someone from their group became ill or had to travel away from the plant. In addition, the members became intolerant of what they began to call halfway measures. By using the term "halfway measure," the group enforced the emerging idea that each member was to do his or her best on every assignment. "Just good enough" would not be good enough for any member of the group.

In time, the members decided that it would be wise to double-check one another's written work. They read, criticized, and sometimes edited technical reports, major capital requests to management, and the like, as a way of helping one another achieve clear and persuasive writing. The effect was unusually high-quality output by group members, but problems did arise. The double-checking was somewhat time consuming. And the members began to depend on one another for editorial help as a necessary part of the procedure before a member sent a report forward to management. Thus this group of six engineers evolved a group value of quality, and decided on a plan to ensure that quality. Their plan was beneficial in some ways and harmful in others.

Group Norms

One way to define *group norms* is to say that they are standards of behavior that groups impose upon their members. Thus group norms are the group rules—the dos and don'ts that result from the interactions of group members over time. A norm, then, is a standard model, or pattern of behavior. Group norms seem to occur (that is, they evolve out of the group members' trial and error) in at least three areas of group life: social, procedural, and task. Groups learn to work together, in other words, and they develop a history and tradition. They do this as a result of their own interactions. Members learn from one another "how it's supposed to be" as a result of trial and error and from the rewards and punishments that the group can give an individual. Examples of norms in a decision-making group are the understanding about how long an individual should talk, what kind of language members are permitted to use, and how members might be confronted about their unacceptable behavior. Norms evolve out of the trial-and-error process as group members interact. Over time, members of a group learn to conform to these behavioral conventions, some of which are never specifically identified. Norms result from group interaction and they directly affect whether or not a group is successful.

The term *norm* comes from the word *normal*. Behavior is normal if it seems to fall within the guidelines that a particular group accepts as appropriate for itself—guidelines that the group validates by consensus. The important thing to remember about norms is that they evolve only if they receive collective support.

Jack Gibbs[6] describes norms as having three attributes. First, norms include *collective evaluation*. This implies that a group holds a norm if members share a belief that persons ought or ought not to act in a certain way. If one or two members held such a belief, it would not be a norm. This raises the issue of how many members it *does* take to call a belief a collective belief. There is really no rule that can be applied here, but it certainly takes more than a few of a group's members.

A second attribute of norms that Gibbs described is *collective expectation*. Collective expectation refers to predictions that a group has as to what a person *will* do, rather than what he or she *ought* to do. An expectation is created prior to an act. In a group context, the collective expectation of what members will do creates part of the group's "truth." This is different from collective evaluation in that we may believe that people should not come late to meetings, but we actually expect that they may be several minutes tardy. Our belief about the norm is different from our expectation.

A third attribute of norms is that they produce *reaction to a behavior*. A norm exists if a member behaves in a way contrary to it and another member reacts to the behavior. The member reacts and other members support that reaction by either agreeing with it or remaining silent—that is, by not objecting to the member's reaction to the behavior. An example of a reaction to a behavior will clarify this idea. Suppose a group of managers is accustomed to processing problems in quiet and dispassionate terms. We would discover that there is a norm for this if a member objects to the behavior of a new member who believes that loud and passionate opposing argument about ideas and proposals is the best way to air the issues. The norms the group sanctions prohibit loud and passionate advocacy. You can identify the norm by the fact that one member objected to the new member's behavior and no other member countered the objection.

A norm, then, is a socially sanctioned behavioral limitation that evolves out of the interactions of a group on the basis of trial and error, reward and punishment. The norms of a group depend upon the group's willingness to enforce them.

The evolution of group norms is very important to a group, of course. The norms bear directly upon a group's success in meeting its goals. They also make an enormous difference to a member's individual satisfaction in working with the group, and to the group's cohesiveness as well.

But the emergence of norms can also create some dangers to the group—dangers that flow from habit and rigidity, and from loss of creativity.

To illustrate the dangers, consider those six engineers again. Their habit of double-checking each other's written work may seem a good idea for all the reasons of quality that led them to do it in the first place. But every job includes some things that are not very important. For example, engineers often write "for the file." That is, they write to create a paper trail in order to cover themselves and the company in the unlikely event that something goes wrong.

The custom of waiting until each can check the other's written work would probably constitute an unnecessary delay in the case of such a report, written for the file. If this habitual way of doing things were to evolve into a much stronger position— rigid adherence to the custom of double-checking—the group would risk its efficiency even further.

Remember that we said that norms evolve in the areas of procedure and task, and also in the social dimension of a group's life. Suppose a group began to adhere rigidly to customary ways of doing things in the area of procedure. In that case, the group would risk loss of creativity. A glance at Chapter 3 will illustrate this point clearly. In that chapter we discuss a variety of approaches that groups can take to setting and following agendas, and a variety of discussion techniques and methods of deciding. These alternatives are presented precisely because we wish to offer you a broad range of creative alternatives. Clearly, adherence to only one agenda system—adherence to one method of deciding—would stifle a group's creative potential.

If a group evolves a norm that is damaging, what can an individual do to provide leadership? You won't be surprised that we advise you to bring the norm up to the level of talk.

First, identify your concern. Say something like, "I'm worried that we've fallen into a habit . . . ."

Second, ask the group members to discuss their perceptions so that everyone has a chance to become aware of the dysfunctional norm. "I'd like to know if the rest of you think there's a problem with . . ."

Third, ask the group for an agreement to change the emerging norm. "Well, we all agree that this is a problem. Can we also agree to discuss alternatives, and agree on a way to act differently?"

After the group has identified a way to resolve the problem, restate the agreement. "So we're agreed, then, that we'll . . ."

Our point here is a simple one, but very important. Understanding a group's culture can make an important difference to you as a group member, whether you play a participant's role or provide the leadership for the group. It can influence both the efficiency and effectiveness of the group in meeting its task goals, and it can influence the cohesiveness of the group by dissipating tensions and fostering member satisfaction. The group's notions of how it's supposed to be, however, can also create very serious problems for the group—problems that have to do with habit, rigidity, and the consequent loss of creativity.

Tasks and Relationships

If you examine a communication event closely, you will discover that it has two dimensions.[7] In one dimension the participants work on some object, phenomenon, or event of the real world. You will discover that the communication event deals with topics or tasks. The *task* is the focus of the work of the group, and that work centers around the achievement of the group's goal. In a political action group, the task may be promoting a candidate. In a marketing department, it may be a new marketing approach for a product. In a city government meeting, it might be allocating funds to various departments. In the group's other dimension, sometimes referred to as the maintenance function, the participants work on their relationship—learning it, refining it, nurturing it. The *relationship* focuses on who we are with respect to others and the management of the surrounding circumstances. To illustrate these two dimensions of communication, suppose a friend who owns a sailboat invites you to a meeting of a social group, the Buccaneer Yacht Club. You attend the membership meeting and hear this conversation:

> SUE: "I think that in addition to the race of the thirteenth we should plan a work day."
>
> DON: "I appreciate that idea, Sue. Some of us are a little beyond our racing years. We still want to be included, and the work day is something we can help with."

This exchange illustrates the task dimension of communication. Sue talked about objects, phenomena, and events in her suggestion. The objects were herself, sailing, and a work day. The phenomena include sailing and working. The events include joining together, racing, and meeting new people and old friends.

The task dimension of this talk is the planning of a race and consideration of a work day. Although it is possible to locate a communication event in which there is no task dimension, for our purposes it is sensible to assume that there will always be a task dimension in group communication events.

The example may also be used to illustrate the relationship dimension, but you really have to be there for this to make much sense. Most of the time—and in this case—people in our culture delegate much of their communication about relationships to nonverbal messages. So we must take in this nonverbal behavior to be able to say much about the relationship dimension.

If you were present at the sailing club and were able to examine the conversation carefully, you would discover some interesting facts that normally do not get talked about. Those facts are the components of the relationships that exist between individuals. Typically, a relationship exists in the *observations* we make of one another and the *guesses* we make about what those observations mean. If you think about it carefully, you will discover that observations and guesses are always present-tense phenomena. Moreover, the guesses are always inside your head.

If that second idea seems obvious, it is important nevertheless. If you make an observation and a guess about someone, you are taking data inside yourself and then—but not before then—processing it. You might see someone smile—that is an observation with language attached. What is a smile? What you actually see is a person's facial changes. Perhaps the corners of her mouth rise slightly; perhaps her eyes widen somewhat; perhaps her teeth show between parted lips. These are observations. You take them inside yourself and you call them a smile. You suppose that the smile means something. This is the guess, and it is inside you, too.

A relationship, then, exists in the present, and inside individuals. It consists of observations and guesses. The guesses typically have to do with such things as feelings, wants and expectations, and intentions and images. It is a pity that in our culture we too often seem unwilling or unable to talk about our relationships, so we leave to chance that each of us will be able to interpret accurately the other's nonverbal messages. Worse still, we actually believe that we are able to do this, so we rarely if ever check out the accuracy of our guesses.

That saddening fact provides a most important truth about our communication. We often act on our guesses about what the other person is thinking. But it is obvious that we can never read someone else's mind; therefore, it is important to check out our guesses before we act on them. If we think about this statement in relation to group contexts, it becomes clear that learning to check out guesses is a most basic communication skill.

Task-dimension concerns in group communication In the context of a group meeting, there are always task-dimension concerns. Those that are most compelling (although the list is not exhaustive) include such notions as whether or not to have a meeting, decision making, leadership, and participation. In sum, the appropriate concerns of the task dimension are those that contribute to productivity.

The *productivity* of a group refers to its task-related output. Productivity is what comes from a group's decision-making activities. Productivity is always centered in the tasks or goals of a group, measured against either quality or quantity criteria.

To compare and contrast these criteria you might talk about a particular work group—perhaps a city government planning commission. The productivity of this group might be measured in terms of the quality of its decisions with respect to variances it passes during its weekly meetings. It could be said of the commission: "This commission has exceedingly high standards with very high reliability."

Similarly, it might be said of the commission: "The commission's output, measured in number of decisions per meeting, has increased dramatically over the past few years." That statement would also be about the commission's productivity. It refers to the quantity produced by the commission's members over a given period of time. So a working group might be judged by the number of units it produces or by the quality of each unit.

Productivity, then, is the yield of a group's efforts to accomplish its projects. As such, productivity is something that flows from communication in the task dimension. This distinction can become an important one for working groups, since it is directly related to their goals. One group may say of itself: "We want to be a good group" and mean: "We want to turn out many . . ." Another group might say of itself: "We want to be a good group" and mean: "We want to turn out a few high-quality . . ."

Relational-dimension concerns in group communication In the relational dimension, the one that gives rise to members' attraction to the group, the appropriate concerns are about managing and developing relationships among the members. A list of these considerations would include such phenomena as norms and their evolution, roles and their evolution, power and power use, conflict and conflict management, and of course, the relationships per se. Each of these issues will be considered one by one later in this book.

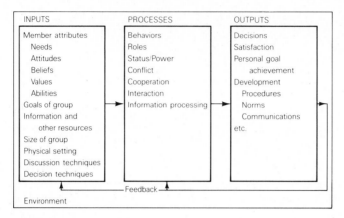

FIGURE 1.2
The Small Group as an Information-Processing System

THE SMALL GROUP AS AN
INFORMATION-PROCESSING SYSTEM

The small groups that are of interest to us can be best viewed as information-processing systems. Figure 1.2 presents the various components of a decision-making group that make up this system. Notice that the system includes inputs, processes, outputs, and feedback loops operating within an environment. People and things are brought together, processes take place, and some products are created. Notice also that the group monitors its processes and outputs and feeds back information related to them as inputs. In other words, the group learns from its experiences, grows, and creates a history that affects its subsequent performances. The environment surrounds the group, providing a basis for both understanding and constraining the group's actions. What happens outside the group may change members' attitudes, change the nature of available resources, change the goals of the group, and so forth. Rarely can a group operate in isolation.

The variables in this model can be classified as either *individual-level* or *system-level* features of a group.[8] The characteristics that individual members bring are individual-level variables; cultural norms, cohesiveness, and the like are system-level variables. An understanding of how these levels affect each other and the group's output is important to an overall understanding of groups. We will address this influence as we take up the variables in subsequent chapters.

The information-processing system depicted in Figure 1.2 serves as the framework for organizing the remainder of the book. It includes and orders the major variables that affect a small group in its decision-making effort.[9] Part II, "Preparing for Group Meetings" (Chapters 2, 3, and 4), considers the variables listed as inputs. Part III, "Participating in Group Meetings" (Chapters 5 through 10), addresses the process variables. Part IV, "Analyzing Small Group Decision Making" (Chapter 11), focuses on observing and measuring outputs. Part V, "Preparing for and Participating in Public Group Meetings" (Chapter 12), provides information and advice about managing the public group presentation.

ETHICAL RESPONSIBILITIES IN SMALL GROUP DISCUSSION

When people engage in group discussion for the purpose of solving problems, they agree that they will give up some of their individual sovereignty so that the group process can work. They become, for a time, interdependent. In doing so, they assume an obligation to one another to live by the highest personal standards of ethical conduct they can manage. Here are some of the important ethical standards for small group participants.

Determine To Do Your Best

As an individual you have a lot to offer. You are knowledgeable and you have ideas and opinions that have been filtered through your own processing system. Your strengths and your weaknesses *are* you when you commit yourself to group processes. You should determine to give the best you have—and you should determine not to hold anything back.

But sometimes individuals do hold back. They avoid taking the leadership role, for example, because so many others are too willing to let them take it. They learn that if they freely offer their skills they will be called on to do that again and again. So they hold back. They do not do it.

If something is worth doing, it is worth doing well. If a goal is worth achieving, it is worth the best efforts of everyone involved in achieving it. If group process is worth participating in, it is worth the most skillful participation you can manage. To choose not to give your best is to violate one of the most profound personal ethical standards that has evolved in our culture.

Determine To Behave Rationally and with the Group's Good in Mind

An individual must sometimes put personal goals aside in order to achieve the goals of a group. An individual must sometimes put aside private convictions in order that the group consensus may come to bear on a problem. An individual must sometimes put private truths in second place to public and group facts and opinions. Determining to behave rationally and to work for the group's good means making a commitment to keep an open mind and to listen to evidence and arguments, even though they may appear to contradict one's own positions. Determining to behave rationally in the group's best interests means, in the end, making a commitment to problem solving and decision making on the basis of the evidence and the group's best understanding of that evidence, even though doing so may leave personal and private agendas unfulfilled.

Such a commitment requires courage and great personal character. It may mean making personal decisions on the basis of facts, and it may mean persuading other group members to open up to those facts even when they are pressuring you to conform. Such a commitment means keeping personalities out of conflicts, examining and accepting or rejecting ideas while valuing the person whose ideas they are. Such a commitment means determining the behavior that is essential if group discussion is to be worthwhile. Group members have a right to expect that commitment from you. You have an obligation to make the commitment.

Make a Commitment To Fair Play

Group problem solving must be understood to be a cooperative event. It is not a debate, because, for the most part, it is not a competition. So determining on fair play means determining to seek and present all the ideas and evidence, whether they seem contradictory or not.

In a debate the opposing sides agree to disagree. In making that decision, they agree further that they will present only the strongest and best arguments and evidence on the side of the issue they represent. They agree to minimize or refute altogether the evidence and arguments of the opposing side. But group discussion is not debate. When groups are working together well, the group goals are the most important individual members' goals. But sometimes individuals lose sight of this simple idea, and they begin to push hard for a goal that is outside of the group's interest.

Every member of a discussion group has a right to expect that you will accept a standard of behavior in which you do not grind your private ax at the expense of the group project. Every member has a right to expect that you will play fairly, just as you have a right to expect that every member will play fairly with you.

Determine To Listen Carefully and To Participate Fully

This standard of personal conduct is, of course, closely related to the others. But it adds one final dimension that every member has a right to expect. When you say something, you have a right to expect that the other members of the group will give you a fair hearing. You have a right to expect that they will listen carefully, provide you with feedback, come to understand what you are trying to say, evaluate what you have said, and treat your ideas seriously. None of this means that they will ultimately agree with you, of course—you would not want total agreement. But you do want others to listen carefully, and to participate fully with you while you are talking.

They want that from you, too, and they have a right to expect it. Listen carefully and fully to other people's ideas. Listen carefully and fully to what other people are *not* saying, too. Participate with them when they are talking, for not to do so is to sabotage the best interests of the group and to endanger the problem-solving benefits of the group process. To do so, on the other hand, will foster group satisfaction.[10]

Take On a Participant-Analyst Role

You must be willing to take on a participant-analyst role. The participant-analyst role requires that you engage in the decision-making process and also direct your attention to observing and evaluating what is happening. No two groups are alike. Therefore, you will need to analyze and make decisions about *what is happening now and in the particular group*. What worked well in some other group in the past may not work now. You must be an analyst to be a good group member. You cannot necessarily fall back on past experiences and what worked before. You must adapt your behavior to what the group needs at that particular moment. And if you cannot personally meet the need, it is in part your responsibility to seek what is needed from others in the group.

SUMMARY

In summary, the study of group communication may be among the most valuable a student can undertake. Personally and socially, the ability to work with and in groups has enormous potential for increasing your success and the success of the people around you—success in reaching goals and success in achieving potential.

A number of important terms were defined as a way of making clear the focus and limitations of the book. The focus is on group communication as opposed to interpersonal communication or mass communication or public communication. That means the scope of this book is limited to the study of communication in contexts where three or more individuals relate to one another out of some common goal. The kind of group that is of most interest in this book is the small decision-making group. Its members are aware of one another's roles and communicate face to face.

Decision making, in this text, refers to a group task rather than an individual task. In this regard, group goals are achieved by means of group choices among alternative behaviors or conceptualizations.

In this chapter, some of the most common group experiences that you are likely to encounter were identified. These ranged from information-sharing meetings to decision-making groups to special-events meetings. In each of these group experiences, there were always certain task-dimension concerns—such things as identifying problems, analyzing data, and testing alternative solutions—as well as relationship issues.

We then discussed the communication process. We drew a model of communication that included a source/encoder, messages, channels, a receiver/decoder, feedback, noise, and situation. We suggested the transactional nature of communication and of the process of assigning meaning.

We also focused upon some basic dynamics of groups. Beginning with the group's evolving culture (ways of doing things that generate from the group's values), we looked at how trial and error and reward and punishment create that evolution. From the evolution a group draws its norms—its behavioral rules. Then, too, behavior within the group develops along both task and relational dimensions.

In large measure, learning to be a good communicator in group contexts means learning to provide leadership in the task and relationship areas. Leadership is not the prerogative of any one individual; rather, leadership is everyone's business. In this regard we defined productivity as the outcome of talk about tasks and cohesiveness as the outcome of talk about relationships—the two dimensions of all group communication. We pointed out that although these dimensions are not easily separated, it is useful to try to examine each. We presented several major concerns that a group member might consider in each area.

We also introduced the notion of small groups as information-processing systems. People and things are brought together, process takes place, and products are created. Feedback about the process and products then becomes input. This model provides the basic structure for this book.

All these concerns led to our argument that people in groups have certain ethical responsibilities to their groups: to do their best, to behave rationally, to play fair, to listen carefully and take an active part, and to take on a participant-analyst role.

We think the study of small group communication is exciting and intensely rewarding. We hope you will think so too.

EXERCISES

1. Consider your experiences in small groups over the past few years. List your strengths and weaknesses as a communicator in groups. Decide on goals to adopt as an action plan for your course in group communication that will help improve areas you judge as weaknesses.[11]

2. Locate other textbooks on small group communication in the school library. Examine the definitions of small group communication from three of these and compare them with the one offered in this chapter. Compare and contrast the definitions. Now decide which definition you find to be most useful. Write a short essay that suggests what your favorite definition is, how it differs from others, and why you favor it.

3. Discuss in small groups the components of the communication model presented in this chapter until they are understood by each member of your group. Now construct a communication model that illustrates the communication process as your group sees it. Once you have developed a model, extend it to describe communication in the small group. Present this model of group communication to the class. Compare your model with others that were presented.

4. Think of the best small group discussion experience you have had in the past year. Write a list of ideas that suggest why this was a good group experience. Compare your ideas with those of your classmates. What are the similarities? What are the differences? How do you account for these? Now try to agree as a class on the qualities or concepts that make a group good.

5. Keep a personal journal of your experiences in the group or groups you belong to in this class over the term. Make an entry for each group meeting as soon as possible after that class meeting is over. Tell what happened, discuss your contributions, and evaluate each of these. On the basis of your observation and evaluation, set a goal for yourself for the next group meeting. After the next group meeting, add to your journal a short discussion of how you did with the goal you set. Be concise and clear in your entries.

6. Identify a group that you and at least two others in your class can observe. Observe the group and write an independent report that you bring to class. Comment on the following:

a. Identify the norms of the group. Give evidence of the existence of the norms you cite. Tell whether the norms were goal productive or not.

b. Identify the task of the group. Then, say on what basis you would evaluate the group's productivity. Give your assessment of its productivity.

c. Consider the social dimension of the group. How cohesive was this group? What evidence do you have to support your judgment? How did the social dimension affect the group's task performance?

Now compare your observations with those of your classmates who observed the same discussion.

7. Think of a group with which you felt particularly frustrated. What norms seemed to be being followed? Can you account for your frustration through an examination of the participation of the other members? What might be done if you encounter similar norms in the future? Answer these questions in a two-page analysis.

8. Consider two groups to which you belong. How are you different in each? Consider your dress, amount of talking, the people with whom you talk, the group's expectations of you, the responsibilities you are willing to take in the group, and your feeling of acceptance in the group. How is the group culture different in each? Can you explain how the particular culture of the groups affected your description of where you are in the group? Write a two-page essay that addresses these questions.

NOTES

1. Robert S. Spich and Kenneth Keleman, "Explicit Norm-Structuring Process: A Strategy for Increasing Task Group Effectiveness," *Group and Organizational Studies* 10 (1985):55.

2. Group membership is important because it satisfies a need. Groups help by providing a mechanism whereby people can make a contribution to something greater than themselves. Thus groups can fulfill the motivation to give. T. J. Larkin, "Humanistic Principles for Organizational Management," *Central States Speech Journal* 37 (1986):37.

3. Abraham Maslow, *Motivation and Personality*, 2d ed. (New York: Harper & Row, 1970).

4. *The Random House College Dictionary*, rev. ed. (New York: Random House, 1984), 325.

5. For an excellent discussion of this idea, see B. Aubrey Fisher, *Small Group Decision Making: Communication and the Group Process*, 2d ed. (New York: McGraw-Hill, 1980), 183–185.

6. Jack Gibbs, "Norms: The Problem of Definition and Classification," *American Journal of Sociology* 70 (1964–65):586–594.

7. We discuss the task and relationship dimensions separately here to make them easier to talk about; they are in fact interrelated and complement each other. See Donald G. Ellis, "Relational Control in Two Group Systems," *Communication Quarterly* 46 (1979):153–166; B. Aubrey Fisher, "Content and Relationship Dimensions of Communication in Decision-Making Groups," *Communication Quarterly* 27 (1979):3–11.

8. Randy Y. Hirokawa and Dierdre D. Johnson, "Toward a General Theory of Group Decision Making: Development of an Integrated Model," *Small Group Behavior* (in press).

9. See Dennis E. Warnemunde, "The Status of the Introductory Small Group Communication Course," *Communication Education* 35 (1986):392, for topic ranking.

10. Beverley J. Hartung Hagen and Genevieve Burch, "The Relationship of Group Process and Group Task Accomplishment to Group Member Satisfaction," *Small Group Behavior* 16 (1985):211–233.

11. Joann Keyton of the University of South Alabama has been working with and refining the use of a journal assignment as a method of teaching small group analysis. She constructed these assignments, which can be collected in a journal. Exercise 1 in each chapter can be used as part of an ongoing journal.

RECOMMENDED READINGS

Larry L. Barker, Kathy J. Wahlers, Kittie W. Watson, and Robert J. Kibler, *Groups in Process: An Introduction to Small Group Communication*, 3d ed. (Englewood Cliffs, N.J.: Prentice-Hall, 1987), Chapter 2, "A Systems Approach to Small Group Communication."

John F. Cragan and David W. Wright, *Communication in Small Group Discussions*, 2d ed. (St. Paul: West Publishing, 1988), Chapter 1, "Introduction to Small Group Communication."

Randy Y. Hirokawa and Marshall Scott Poole, eds. *Communication in Group Decision-Making* (Beverly Hills, Calif.: Sage, 1986).

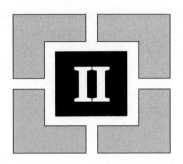

Preparing for
Group Meetings

CHAPTER 2

Preparing for Group Discussion

OBJECTIVES

After reading this chapter you should be able to:

Specify four questions that will allow you to select participants intelligently.

Separate and explain three kinds of discussion issues: fact, value, and policy.

Focus a discussion issue so that it will be conducive to group processing.

State the major questions to be considered in deciding how much structure is needed in a group.

Identify the five key task dimensions.

State in your own language and describe each of the four steps in researching a discussion topic.

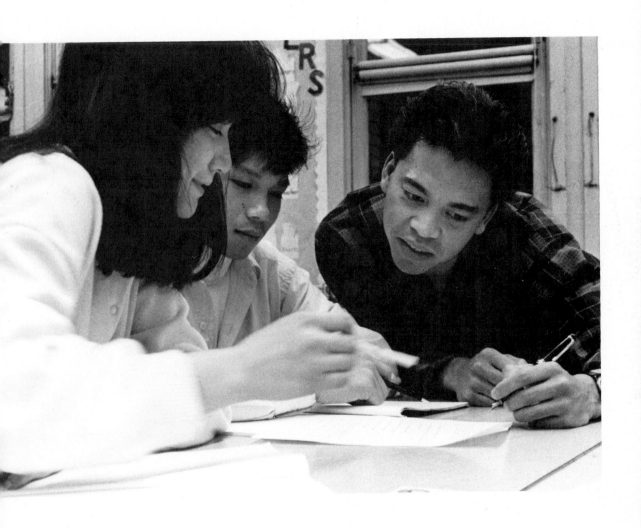

"When I look back on the time that I started to move up in the company, I recall George, then my boss, commenting on how pleased he was at the active role I took in departmental meetings. It hadn't started out that way. I had to learn how to be productive in conferences," commented a 45-year-old area manager.[1]

"Sometimes I feel like I spend half my workday in meetings. And sometimes I'd like to just get up in the middle of one and leave. Too many people don't know how to run a meeting. That kind of consultation is important, but I don't want someone to waste my time. That's why anyone in a leadership position around here needs group skills." This comment was made by a 47-year-old senior vice president of a large manufacturing firm.

"Being seen as a team member is a critical factor in my business. If you don't know how to pull your weight in the group, it's noticed," said a 29-year-old sales representative from New Orleans. He was among the top several representatives of his company's southeast district.

"I was never so embarrassed in my life. On my first job the boss asked me if something was wrong as we were coming out of a meeting. He was concerned that I didn't have much to say. I've learned a lot since then. If you want to move up in your career—and you do not have to stay in one company to do it—you have to learn how to help the group along with its goals." That was a 39-year-old middle manager from Dallas who works in the hubbub of advertising.

Each of these individuals is well qualified to make suggestions to people who are studying toward a career objective in the business community. Each has suggested that in order to be a successful professional you have to know what to do in group situations. The purpose of this chapter is to focus attention upon those behaviors that will help you prepare effectively for group situations.

This chapter focuses on preparing for group meetings. It begins by addressing issues related to selecting participants. Then it examines the problems of posing a discussion issue and selecting an appropriate structure for the discussion situation. Finally, the chapter provides guidelines that will help in securing, evaluating, and preparing information. You will want to keep these ideas in mind as you prepare to be a productive group member.

SELECTING THE PARTICIPANTS

The first step in planning for a meeting is to select the participants. When you are in control of the meeting, identifying the participants is a relatively easy thing to do. When you are not in charge, there are still important considerations to be made about identifying the participants.

But suppose you are in charge of the meeting. It is often surprising to new employees that they are called on to plan meetings. You should know from the outset how to do that, because you will probably continue to plan meetings throughout your career.

In general, how you go about identifying participants will depend upon the context. For instance, in many organizational settings, identifying participants is easily accomplished by looking for those who are interested in and have the expertise related to the particular problem.

Notice, however, that interest in a particular problem area does *not* imply agreement among the members. One individual may be very liberal in her views about the economy, population control, and local politics; another may be on the conservative side of these issues; both may be equally motivated to join a discussion about such topics. Disagreement can be healthy for a discussion. It helps a group to weigh evidence more carefully and to evaluate its conclusions more fully and carefully.

Sometimes the membership of a group is predetermined, and those who are in charge of planning the meeting will not select the participants. Regular Monday morning meetings, conducted in many work groups in business and industry, provide a simple example of this kind of group. Planning for such a meeting does not include selecting the individual participants. Rather, it focuses upon the agenda items, the priority among those items, and such concerns as the raw data from which conclusions will be drawn.

Of course, some groups that meet regularly *do* invite outside participants to their meetings. Consider, for example, the weekly meeting of a group of department heads in a public relations agency, at which they exchange notes and ideas and coordinate their efforts for the firm. During one meeting, the group discussed the allocation of space in a building acquired by the company, and ways to make maximum use of the new building. They invited to this meeting an architect/builder, an accountant, and someone from upper levels of management. Whom to invite will depend upon the expertise needed and the specific subject matter under discussion. Significant "political" ramifications might determine some of the individuals to be invited. Of course, you will not always be able to control who attends a meeting. Still, it seems a good idea for you to influence membership in a group where that makes sense. For example, you might want to suggest a couple of members whose views would add to the richness of the discussion. Keep in mind, though, that there is an important balance between enough similarity to work together and enough difference to consider an issue from a variety of perspectives.

Good groups do not pool their ignorance. Rather, they pool their information. They identify what they do not know and how to go about finding out what they do not know, and then they approach the problem. So, in the selection of group members, a sensible set of questions would include:

1. "Is there anyone who should participate in our group because of special qualifications or expertise?"

2. "Is there anyone who should participate in our group because of the political sensitivity of the subject matter?"

3. "Have we duplicated ourselves in any way that may inhibit the group—or inadvertently damage the organization of which the group is a part?"

CONSIDERING DISCUSSION ISSUES

Kinds of Discussion Issues

Generally speaking, groups talk about three kinds of issues: fact, value, and policy. In groups in the real world, these kinds of issues are frequently found together, although one may be the primary focus. Here we will discuss them separately for clarity. Some of the issues discussed by groups that meet regularly are primarily questions of *fact*. For example, groups in the business community might worry about the question "Are we going to make a profit in the next quarter?" Similarly, a business group might discuss the question "What level of output can we expect this quarter for this production line?" Questions of definition are questions of fact: "What do we mean by poverty?" "What are the limits of a certain acreage?" "How many units of production constitute an optimum number?" So are questions of cause, although we may not always be able to discover the cause: "What caused this override of our cost estimate?" "Why did this well-planned strategy fail?" "How did this problem occur?" Sometimes we guess at causes when we are unable to collect data.

Typically, issues of fact do not lend themselves to classroom discussion because the level of detailed information necessary to answer them is beyond the resources of a classroom group. But issues of fact are very common in business and organizational settings.

Issues of *value* are questions about the goodness or worth of something. Issues of value often call for the group to make a judgment or to make statements about broad philosophical issues. For example, these questions come from issues of value:

1. "What is the value of a liberal arts education when compared with a business education for our management trainees?"

2. "What is the future of the labor movement?"

3. "Will the information age truly benefit humanity?"

4. "Which will be a better value—the Commodore or the IBM computer?"

As a rule of thumb, issues of value are more difficult for a group discussion because they require the group to establish and apply evaluative criteria as members identify broad philosophical or social goals. *Criteria* are standards of judgment. A person's value system provides standards for judging what might be a good answer to one of these questions. Of course, problem-solving groups very often consider value issues, as well as factual questions, when they are working on problems and solutions.

Issues of *policy* are questions that invite the group to some action—some course of behavior. As problems occur, people address them and focus upon and identify solutions. These may be characterized by the words "should do." For example, each of the following questions was generated from an issue of policy—each calls for individual or collective action:

1. "What should we do to reduce our overhead expenses?"

2. "Is there anything our company can do to further the cause of freedom and equality for minority members?"

3. "What should the position of this company be on State Bill No. 55-673?"

4. "What should we do next?"

Issues of policy provide the richest opportunities for groups to work together toward some common goal. They are by far the most common form of discussion question that people ever confront. Skill in managing issues of policy may be one of the most potent tools an ambitious person can have.

Focusing the Discussion Issue

An issue for discussion can be so broad in scope that the group cannot manage it. When the possibilities for problem identification and solution are virtually limitless, you know the issue needs to be focused and delimited. Typically, most discussion groups discover that they must focus and narrow their concerns to manageable limits. You will see at a glance that these issues are too broad for any meaningful discussion to occur:

1. "What should be done to strengthen the world economy?"

2. "What should be done to prevent teen-age pregnancy?"

3. "What should be done to raise the educational level in the various states?"

4. "What should be done to secure the quality of life of all employees?"

Each of these issues might be focused and narrowed to manageable limits, of course. If a group wanted to focus upon poverty and ignorance, how might members go about narrowing the issue? An obvious first step is to identify the amount of time available for the discussion. An hour-long meeting could treat only a small fraction of the large problem area—poverty and ignorance. Perhaps the first inclination might be to address the question: "What should be done to interrupt the poverty-ignorance cycle in America's urban centers?"

Such a question focuses the issue somewhat. Nevertheless, a group could work for years and years attempting to answer it. But notice that the range of the issue may be cut to manageable proportions merely by focusing it upon a single problem: "What should be done to reduce poverty in America's urban centers?"

Better yet, the issue could be focused still more by identifying just one agency, or just one geographical area for consideration: "What actions, if any, could our organization take to reduce poverty in our city?" Even with this narrow focus, the issue remains complex, but a group could manage a discussion of the topic. If the larger issue needs to be discussed, it might be divided into several questions to be taken up in several meetings.

DECIDING ABOUT STRUCTURE

How structured does decision-making activity need to be in order for a group to do its job efficiently? There is no easy answer to this rather simple question. The leader of a group—and even the group itself—must weigh a number of factors to answer this question. Some of the important considerations in making this decision are:

1. Order—How much order (or disorder) is needed?

2. Time—How much time does the group have to carry out the task?

3. Group size—How many people will be present to give information?

4. Group sentiment—How strongly do group members feel about the topic and each other?

5. Task—What is the nature of the task?

The following paragraphs address the issues represented by these questions.

Need for Order

Observation suggests that different people need varying amounts of order in their lives. Consider your own experience in growing up in your home. Did it seem that different members of your family could tolerate different levels of clutter? The amount of orderliness needed differs from person to person. How about planning the family vacation? Did you discover various needs for organization? Maybe your mother needed to know precisely when and where you were going—hour by hour—but perhaps your father would have been satisfied with just knowing that you would spend Tuesday on the beach at Gulf Shores.

This same variety in need for orderliness and organization is experienced in group contexts. Our experience in groups verifies that some members are content to have a rough agenda to follow. Others seem to thrive on more structure. They want to know what issues will be covered, the order in which these will be addressed, the specific role they are expected to play, and so forth. You can be sure that this need is real for them. If you check other areas of their lives, you will probably find the need for order there also.

On the other hand, you may discover that some group members are stifled by too much structure. They feel restricted and much less spontaneous under circumstances with too much structure. It may be really difficult for these people to adapt. Task leaders should take these desires into account when planning agendas. If you are a task leader and have both types of people in your group, you may have to take the middle ground to satisfy both of these divergent needs. Yet there may be other determinants that, when considered, will cause you to introduce either more or less structure. These factors include the time available to carry out the task, the number of group members involved, the social climate of the group, and the nature of the task.

Time Considerations

Consider how time relates to structural options for a group. Imagine that you belong to a community service group—a member of a neighborhood homeowners' association. The city council has decided to install new streetlights. It needs a recommendation from the residents as to locations for the lights by Monday of next week. Your group has scheduled a Thursday night meeting. Do you, as leader of the group, try to set a specific agenda? Or do you let the group proceed without any plan for structuring its interaction? The time limitation may present a need for more structure. Most of the members are busy people and are not likely to want to meet several times to resolve this issue. If you do not set a specific agenda, group members may find it impossible to make a decision within a single meeting—and within the hour or two they each have allotted. On the other hand, if they had several meetings to complete their task, the members might approach the problem in a more spontaneous fashion.

Group Size Considerations

Consider again the meeting of your neighborhood association. Will you have fifty of your neighbors present? Twenty? Fifteen? Ten? Five? Certainly if you want to ensure the opportunity for participation when the group is large, you will want to provide more structure, thereby providing a greater chance for everyone to talk. Structure can limit the freedom to move to side issues and personal agendas. Formal procedures may restrict the amount of time any one member is permitted to talk. This can allow the less aggressive person an opportunity to participate more fully. In a smaller group it is possible to allow for more lengthy comments and a greater degree of spontaneity. The larger group restricts this behavior. The size of the group can help you decide how much structure you need to impose.

Group Members' Emotional Involvement

Groups whose members are emotionally involved in the task may need more structure. Suppose that an older member of your neighborhood association is terrified because his property is dimly lit. His emotional involvement in the topic may cause him to dominate the meeting. He may even try to obstruct progress if he does not seem to be getting his desired outcome. If others are also emotionally involved in this issue, the group may not be able to think rationally without some agreed-on agenda.

Hostility among group members can cause problems. Members may move outside the task as they express hostility. This failure to come to direct contact can be disruptive to task completion, especially when the group has some deadline. Securing agreement to an agenda may limit this kind of behavior. For example, as the leader you can remind group members that they have an agreed-upon agenda and ask them to try harder to stick to it.

Nature of the Task

Tasks differ in ways that affect the need for organization. Marvin Shaw[2] used a step-by-step procedure to identify task dimensions within a set of 104 tasks. From this work, five task dimensions that are of interest can be identified: task difficulty, solution multiplicity, intrinsic interest, cooperation requirements, and population familiarity.[3]

Task difficulty suggests the amount of effort required to complete a task. A task may require more effort because it is complex and/or requires considerable knowledge. Some tasks are simpler than others—they involve less data, fewer causes, less complex solutions, and the like. The neighborhood association's consideration of the placement of streetlights might be such a task. But suppose that the association wants to deal with a problem of declining membership. This problem may require collecting data by survey and analyzing complex causes. Because of the task complexity, it may best be handled by a more structured approach to organization. For such a task, you might propose that the group follow one of the agendas presented in this chapter.

Solution multiplicity refers to the number of reasonable alternatives available to solve a problem. Some problems are high in solution multiplicity because they have many alternatives that cannot easily be demonstrated as correct. Research findings bear indirectly on this issue and on the need for organization. For example, Shaw and Blum[4] studied solution multiplicity with respect to particular kinds of leaders—directive and nondirective. They rated three tasks as differing on the basis of multiplicity. In the first, group members were asked to list the five most important traits needed for success in our culture. In the second, the group was asked to select one of five solutions for a young politician with an alcoholic spouse. The third task required the group to play the parlor game twenty questions.

These tasks are presented to show why research can be viewed only as an indirect indicator. Notice that the three tasks are very different from what decision-making groups are usually asked to do. The first does not ask for a single decision. The second provides the answers and asks for a selection process. The third is a parlor game. But the findings might generalize to other decision-making tasks. Shaw and Blum found that directive leadership was more effective in groups with low solution-multiplicity tasks, but nondirective leadership was more effective on the mid- to high-range multiplicity tasks. The measure of effectiveness here was time needed to complete a task.

Intrinsic interest refers to the interest generated by the task itself. This level of interest is related to attraction and motivation for the group. Leonard Berkowitz[5] studied preferences for shared leadership in small decision-making groups. He found that members who were extremely involved in the task—high attraction and interest—were more interested in sharing procedural control. The opposite held for tasks that were less interesting. The members preferred strong procedural control by the leader.

Consider again the neighborhood association and its decision about streetlights. Suppose you have a strong interest in the issue. Would you want the leader to dictate the agenda and procedure? Or would you want to have a part in deciding how the group will proceed? We think you are likely to want to be involved in this decision.

Cooperation requirements are defined as the degree of coordinated effort necessary to complete the task. Much of the decision making we experience in our professional lives falls into this category. Suppose that a management team of a company that manufactures electronic equipment is trying to make decisions about moving into manufacturing telephones. The complexity of the problem and the need for a coordinated effort are both inherent in this context. A published agenda for the discussion of this issue will give members the best opportunity to come to the meeting prepared to provide input and coordinate their efforts. A meeting that follows a published plan can lead to greater productivity and efficiency in handling the issue.

Population familiarity suggests the extent to which the group has had experience with a task. Groups that are highly familiar with a task tend to do better with it.[6] But there is also a very clear danger with high task familiarity. Groups with long experience are likely to be less critical and creative because of that experience. You can imagine a member saying, "Oh, I see. This is the same problem we settled last month. I know exactly what to do." Because of this tendency, high-familiarity groups probably need procedures that will ensure that members look carefully at a problem. They must look for the unique and be prepared to go beyond the usual solutions. Brainstorming is one procedure that has been shown to be effective in combating such tendencies.[7] Group discussion techniques are addressed in the next chapter.

Should groups follow structured decision-making agendas? It depends. You can see from this discussion that the question has no easy answer. The guidelines presented for making this decision will help you. But in the final analysis, either you or the group has to weigh these factors and decide.

SECURING INFORMATION

An essential part of planning and preparing to talk about some problem or topic is becoming informed about that problem or topic. Such a statement seems obvious. Amazingly, though, many individuals in many organizations appear to believe that knowledge of a subject is not a relevant qualification to discuss that subject. In one group discussion observed in an executive workshop, a well-paid junior executive made this remark:

> I am surprised that I have always done so little to study questions before we sat down to discuss them. I suppose I thought that the purpose of a group meeting was for others to inform me about the subject matter so that I could offer my opinions. Of course, I always try to know what I'm doing when I have to make the decision, but I really have not made

much of an effort to know what I'm doing when a group is supposed to decide. I can see now that the group decision suffers.

This individual's statement received quite a bit of support from others in that workshop. Consider these fragments from their tape-recorded conversations:

> Yeah. I can't say that I leave it all to other people, but I sure have done that, too. Once I went to a meeting—last week, I think it was—when I didn't know much more about the subject than that the company was thinking of working on it. I guess I didn't understand what I was supposed to accomplish at that meeting. I wasted my time by not being informed.

> I don't always have much time . . . [chuckles from the others] . . . I don't always take time to look into things. In fact, I guess that I depend on the group members to do my initial thinking for me. Of course, when I get involved, I try to study the matter. . . .

Such comments suggest that some individuals in responsible positions attend group problem-solving meetings without preparation.

What do you do to get ready for a problem-solving discussion? How do you identify and find information? Answers to these questions follow.

Conducting an Inventory and Analysis of What You Know

Personal knowledge is probably the most significant single source of information in any group member's repertory. Review what you know in some systematic fashion. Have you taken any courses related to the subject matter? Have you had any direct life experiences in the area? Have you written any papers on the subject or related to the problem? Have you read any books? Have you studied any articles? Have you had any conversations with anyone about the subject matter? Make some notes as you work through this set of questions. After you have answered the questions, organize this information using one of the problem-solving agendas found in Chapter 3. If you spend time retrieving the loose ends and bits of information that you have already acquired about the subject—and often you know much more than you might imagine—you will save yourself a good deal of research time.

Gathering Additional Information

Interviews   Depending upon the subject matter, there are many individuals in your community who can be counted on to provide you with information. A knowledgeable person will be able to suggest additional sources of information. He or she may well be able to provide you with pamphlets, brochures, and books directly related to the subject matter. An individual who knows about the subject area may be able to help you clarify the issues, and may lead you to sources of information that would require hours of exhaustive research to find on your own. Even an individual who is not an expert may well be able to ask questions or provide suggestions and leads to sources of information you would not have thought of.

It is wise to enter each interview with your eyes open. Not everyone on the staff of the chamber of commerce knows enough to be a good source of information on attracting new industry to the community. Not every person who works at the local bank knows about the economy. Not every police officer knows about the incidence of drug abuse in the local schools. Temper your conclusions on the basis of the information you pick up in the interview.

At a second level, we recommend careful planning of each interview so that you have a clear focus upon what you want to discover, and so that you do not waste anyone's time. Get an appointment at a convenient time, try to agree on a specific amount of time for the interview, get there punctually, and end the conversation within the allotted period. During the interview, try very hard to keep the conversation on the subject matter. Use the problem-solving agenda to help plan your questions. Let those questions provide the agenda for the conversation. Submit the questions to the informant in advance if possible, so that you can find out if he or she knows enough to provide you with useful information.

Your group may want to collect data about the issue you will discuss. A *survey interview* will allow you to do this. It is a structured interview in which each respondent is asked the same set of questions, with the responses pooled so that conclusions can be drawn about the group that the interviewees represent. A scientifically designed sample of the overall group to be polled is a must if the results are to be valid. You can get a rather distorted picture if the sample is not truly representative. If you do collect data through a survey, it is wise to consult someone who has been trained in survey research to help ensure that correct survey procedures are being followed.

Library research An expert will be able to give you information and ideas. An expert will also be able to direct you to other sources of information, and may even provide you with materials related to the subject area. This fact suggests that another major source of information is your own reading behavior.

Books, magazines, brochures, pamphlets, a variety of government documents—all are sources of information a reader may find useful. Reference works (encyclopedias, both general and topical) can provide ideas. They can identify other sources of information (a bibliography or bibliographies). They can give you precise definitions of a wide range of complex and technical terms (dictionaries, both general and topical). And, of course, they can provide you with in-depth treatment of the subject area in general and in its particular aspects.

You may be able to find help in locating sources of information by consulting bibliographies of bibliographies. Among the ones you are likely to find in your library are A *World Bibliography of Bibliographic Catalogues, Bibliographical Index,* and *Bulletin of Bibliography and Magazine Notes.* Of course, bibliographies are often found at the end of many books, doctoral dissertations (locate these in *Dissertation Abstracts*), and research articles.

You can consult periodicals indexes to locate information in magazines, journals, and newspapers. Some of the more common ones found in the library are *The Reader's Guide to Periodical Literature, Applied Science and Technology Index, The Education Index,* and *The New York Times Index*. Also check with your librarian for government documents that may be of help. Use the *Monthly Catalog of U.S. Government Publications* and the *Monthly Checklist of State Publications* to aid you in your search.

Magazines come in general form (*Readers Digest, The New Yorker*) and in more specialized form (*American Photography*). There are special and professional publications (*Quarterly Journal of Speech, Academy of Management Journal, American Journal of Sociology*). There are also many special-interest magazines (*Business Horizons, Mechanix Illustrated, Consumer Reports*). Indeed, for every subject that bears on any relevant subgroup in our society, you will be able to find several specialized publications. Involve a reference librarian in your search if you are not familiar with possible sources.

Special-interest groups and special-interest agencies within larger organizations publish an enormous number of pamphlets and brochures about topic areas that a discussion group might want to explore. Of course, the largest publishing company in the world—larger than any in the private sector—is the federal government of the United States. The Government Printing Office has almost certainly published something on any subject you are likely to discuss. All you have to do is a little reading. Be sure you read sources that present all sides of the issue.

Direct observation   Some topics lend themselves to the most direct kind of research. If a group is about to discuss some condition in the local community—for example, the willful littering of the highways and byways of Baldwin County—knowledge of that subject may mean taking a photograph or two of the hundreds of beverage cans and bottles tossed out by careless motorists as they drive down the roads. Observations usually result in enthusiastic reporting; an individual who gets firsthand information is likely to have developed a strong emotional involvement in the subject. Because this is true, use caution. Direct observation has three common pitfalls.

First, untrained observers often do not see things accurately or objectively. An individual observer may record a distortion simply because he or she was not at the scene long enough to get a complete understanding of conditions there. Also, observers are likely to place themselves physically in a location that may create a distorted image. A well-traveled highway is likely to have more roadside trash than a barely traveled country lane. Observation of only one of these would probably yield distorted conclusions.

A second pitfall into which the amateur observer often falls is inaccurate reporting. Careful use of descriptive language (as suggested in Chapter 4) is the most obvious single security against false reporting. This also includes specific rather than general words. If a reporter says, "The city council was in disarray today," she leaves an impression of a problem, but gives very little information. If she chooses to be more accurate in reporting her observation, she might say, "I spent two hours observing the city council meeting today. The president began by asking members to add to an already published agenda. Then, he shuffled the agenda so that an issue that was to be considered later was considered first. Consequently, those who wished to speak about it were not present. Then he allowed discussion of a seemingly minor issue to go on for almost an hour. The result of the apparent disorganization and lack of control was completion of only half of the agenda items."

Biased reporting is the third and perhaps the most dangerous pitfall for amateur reporters. The major problem is not usually evil or deceptive intent—it is that inexperienced reporters tend to observe what they want to observe. Consider the city council illustration a final time. An individual who has developed an antagonistic relationship with the city council chair is likely to report observations of the council meeting in more biased and stronger language. We might read "The city council meeting was disorganized and out of control today. Again the council president lost perspective when . . ." If a member of a group reports information couched in this kind of bias, the group's recommendations may reflect this bias too.

Thus securing information about a subject area involves knowing yourself, talking with others about the subject, reading as widely as the limits of time and energy allow, and studying the problem firsthand. What do you do with the information after you have secured it?

Evaluating the Information

Clear thinking is an essential part of planning and preparing to talk about problems and topics. The quality of your thought, of course, depends on a large number of variables, including the accuracy of your information and the logic you apply as you drive toward conclusions on the basis of the information collected. One particularly important distinction to keep in mind as you gather and analyze data is the difference between facts and inferences.

A *fact* is a statement about an observation that can be demonstrated to be true. It can be shown to be true through verification. Statements about past events cannot be verified, so a different kind of test is applied to them. Such statements are assumed to be true if several independent observers have reported the same information. An *inference* is a conclusion that is made about an observation. The conclusion is one person's opinion, based on his or her reasoning, about what is or has been observed. Our faith in an inference is often a function of the credentials and training of the person making the statement and the number of others who share that opinion.

Examine those data you have identified as facts. Can you verify them? Are the facts reported similarly by several sources? Who is reporting the facts? Are they being reported by someone who is without bias and who has the expertise to collect data accurately? Now look at the statements you have identified as inferences. Is the person making the statement recognized as an expert? Do other experts agree with the person? Does the person making the statement have a vested interest that might bias his or her conclusion? Can you identify evidence (facts) that support this conclusion? Does the reasoning used make sense to you?

In a group situation, two features of straight thinking are especially important. It is important to think for yourself, and it is important to think tentatively.

Thinking for yourself means that you must avoid following a group that is not thinking carefully and critically. Some groups get caught up in a solution and stick with it in spite of the fact that certain members have personal misgivings about it. These members keep their doubts to themselves for the sake of group unity. This phenomenon, *groupthink,* is so important that we devote a major part of Chapter 8 to it.

Thinking for yourself also means that you watch out for the tendency—especially among individuals who are not experts—to accept uncritically the ideas and opinions of individuals who claim expertise. And, more subtly, there is always the tendency among individuals to accept a basic orientation toward the world—an orientation that derives from family and friends, and from the mores and attitudes of such influential organizations as the church and the local school. If there is a general climate of opinion in a place, the people who live there are likely to conform to that general climate. And they do so without consciously thinking about it. Clearly, thinking for yourself implies reminding yourself continually of these pitfalls. You might want to ask yourself the following questions from time to time as you consider the information you have gathered:

1. "Do I have any built-in bias about this information? From family? From friends? From school? From church? From some special other person?"

2. "Have I accepted this idea because the information justifies it? Or have I accepted the idea because I trust the individual who gave it?"

Without clear thinking, the individual who engages in group discussion runs the very serious risk of accepting wrong conclusions. Beyond that, there is always the risk that an uncritical thinker may influence the group toward a wrong conclusion.

Thinking tentatively means remembering that the entire purpose of group discussion is for members, collectively, to supply a better base for decision making than any individual might provide. If you go into the discussion with your mind made up, you cannot contribute to that group effort. It follows that thinking tentatively means holding final judgments in abeyance. It does *not* mean that you should not be sure that your ideas are credible and that there is logic in them. It means that as a good discussant, after you have considered the matter, you will submit that thinking to the scrutiny and evaluation of the other group members. Do not commit yourself to a conclusion. Keep your thinking tentative.

Preparing the Material for Use

You must prepare the information you have collected through your research so that it is in a form you can easily retrieve when you are interacting in a group. The most effective way to do this is to integrate the information into a tentative outline that follows the decision-making agenda you plan to use. (You will learn about several alternatives for decision-making agendas in the next chapter.) The agenda will pose questions that your information will help answer.

Consider the major headings and subheadings in your outline as main issues that the group will take up. Major issues might be "those affected by the problem," "seriousness of the harm," "contributing causes," and so forth. Now, mark in the margin of your notes the issue to which that particular material pertains. Group the material for each issue and record it on your outline. The outline will prepare you to make significant contributions to the content and orderliness of the group's deliberations.

What we have said so far is that preparing to talk about problems and topics involves overcoming resistance to personal planning. It involves focusing the problem area. It involves identifying the participants. It involves understanding your problem with regard to the classification of fact, value, or policy, and understanding the wording of a discussion question. The problem should be open to alternative solutions and be stated briefly and concisely.

Part of planning and preparing involves securing information and, of course, thinking clearly about the information once it is secured. All these things occur before discussion begins. But you will notice that they are all task and topic related. That is, they focus upon the problem area and the relationship of that problem area to the individual who will discuss it. That individual must know something about the subject and know it well. But an able discussant must have far more than mere subject-matter expertise. A good discussant needs to understand that his or her behavior during the group discussion is as important as the behavior involved in prior planning.

SUMMARY

An initial step in planning for a meeting is selection of participants. You can identify certain participants by looking at special qualifications or expertise. Other participants may be invited because of the political sensitivity of the subject matter. Check also to see if there is any unnecessary duplication in the membership that might inhibit or inadvertently undermine the group's deliberations.

Next, consider the discussion issue. Is it an issue of fact, value, or policy? Issues of fact are answerable by securing needed information and, therefore, are rarely issues for decision making. Issues of value are questions about the goodness or worth of something. These call for a group to make a judgment. Issues of policy are questions that invite the group to some action. These issues provide the richest opportunity for groups to work toward some common goal. Whatever the nature of the issue, the group must focus it into manageable limits before it proceeds.

The decision about how much structure is needed in a decision-making group is a complex one. When deciding, the leader—or perhaps the group itself—must consider several questions:

1. How much order is needed to allow group members to feel comfortable?

2. How much time does the group have to carry out the task?

3. How many people will be present to give input?

4. Do the group members have strong feelings about the topic or about one another?

5. What is the nature of the task?

Tasks can be classed by their difficulty, solution multiplicity, intrinsic interest to members, cooperation requirements, and population (member) interest.

A final step in preparation is securing of information. Begin by conducting an inventory and analysis of what you know. Next, gather additional information to supplement your knowledge through interviews, library research, and direct observation. Once information is gathered, it must be evaluated and organized in order to be ready for use.

EXERCISES

1. Identify a group experience from your past that was not as successful as you had hoped. Analyze what went on in the group on the basis of the five criteria presented under "Deciding About Structure," pages 36–39. Did any of these factors contribute to the group's problems? For those factors that affected the group, be prepared to suggest how they did so. Be prepared to report your analysis in class.

2. Check your understanding of how to word a question on a discussion issue by preparing a short critique of the following items:
   a. Should students who have an A in a course going into the final examination be required to take the exam?
   b. The federal government should provide help for job-training programs.
   c. What can be done to promote world peace?
   d. The federal government should give tax credit to parents who send their children to private schools.
   e. What should the fraternity do for its spring event?
   f. How much money should be allocated to repair county roads?
   g. What can be done to improve the student health service?
When an item is poorly worded, write an alternative question. Share your work with a small group of classmates. Do you and the other members of your group agree about the questions?

NOTES

1. This person was using the word "conferences" to refer to business meetings of a small group of staff members from across his organization. Typically, the group included the heads of six departments and three or four other carefully selected individuals, who were there because of their special expertise.

2. Marvin E. Shaw, "Scaling Group Tasks: A Method for Dimensional Analysis," *JSAS Catalog of Selected Documents in Psychology* 8 (1973): M.S. 294.

3. See Randy Y. Hirokawa, "The Role of Communication in Group Decision Making: A Task-Contingency Perspective" (unpublished manuscript, University of Iowa, 1987), for more on tasks and decisions about organizing.

4. Marvin E. Shaw and J. M. Blum, "Effects of Leadership Styles Upon Group Performance as a Function of Task Structure," *Journal of Personality and Social Psychology* 49 (1965):238–242.

5. Leonard Berkowitz, "Sharing Leadership in Small Decision-Making Groups," *Journal of Abnormal and Social Psychology* 48 (1953):231–238.

6. James H. Davis, *Group Performance* (Reading, Mass.: Addison-Wesley, 1969).

7. Alex F. Osborn, *Applied Imagination: Principles and Procedures of Creative Thinking* (New York: Scribner's, 1953).

RECOMMENDED READINGS

Earl R. Babbie, *The Practice of Social Research*, 4th ed. (Belmont, Calif.: Wadsworth Publishing, 1983). Chapters 7 and 9 explain survey research.

Marvin E. Shaw, "Scaling Group tasks: A Method for Dimensional Analysis," *JSAS Catalog of Selected Documents in Psychology* 8 (1973):M.S. 294.

Gerald L. Wilson and H. Lloyd Goodall, Jr., *Interviewing in Context* (New York: Random House, 1990).

CHAPTER 3

Decision Making in Small Group Meetings

OBJECTIVES

After reading this chapter you should be able to:

Analyze a situation and assign the decision to the appropriate decision maker(s).

Specify the steps involved in using an agenda based upon reflective thinking.

Contrast the Brilhart-Jochem creative problem-solving sequence with an agenda based on Dewey's reflective thinking process.

Construct a decision-making agenda that follows the ideal solution sequence.

Suggest how a decision-making group might follow an agenda fashioned after the single question sequence.

Tailor an agenda to a group's needs.

Utilize a variety of discussion techniques: brainstorming, nominal group technique, buzz groups, quality circles.

Explain the circumstances and implications for decision making by consensus, compromise, majority vote, the leader, and arbitration.

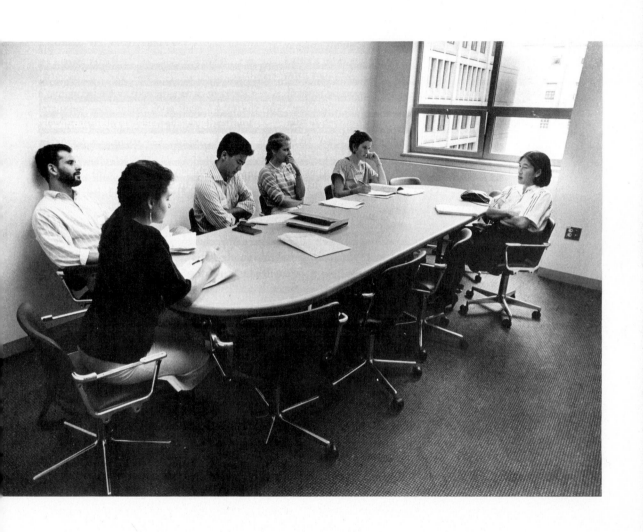

A steering committee for the annual financial pledge campaign for a local church was meeting to organize the effort. Jerry, who heads the finance committee, is chairing this specially appointed group. Other members of the committee are Dan, Gail, Jean, and Calvin. Notice the interaction as they meet for the first time.

> JERRY: I guess we are all here. Let's get started. It seems to me that our first task is to lay out a plan as to how we will get ourselves organized. We have to work so we will be ready to kick off the program by November first. Some of you worked on the campaign last year. Let's list the tasks that need to be accomplished.
>
> GAIL: We will need to recruit captains to lead groups to visit members.
>
> JEAN: I believe we also had co-captains. We'll need to recruit these people too.
>
> JERRY: Right. And what else do we need to worry about?
>
> DAN: We'll need to work up material describing the church's plans for the program.
>
> GAIL: And we need a budget and discussion about the areas in which we're expecting an increase.
>
> CALVIN: As I remember, we worked up some examples of ways of answering questions that people might have about the program. We'll need to get someone from programming to work on this right away.

You can tell by the direction that Jerry is leading this group that he has begun the process of organizing. He has asked group members to define what it is they have to do to accomplish their task. We can imagine that Jerry will continue the process of defining the task and then set the agendas for a series of meetings. This kind of planning is an important step if the group is to accomplish its goals in a timely manner. We had an opportunity to watch this group organize and carry out one of the most successful financial campaigns in its church's history. Understanding how to set and follow an appropriate decision-making agenda was a key factor in the group's success.

We begin this chapter by discussing individual versus group decision making. Then we present several agendas for your consideration. Each is useful under certain circumstances, so we suggest how each agenda might be used and also adapted to meet a particular group's needs. Next, four special discussion techniques are examined to help groups meet special problems. Finally, several decision-making methods are presented, along with the circumstances under which each is most likely to be useful.

INDIVIDUAL OR GROUP DECISION MAKING?

Each time a problem is uncovered, a judgment must be made as to who should make a decision about it. Should the problem be turned over to an individual or to a group? This is a complex problem with no simple answer. In fact, Victor H. Vroom and Arthur G. Jago have developed an elaborate plan for making a judgment about who should make a decision.[1] Here we wish to provide some of the most important questions to be considered in making the judgment about who should wrestle with a problem. Our discussion is based on Vroom and Jago's work as well as that of others.

1. *Is there one person who is truly an expert and the group is clearly not?*
   The expert should probably make the decision.

2. *Is there a severe time constraint on making a decision?*
   Turn the problem over to an individual who possesses the needed information and expertise to make a decision. Groups usually move more slowly than individuals. If the problem is given to a group, a leader can help the group move more quickly by imposing structure and holding the discussants to the time limits.

3. *Is the problem complex?*
   A complex problem usually requires a variety of views and expertise. A group is more likely to have the needed knowledge and expertise. Turn the problem over to the group, provided there is no time constraint. If the problem is simple and noncontroversial, turn it over to an individual who has the expertise to make the decision.

4. *Is it important that the group accept the decision?*
   If the problem is such that what needs to be done is clear and the group is likely to accept the decision, turn it over to an individual. If the group has to live with the decision and/or must implement it, and especially if the issue is controversial, turn the problem over to a group that has the knowledge and expertise to make a decision.

AGENDAS FOR SMALL GROUP DECISION MAKING

Agendas Based On Reflective Thinking

Suppose that you are enrolled in a philosophy class at your college or university. Your instructor is Professor John Dewey. He is interested in discovering how people think when they solve problems, so he asks you and several others to describe in detail how you solve problems.

Professor Dewey collects all your statements about problem solving and analyzes them for common characteristics. He is asking two questions:

1. Are there commonalities in the way these students think when they solve problems?

2. If so, what would a problem-solving agenda look like if it were based on these commonalities?

Dewey finds enough similarities to be quite confident that he is onto something important. He decides that the similarities are so significant that he will write a book to let others know of his discovery. This is in fact what a professor named John Dewey did. He published the results of his effort in a book entitled *How We Think*.[2]

Dewey believed that thinking reflectively obligates a person to adopt an attitude. The person must begin the process with a desire for "active, persistent, and careful consideration of any belief or supposed form of knowledge in the light of the grounds that support it and the further conclusions to which it tends."[3] Dewey is suggesting that the person must be committed to "active, persistent and careful consideration" of beliefs. Also, the person must carry this commitment to an examination of the "support" and "conclusions." All the while, group members must remain flexible in applying the decision-making process. This means a group should be prepared to modify the agenda to suit its purposes.

Below is a decision-making sequence generated from the ideas that John Dewey discovered in his research. The agenda, highlighted by italic print, is illustrated with an outline that a housing authority used to consider what to do about security in one of its buildings. As you read the agenda, first scan the italicized sections. Then go back and read the full text.

I. *What is the nature of the problem?*
There has been a 5 percent increase in crime in the Hillsdale Building. There were ten burglaries, two rapes, and two cases of vandalism in the past three months.

A. *What are the particulars of our group's assignment?*[4]

1. *Given this statement of the question, is it what we all understand to be the nature of the problem?*
Yes, we agree.

2. *Do we understand all the terminology related to the question?*
What is meant by burglary?
The breaking and entering of a premises and taking of possessions of another person.

3. *What kind of outcome is expected from the group? Discussion of the problem? Presentation of alternative solutions? A decision?*
Discussion of the problem and the presentation of a plan to the executive director for implementation.

B. *What harm is present in the current situation?*

1. *What is the harm?*
The pain and suffering of the individuals.
Loss of property valued at $4,500.
Image of the housing authority as providing safe living arrangements for the citizens of the county.

2. *Who is affected?*
The residents of the Hillsdale Building.

The employees of the housing authority who work in the building.
All the housing authority board members and employees, indirectly.

3. *How serious is the harm?*
Crime is on the increase.
The loss and the personal injury involved are substantial.

4. *How widespread is the harm?*
People on nearly every floor have been victims or know victims.
Residents of other buildings have complained of an increase in security problems.

C. *What seems to be causing the problem?*

1. *What factors if removed or changed would remove or lessen the harm?*
Vacant apartments seem to attract vandalism and crime.
Residents do not report suspicious people who hang around.
Residents often leave doors unlocked.
Many residents do not have telephones, so they have no good way to call for help.

2. *What are the obstacles to successfully removing the causes of the harm?*
It may be difficult if not impossible to rent all the units in this building.
Residents do not have funds to have telephones installed, and board policy prohibits payment for private installation.

II. *What criteria should we set?*

A. *What are the important conditions—criteria—that an effective solution must meet?*
We cannot break existing board policy.
We cannot spend over $5,000, the amount allocated for this project.
We must not approve a plan that advantages particular residents of the complex over other residents.
The plan must be such that it can be implemented in other buildings where security problems are beginning to surface.

B. *Are some criteria more important to use than others? Can the criteria be rank-ordered in terms of importance?*
Yes. We must treat all residents equally. We cannot go over the $5,000 allocated. Board policy might be changed, but only if absolutely necessary.

III. *What available alternatives might meet the causes of this problem and alleviate the harm?*

1. Install an emergency alert system on each floor.

2. Increase outside lighting.

3. Replace locks on doors with double-bolt-type locks.

4. Install peepholes in doors.

5. Offer incentives for residents to move to empty apartments, closing off the top floor temporarily.

6. Organize a crime watch among the residents, offering cash rewards for making a report that results in apprehension and conviction of criminals.

7. Hire a private security system.

8. Attempt to get increased county police surveillance.

IV. *What is the best solution for this problem?*

   A. *Which of these or what combination of these solutions seems most likely to counter the causes of this problem?*
   Better locks and peepholes would help keep criminals out.
   Elimination of empty apartments would allow for more people to be around to discover the crime.
   A private professional security service would provide the most reliable protection.
   Increased outside lighting would most certainly discourage crime.

   B. *Of the solutions that seem likely to be effective, which ones meet the criteria that were set?*
   Moving residents might not be fair. Some residents have lived in their apartments for fifteen years.
   Cost is a factor. The funds will not allow for a private security company. Perhaps the county police are an alternative.
   Cost of the other items is probably within the $5,000.

   C. *Given solutions that are likely to counter the causes, and meet the criteria set, what seems to be the best solution?*
   All the solutions seem likely to work, except moving people and the crime watch. Residents are unlikely to respond to an effort to organize them. They haven't been known for community responsibility and pulling together.

V. *What plans will we set in order to implement our solution?*

   A. *What needs to be done?*
   Turn the plan over to the executive director for action.

   B. *In what order?*
   Ask the director to begin with lock installation, immediately.
   Contact the county police and ask them how they can provide increased patrolling of the Hillsdale Building.
   Then a contract for upgrading lighting needs to be made.

   C. *By whom?*
   The executive director will carry out these plans and report back to us within thirty days.

VI. *How will we evaluate the effect of our solution?*

    A. *What observable evidence will we monitor to evaluate the effect of our solution?*
       We will collect crime reports and residents' complaints.

    B. *Who will be responsible for follow-up evaluation?*
       The executive director.

Several scholars have provided variations on this general scheme for decision making to adapt it to particular group and situational needs. We present three of these below. The first, the Brilhart-Jochem sequence, is especially useful if the problem is such that multiple solutions are possible and creativity is important. The second, the ideal solution sequence, is appropriate when the views of various segments of an organization need to be considered. The third, the single question sequence, is useful when a group is beginning its decision process without knowing what issues might be involved in the problem at hand.

Brilhart-Jochem Ideation Criteria

An alternative agenda was developed by John Brilhart and Lurene Jochem.[5] Brilhart has called this the creative problem-solving sequence,[6] as it makes use of a well-known principle of creativity. The idea behind the Brilhart-Jochem scheme is that in limiting one's perspective, a person limits what he or she is able to think about a problem.

Suppose a student group is trying to make a decision about what to do about safety on its campus after dark. Suppose again that they are told that there are no funds available to use in whatever solution they decide to adopt. This limits the kinds of ideas they might consider for dealing with student safety at night. Now suppose instead that they consider solutions without concern about the amount of money they might have. Maybe John would suggest a few safety lights at key locations. We might imagine that that would cost several thousand dollars. Now perhaps Linda suggests merely moving some lights from locations where they are not needed. The cost of this plan, assuming use of already paid-for university maintenance, is only $500. Perhaps "no funds" does not really mean that absolutely no money is available. Five hundred dollars might be a realistic possibility. Here is the point: If the group had begun its consideration of solutions with an affirmation that there was no money for the project, John would probably not have made his lighting suggestion. If John had not suggested the lighting idea, do you suppose Linda would have thought of moving the lights? Of course, we do not know whether she would have done so or not. But perhaps it was John's idea that helped Linda to think of hers. This reasoning would suggest that limiting the scope of the group's thinking—that is, in this case telling themselves that they had no money to spend—limits their ability to think about solutions. It limits their ability to be creative in generating solutions about this problem.

Brilhart and Jochem provided a plan to help a group to avoid this limitation of their creativity. The first point where a limiting factor comes into play in Dewey's original scheme is in setting criteria. When a group sets criteria it limits the solutions it is willing to consider—and this is why groups set criteria. In fact, Brilhart and Jochem suggest that you do this, too. However, they argue that the time to set criteria is after the group has generated as many solutions as it is able to discover. So Brilhart and Jochem shuffled Dewey's sequence a bit to form their own five-step creative problem-solving agenda.

1. What is the nature of the problem facing us (present state, obstacles, goals)?

2. What might be done to solve the problem (or the first subproblem)?

3. By what specific criteria shall we judge among our possible solutions?

4. What are the relative merits of our possible solutions?

5. How will we put our decision into effect?[7]

You can see that the main difference between this agenda and the one that was just presented is the reversing of steps 2 and 3. Criteria, originally step 2, comes after suggesting solutions, originally step 3. Each of the agenda items for these steps asks for the same kinds of considerations as addressed in the previous agenda. To help you visualize the kinds of subquestions that will help you process these main questions, a full discussion outline using the Brilhart-Jochem agenda is presented here.

I. What is the nature of the problem facing us (present state, obstacles, goals)?

    A. What are we talking about?

        1. Is the question or assignment clear to us?

        2. Do we need to define any terms or concepts?

    B. What is our area of freedom?

        1. Are we to plan and take action, advise, or what?

        2. What sort of end product should result from our discussion?

    C. What has been happening that is unsatisfactory?

        1. What is wrong? How do we know?

        2. Who is affected, how, and under what conditions?

        3. How serious do we consider the situation to be?

        4. Have any corrective actions previously been tried that did not work?

        5. What additional information do we need to assess adequately the extent and nature of the problem?

    D. What is the desired situation or goal we hope to achieve?

    E. What factors seem to have caused this problem?

        1. Are there any causative conditions about which we can be certain?

        2. What obstacles must we remove to achieve the desired situation?

    F. How can we summarize the problem to include the present situation, the desired situation, the difference, the causes, and the obstacles?

      1. Do we all agree on this statement of the problem?

      2. Should we divide it into any subproblems?

        a. If so, what are they?

        b. In what order should we take them up?

  II. What might be done to solve the problem (or first subproblem)? (Here the group brainstorms for possible solutions.)

 III. By what specific criteria shall we judge among our possible solutions?

    A. What absolute criteria must a solution meet?

    B. What relative standards shall we apply? (List and rank these values and standards by group agreement.)

 IV. What are the relative merits of our possible solutions?

    A. What ideas can we screen out as unsupported by uncontested facts?

    B. Can we combine and simplify our list of possible solutions in any way?

    C. How well do the remaining ideas measure up to the criteria?

  V. How will we put our decision into effect?

    A. Who will do what, when, and how?

    B. Do we need any follow-up or check procedures?[8] (If the answer to V-B is yes, then complete Step VI.)

 VI. How will we evaluate the effect of our solution?

    A. What observable evidence will we monitor with respect to the problem?

    B. Who will be responsible for the follow-up evaluation?

Ideal Solution Sequence

Sometimes we encounter a problem that we know can be solved by a variety of solutions. Often various groups are affected by the decision directly, so that each of these groups has its own "ideal" solution. Carl Larson discussed a decision-making sequence that takes these factors into account.[9] This plan asks the group to take into account the various ideal solutions the involved parties might favor.

    It is easy to imagine a group with such a problem. Consider this special committee that was appointed by the vice-president of a university to consider a change in the between-term break in December. Follow this outline of how the group approached the situation using the ideal solution sequence and you will see how the group took into account the views of various segments of the organization.

Larson lists these four questions in the ideal solution sequence:

I. Are we all agreed on the nature of the problem? (This involves stating the problem and understanding the nature of the problem. It can be developed as any of the first steps outlined above.)

I. We have been called together to make recommendations as to when the Christmas break should be taken. Do we all agree that is our goal? (Here the problem would be analyzed as the first step in the reflective thinking pattern or Brilhart-Jochem pattern.)

II. What would be the ideal solution from the point of view of all interested persons or groups involved in the problem?

II. The students want more time to work prior to Christmas. They would like to be out at least two weeks prior to Christmas. The people in the registrar's office and other administrative personnel want to have more time after Christmas. The faculty senate has passed a resolution urging this committee not to split the term. They do not want to come back after the break and still have a term to complete. The ideal solution from the view of all parties would be to complete the term before Christmas, returning for the new term on January 2.

III. What conditions within the situation could be changed so that the ideal solution might be achieved? (Here is where the group members consider proposals for change. They are concerned with finding the change—solution—that will deal most effectively with the harm. But they also might discover obstacles that cannot be changed. With this in mind, they are ready to find the best possible solution.)

III. No, a two-week break before Christmas would not allow time to cover the course material. Could we start the term earlier, so that it could end two weeks before Christmas? Yes, I think so.

IV. Of the solutions available to us, which one best approximates the ideal solution? (Groups often approach this task by trying to incorporate elements of the various groups' solutions into an ideal solution.)

IV. We could extend the term break so that students would be able to work for two weeks prior to Christmas. The extended break would allow administrative personnel the time they want to be with their families. It would not break up the term.

Single Question Sequence

In research he conducted on group problem solving, Carl Larson found that this pattern, like the ideal solution sequence, produced more choices of best alternatives than did the reflective thinking pattern.[10] This sequence was formulated to help groups identify issues that flow from a particular problem. Once they have identified the issues, they are asked to resolve them—phrased in the form of subquestions—and then to identify the best solution to the major question. The questions that led the governing board, which was deciding about adding new programs, through this procedure are these:

I. What is the single question whose answer is all the group needs to know in order to accomplish its purpose?

I. How many programs can we provide with the 10 percent increase over our current budget?

II. What subquestions must be answered before we can answer the single question we have formulated?

II. What programs should be instituted? How much will each cost? What cost will we incur for personnel and equipment? What is the anticipated participation in these programs?

III. Do we have sufficient information to answer the subquestions confidently?
A. If yes, answer them.
B. If no, continue below.

III. The answer is no. We continue with IV, below.

IV. What are the most reasonable answers to the subquestions? (Notice that the language here asks for the "most reasonable." Circumstances might be such that some issues cannot be fully resolved, and therefore the group must accept the most reasonable answer.)

IV. We cannot agree as to which programs we should initiate next year. We did agree to poll the membership and go with some of their suggestions. The average cost of each program last year was $11,000. The miscellaneous costs associated with each program were $2,450. The receipts from membership fees increased 12 percent.

V. Assuming that our answers to the subquestions are correct, what is the best solution to the problem?

V. Assuming that these figures hold, we should be able to fund two new programs at an estimated cost of $27,000.

From here the group might move to deciding how to implement its decision.

A word of caution: Merely applying an appropriate agenda for decision making is not enough. Decision quality rests with how the agenda is applied. Randy Hirokawa found that *careful* analysis and understanding of the problem and *thorough, vigilant* appraisal of solutions were necessary for quality decisions to result.[11]

Groups need to remain vigilant in following decision-making procedures. What this means in practice can be discovered by considering further research by Randy Hirokawa.[12] Vigilant decision making requires retrospective questioning once choices are made. In practical terms, this means going back to look at the decision once it is made and asking, "What if we implemented our decision? How would it play out?" Also, it means that groups must thoroughly and accurately understand the problem, consider a variety of acceptable alternatives, and evaluate each alternative carefully.

Careful evaluation means considering both positive and negative consequences associated with each alternative. Thus the importance of critical thinking cannot be overestimated.

Adapting the Agenda to the Group's Needs

Selecting an agenda is only a starting place for a group. A wise group leader is likely to modify the particular agenda to fit the group's immediate need. John K. Brilhart[13] has presented a useful scheme for modifying agendas according to problem characteristics. He suggests how these agendas might be tailored to use the best agenda, the best stage of an agenda, and/or combination of stages from different agendas. Brilhart's suggestions are found in Table 3.1.

Beyond special needs that might be presented by the characteristics of the task at hand, you should consider the impact of your particular group. Ask these two important

TABLE 3.1   Problem Characteristics Matched to Agenda Steps

Problem	Solution(s)
1. Difficulty of problem is high.	1. Problem mapping, as presented in single question format, or Step I of reflective thinking and creative problem solving formats.
2. Multiple solutions to the problem are possible.	2. Ideation, Step II of creative problem-solving sequence, possibly including "brainstorming."
3. Intrinsic interest in the problem is high.	3. A period of "ventilation" before a systematic problem-solving sequence.
4. Corporative requirements for deciding about the problem are high.	4. If not already clear to all, a "criteria" step may be helpful, as in Step III of creative problem-solving sequence.
5. Member familiarity with the problem is low.	5. Many subquestions will be needed in Step I to thoroughly map out the problem. The single question format may be especially appropriate.
6. A high level of acceptance for the solution is required.	6. Be sure to include Step II of the ideal solution format.
7. A high level of technical quality is required in coming to a decision.	7. The reflective thinking sequence may be most suitable.
8. Area of freedom is such that the members are responsible for every aspect of the problem-solving process.	8. Any complete problem-solving sequence, depending on other characteristics.
9. Area of freedom is limited to advising on one or a few aspects of problem solving.	9. The sequence should be shortened to emphasize only those steps in which the group has authority.

questions about the group to help you decide on your agenda: How long have members been working together? Do they have experience in working with this kind of task?

Groups that have been working together for a long time have very often developed their own agenda system. They have developed a particular way of working with problems with which they feel comfortable. It works well for them. If their own agenda system works for them, and if it allows reasonable consideration of the problems they address, then it may be a mistake to impose an unfamiliar agenda on them.

But how do you know if an agenda "allows reasonable consideration of the problems they address"? There are two tests you can apply. *First, do the decisions the group implements seem to work?* Does the decision alleviate the harm? Are the people affected by the decisions satisfied? *Second, does the group have difficulty coming to decisions?* Some problems are difficult and very controversial. We expect groups to engage in considerable conflict about their ideas in these cases. But if the group has difficulty with decision making on a regular basis, then the difficulty may be a function of their agenda.

Perhaps a more careful analysis of the problem is needed. Sometimes too few solutions are considered. At other times the group is so diversified in member attitude that it needs to recognize and consider the ideal solutions for the different groups involved—Step II of the ideal solution sequence. Decision-making difficulty can be a function of failure to discuss criteria—especially if the problem revolves around values. The group's own agenda might need to be modified to take one of these problems into account.

Using the Agenda Effectively

Five important rules will help your group make more efficient use of an agenda.

First, do not keep the agenda secret.   Some leaders bring their agenda to the group's meeting, pass it around to the group's members, and expect the members to make good use of it. This type of behavior does not allow group members to prepare for the meeting with the agenda in hand. As you can imagine, informed preparation is usually better than uninformed preparation. Publish the agenda several days before the meeting, and make it clear to the group that they will be given a chance to modify it if they wish.

Second, tailor the agenda to the specific problem.   This means that you should formulate specific questions for the agenda in terms of the problem. This will also focus the group members' attention. Notice that specific questions have been formulated for the agendas presented above. These help to focus the group's attention in a way that would not be possible if your agenda were published with the more general questions—the ones used in the presentation of the agenda itself. Help in writing specific discussion questions is offered in Chapter 2. Be sure to look at that section before you write questions for your group's agenda.

Third, ask the members at the start of the meeting if they wish to amend or modify the agenda.   Group members may not be satisfied with the particular plan. They need to be able to change it. When they seem satisfied, get verbal agreement. This constitutes public agreement of the agenda as a rough statement of the group's goals.

Fourth, post an abbreviated form of the agenda where the group can see it.   This will help keep the group oriented. It also serves to remind the group of its progress as it moves through the agenda steps.

Fifth, use the agenda to go back and check on the quality of the process and decision.   Did the group conduct a careful analysis of the problem? Does the solution seem to eliminate the causes that were uncovered? Does the solution meet the criteria? Does the group's plan allow for careful monitoring of the implementation of the decision and its results? Has the group considered contingencies that can be put in place if necessary?

DISCUSSION TECHNIQUES

Professors who have been consultants to business and other organizations have developed a number of techniques designed to fulfill certain specific functions.[14] The first two of these, brainstorming and nominal group technique, usually serve as idea-generation facilitators. For example, they can be used to generate a large number of creative solutions. The third technique, the buzz group, serves the purpose of gaining input from a large group meeting. The fourth, the quality circle, involves employees in decisions about their work.

Brainstorming

Brainstorming is a procedure that asks participants to propose ideas but not to criticize them as they are being presented. (Generally someone in the group will record all suggested ideas.) The leader will encourage group members to produce ideas, while discouraging discussion and criticism of the ideas. The underlying assumptions of the system are that criticism restricts the flow of ideas and that discussion of those ideas distracts the group from the task of idea generation. A group that forces itself to generate a large number of ideas will generate some good ones. Further, creative thought is fostered by the stimulation of hearing others' suggestions.

Alex Osborn, co-owner of an advertising agency, first discussed this procedure in his book *Applied Imagination*.[15] Osborn sought some way to help his staff become more creative in their attempt to develop marketing strategies. The assumptions about the generating of ideas and creativity yielded four rules that are calculated to guide a group toward this goal.

I. All evaluation and criticism of ideas is forbidden.

II. Wild and offbeat ideas are encouraged.

III. Quantity, not quality, of ideas is the goal.

IV. New combinations of ideas are sought.[16]

This technique can be used in a variety of ways in a decision-making task. For example, a group might use brainstorming to answer any of these questions:

Where can we find information?

What kind of information do we need to solve the problem?

What solutions might we consider?

What criteria are important to us?

What are the various ways we might implement our decision?

As you can see, a decision-making group can use brainstorming at many points in a discussion. The most usual point for its use, however, is in generating solutions. Of course, regardless of the use to which brainstorming is put, it is only the first step in making decisions. The ideas must be judged as useful and then combined and refined.

Groups that are not experienced in using the brainstorming technique may find they have problems with it. One problem comes from the natural tendency for people to support their own ideas. A person who presents an idea wants to elaborate on it. Someone who thinks that her idea is better wants to tell the group why it is better. So a group that is using brainstorming for the first time will need a leader who can supportively curtail the group members' desires to evaluate and elaborate.

Groups may also get stalled after they have a list of several items. The leader can help here also. Encouragement is needed. The leader might say, "Can we think of three more ideas?" Sometimes it helps the group to get started again if the leader reads the list of suggestions already made. The leader might say, "As I read this list, try to think of ideas we have missed."

Another problem is the tendency for some members to stifle the flow of ideas through their nonverbal communication. For example, a member may frown with disapproval at an idea that he or she does not like. The frown may discourage the contributor's willingness to continue providing ideas. The leader may need to caution group members about this tendency and perhaps invoke some prearranged signal if these kinds of nonverbal messages seem to be affecting the free flow of ideas.

Nominal Group Technique (NGT)

Sometimes more alternatives and higher-quality decisions can be achieved through a technique that is not actually group discussion. *Nominal group technique* (NGT) is a procedure for generating ideas and making decisions in which members work silently— but in one another's presence—to generate ideas. They then pool their ideas, clarify them, rank-order them, and then may move to a discussion of the ideas, and a decision.

This procedure has been labeled *nominal group* because it is not necessary for the group to engage in the type of interaction that is considered important for groups. In fact, in a version of this technique called *Delphi,* participants generate a decision without ever meeting face to face. Delphi requires that the whole process be conducted by mail. The participants generate a list of ideas and are then asked to rank-order a master list; a decision is reached by noting which ideas are most favored.

The procedure was created to avoid two problems caused by group interaction. First, some members are reluctant to suggest ideas because they are concerned about being criticized. Second, some members are reluctant to create conflict in groups. Perhaps they are concerned about maintaining a pleasant social climate. NGT overcomes these problems. In fact, there is some evidence that it produces better performance than do techniques involving group discussion.[17] Here is how André Delbecq[18] describes the procedure:

I. *Silent generation of ideas in writing.* The first step in NGT is to have the group members write key ideas silently and independently.

II. *Round-robin recording of ideas.* The second step of NGT is to record the ideas of group members on a flip chart visible to the entire group. Round-robin recording means going around the table and asking for one idea from one member at a time. The leader writes the idea of a group member on the flip chart and then proceeds to ask for one idea from the next group member in turn.

III. *Serial discussion for clarification.* The third step of NGT is to discuss each idea in turn. Serial discussion means taking each idea listed on the flip chart in order, and allowing a short period of time for the discussion of each idea. The leader points to Item 1, reads it out loud, and asks the group if there are any questions, statements of clarification, or statements of agreement or disagreement. . . . [The leader should] not allow discussion to: (1) unduly focus on any particular idea; or (2) degenerate into argumentation. [Note: The idea here is not to interact about disagreement, but to present the reasons for agreement or disagreement without engaging in a clash with other members.]

IV. *Preliminary vote on item importance.* The average NGT meeting will generate over twelve items in each group during its idea-generation phase. Through serial discussion, group members will come to understand the meaning of the item, the logic behind the item, and argument for and against the importance of individual items. In some manner, however, the group must aggregate the judgments of individual members in order to determine the relative importance of individual items. [One method of doing this is to have group members rank order their choices in terms of acceptability. These can then be tabulated and the results tallied. An idea may clearly emerge from this process. If no idea emerges, the group can then engage in discussion and attempt to achieve an agreement.]

NGT has the clear advantage of minimizing differences and ensuring relatively equal participation. It may also in many cases be a time-saving technique. Susan Jarboe's research suggests that NGT also decreases the tension and hostility a group might normally experience relative to its decision making.[19] But Delbecq and his colleagues suggest that it is best used in meetings that are concerned with *judgmental* decision making. These are meetings that involve *creative* decision making.

The type of questions that such groups would consider are: "What should be done about employee absenteeism?" "What policies should be established to provide for efficient and profitable management of the auditorium?" "What activities should be planned for the fraternity in the next six months?" "What kind of marketing plan should we adopt for this new sport shoe?"

Delbecq makes the point that the technique is not suited to routine meetings. For Delbecq, the routine meeting is a "situation where members of the group agree upon the desired goal, and the technologies exist to achieve this goal. In such a meeting the focus is on coordination and information exchange, and the meeting is 'leader centered.' "[20] (These meetings are also called programmed decision situations, since no real decision making is taking place.) So a meeting to report on production quota and to set new goals would not be suited to Delbecq's nominal group technique.

Buzz Groups

The *buzz group*—sometimes called Phillips 66—was created by J. Donald Phillips to maximize the input of members in a large group meeting.[21] The large group is divided into subgroups of six persons. Each of these groups discusses a designated question for a specific length of time and reports its conclusions back to the large group's leader. The leader collects the results and then displays them for the membership.

The technique involves six steps:

1. The chairperson of the group presents a carefully formulated question to the group. This must be concise and limited in scope so that the groups will be able to manage it in a brief period.

2. The large group is divided into smaller groups of six members. These groups are provided tables if possible. If this is not possible, they must be given enough space to have some privacy. (Usually a large auditorium is used if available.)

3. Appoint a spokesperson for each group. This person will chair the meeting and report back the results to the larger group. The leader should understand the rules: (1) All ideas are to be recorded, and (2) the group is to rank-order them according to the most preferred. Provide cards for recording ideas.

4. Ask the group members to follow this procedure: Propose ideas for five minutes; then devote one minute to deleting duplicates and ideas the group does not want to pass on; then rank-order the remaining ideas. (This is where the procedure gets the name Phillips 66: Six members discuss for six minutes.)

5. Notify the groups when they have consumed five minutes. Give them an extra minute to finish their listing; then ask them to evaluate and rank-order.

6. Now ask each spokesperson to read their group's first suggestion in a round-robin fashion. These can be listed on a chalkboard or overhead projector for

all to see. Of course, duplicates will not be read. Instead, the spokesperson should read the next item on his or her list.

The conclusions from this process can be evaluated by some appropriate subgroup of the membership, such as the group's executive committee or an ad hoc committee appointed for the task.

This technique can be used in a variety of contexts. Political, social, and fraternal groups can wisely use it to get their members involved in the group decision-making process. You can imagine that it helps to overcome some of the problems associated with too large a group trying to engage in decision making.

Quality Circles

A popular strategy for managing people is to involve them in decisions about their work and work environment. We know that people are generally more willing to do their jobs and to make an effort to change their performance when they are taken into account. One very effective way of taking subordinates into account is to talk directly with them about problems and allow them to help make decisions. Direct involvement allows individuals to agree and to make a public commitment to a decision. When that happens, subordinates are more likely to make that decision work.

Perhaps the *quality circle* is the clearest example of a participative management group. Quality circles evolved in Japanese firms through the efforts of an American consultant, Dr. Joseph Juran, who advocated participative decision making as a method of achieving quality control. In 1961 the editors of the Japanese magazine *Quality Control* took up this idea. They believed that involving first-line supervisors in quality control would increase productivity. The result of their advocacy was a new publication called *The Foreman and QC*. Participative management groups became popular in Japan and, consequently, came to the attention of American business and industry.[22] Firms such as Lockheed Corporation, J. C. Penney, Uniroyal, General Motors, Firestone, Chrysler, Ampex, R. J. Reynolds, Bendix, and many others instituted quality circles.

How does the participative management group work?   Participative management groups seek to improve production through employee problem solving. The supervisor of such a group delegates the authority to make decisions to a group of subordinates. Some members of a department *voluntarily* meet to discuss work problems and make decisions. The theory is that the employees are in the best position to know about some problems, *and* when they are involved in decision making, they will be more committed to the outcome. But workers usually need help if they are to be successful participants. We think you can provide that help regardless of your rank in an organization. You can help to build the appropriate climate and to direct and facilitate the group effort.

The supervisor of a participative management group serves as a guide rather than as a boss who imposes a decision. Thus this person is in an unenviable position. Once a group recommends a course of action, the supervisor must either accept the idea or reject it and thereby demoralize the group. And when the decision is implemented, it is the supervisor who must assume responsibility for the outcome, not the employees. For this reason a supervisor should be careful in selecting the problems he or she turns over to a participative management group for resolution.

Recognize also that participative management may not work well in certain situations. If a supervisor asks subordinates whose egos are highly involved in an issue to solve a problem related to it, they may not be objective enough or flexible enough to reach a quality decision. Further, a person who is highly apprehensive about communicating or is low on assertiveness is not likely to be a productive group member. Also, a participative management group may not be successful if no member is willing to engage in leadership behaviors. A manager can guide a group but must rely on some group member for leadership too. Otherwise the manager may have to take too large a role in the group and run the risk of being perceived as manipulative. Finally, recognize that quality circle participants must have top management support, a willingness of superiors to accept suggestions and criticisms from subordinates, and training in task and social decision-making skills.[23]

How do you structure the meeting?   We presented a good format for the participative management decision-making activity in Dewey's problem-solving agenda in the preceding section. Perhaps you can see that the following agenda is similar. We will assume in what follows that you are responsible for planning a participative management meeting.

1. *Discover the problems.* It seems clear that the group will have to discover the problems to be addressed before it can spend time discussing them in detail. Ask people to bring a list of things that keep them from doing their jobs well. Combine the lists on a flip chart and ask the group to rank-order the items from most to least serious.

2. *Gather the relevant data.* You and other group members need time to gather relevant information. Spend some time asking what information group members will need in order to make a quality decision. Ask for volunteers to bring the appropriate information.

3. *Discover why there is a problem.* Remember that many groups are too solution-oriented. Try to get the group to discuss the causes of problems if you can. Point out the relationship between causes and solutions. The solution ought to remove the causes.

4. *Brainstorm for solutions.* It is a good idea to get all imaginable solutions the group might consider on the table *before* a group tries to compare the alternatives. The group needs to know what its options are. Beyond that, brainstorming usually causes a group to consider a greater number of alternatives. Ask members to withhold their comments about the ideas until they have listed as many solutions as possible.

5. *Make the decision.* After alternatives have been recorded, evaluate each of the ideas. How does each compare with the others? Which ideas do not remove

the causes? Which can be eliminated? Which ideas might be combined to make a more comprehensive solution? What would happen if a particular decision were implemented? Is the proposed idea a practical one? These are all questions your group might consider in making a final decision.

METHODS OF DECIDING

The output of the process of decision making is often affected by the way the group comes to its decision. Member satisfaction, willingness to work toward carrying out the decision, and even the quality of the decision may be affected by how the members decide. This potential impact is important and you need to understand the possible outcomes of the various kinds of decision making. Five methods of deciding will be considered here: consensus, compromise, majority vote, decision by leader, and arbitration.

Consensus

Consensus literally means that all group members agree. In decision making, however, we usually mean that all members genuinely agree that a decision is acceptable. Groups are often encouraged to aim for consensus.[24] This does not mean that they are completely in favor of something. As you might imagine, such a decision is difficult for groups to achieve. This is particularly true if the members of the group are personally involved in the situation being discussed. Imagine, for example, an office manager calling her workers together to decide on the allocation of a new self-correcting typewriter. Tracy's involvement in the situation is quite understandable. He is the senior member of the department. Thus he is inclined to argue vigorously for the new typewriter because he knows he ought to be first in line because of his seniority. Sally believes just as strongly that she would receive one of the new typewriters. She has the oldest machine in the department. She believes that receiving the new typewriter would give her the best opportunity to show how good she really is. Others have their arguments, too. In this case consensus is unlikely, unless the group has a strong need for consensus. Such a need can lead to a norm to agree.[25] This group is more likely to have to move to some other method of deciding, perhaps to compromise.

Compromise

Compromise decisions are those in which the people involved give up some of what they hoped for in a solution so that the group can come to a decision. Compromise represents the "best solution" the group can achieve given the diversity of opinion of its members. In the case of deciding about the typewriter, Tracy may agree to wait for the next allocation of new typewriters. But again, if Tracy feels that he really needs a new typewriter, then he is likely to be unhappy with a compromise decision. Others, such as Sally, may also be displeased with the results. This is why a compromise decision is called a lose/lose situation. And if the implementation of your group's decision requires the active, enthusiastic participation of all its members, a problem has been created. Sometimes compromise cannot be avoided. But when compromise is necessary, the group's leadership needs to be aware of the possible difficulties.

Majority Vote

Majority vote differs from compromise. Here members indicate their preferences and the majority will prevails. Most Americans are quite willing to abide by what the majority decides because—at least in the abstract—they believe in this basic tenet of democracy. But if we put it in terms of the decision about the typewriters, the difficulty with this method of deciding becomes clear. Suppose the group has seven members. Four members vote to allocate the typewriters on the basis of seniority, and three members vote to give them on the basis of need. Sally believes that she is being held back by an old piece of machinery. How does she react? She says, "I've lost a big one. I have a knot in my stomach. And I'm really angry." Majority vote is a win/lose situation. The majority has "forced" its decision on the rest of the group. Sally and perhaps others are very unhappy.

In ongoing groups that make use of majority vote, different segments may win at different times. This makes losing somewhat easier for members. Most of us feel better about the situation if we get what we want some of the time. In contrast, if a certain segment of an ongoing group loses most of the time, cohesiveness and group morale will be likely to suffer. Julia Wood noted that people become anxious to take a vote and achieve closure on an issue. She concludes that the vote is often taken at the expense of group harmony and equal representation of the differing points of view.[26] Again, if the majority needs the minority to help implement their decisions, the minority may not be willing to help. They may resent the majority and secretly drag their feet when it comes time to help.

Decision by the Leader

Sometimes by virtue of the leader's position, he or she can impose a decision on the organization or group. In these cases it appears that the group is being asked to make a decision and that it has been given the power to make the decision, when the leader has actually retained that power. Usually the decision is announced after the group has discussed the problem and some solutions. Sometimes, though, the leader may argue in such a way that it is clear that only one solution will be acceptable. The leader might say, "Joe, that's an interesting idea. But I don't see how I could recommend that to the boss. Let's consider this other suggestion again." In still other cases, the leader may merely thank group members for their efforts and then dismiss them. She might say, "I appreciate your ideas and input. Thank you for your help. I'll write up a report and make a recommendation."

Group members' reaction to a decision by the leader depends on the circumstances.

If members have been misled into thinking that they are to make a decision and have the power to do so, they are likely to feel betrayed and resentful. If they know that they are only providing input, and if they believe that they are actually being listened to, then they may engage in worthwhile discussion. If the group members know that their interaction is only a show—that the decision is already made—they may merely go through the motions of discussing and resent the waste of their time.

Imagine again the group that is deciding about the typewriters. It reaches a decision, only to find that the typewriters have already been pledged. Or perhaps the office manager plays an active role in the group, objecting to every type of decision but the one she wants. Since the manager has power, she can impose a decision. The result, however, is resentment and disillusionment.

Arbitration

Sometimes groups are unable to make a decision and do not want to take a vote on the issue. They would prefer that some disinterested third party make the decision, a process called *arbitration*. Generally this third party makes a decision that allows each faction of the group to win some issues while losing others. Labor-management negotiations are typically subject to decision by arbitration when the two sides think they have reached a stalemate and they want to settle the terms of their contract. Since group members are reluctant to give up some of what they wanted in a decision, this method of deciding may also create disappointment and lack of interest in implementing the decision.

Each of these methods has advantages and disadvantages. Probably the method with the most advantages is consensus. Beyond achieving consensus lie the other methods, each with its disadvantages. Be aware of the differences, and the consequences of the method your groups come to in making decisions. Sometimes groups have neither the time nor the ability to achieve consensus. In these cases, pay careful attention to the implementation of the decision. Not all the members of your group may support the effort enthusiastically.

SUMMARY

An important decision to be made when a problem arises is whether it should be handled by an individual or a group. We discussed questions that are useful in making this decision. Several agendas for decision making were proposed. John Dewey suggested a reflective thinking process from which a five-step agenda has been generated. The five steps are: (1) What is the nature of the problem? (2) What criteria should be set? (3) What alternatives are available that might meet the causes of this problem? (4) What is the best solution for this problem? (5) What plans will be set in order to implement the solution? We suggest a sixth step: (6) How will the effect of implementing the solution be evaluated?

John K. Brilhart and Lurene Jochem suggested a modification to this basic agenda.

They suggested what they called the creative problem-solving sequence. Their suggestion is that step 2 should be "What alternatives are available that might meet the causes of this problem?" Step 3 should be "What criteria should be set?" They argued that reversing this order helps generate more creative solutions.

The ideal solution sequence focuses on what a variety of identifiable groups might consider to be their ideal solutions. Its steps are: (1) Are we all agreed on the nature of the problem? (2) What would be the ideal solution from the view of all interested groups? (3) What conditions within the problem could be changed so that the ideal solution might be achieved? (4) Of the solutions available, which one best approximates the ideal solution?

The single question sequence offers an alternative agenda. It has as its focus the identification of issues that will lead to a decision about the major problem. The steps in this agenda are: (1) What is the question whose answer is all the group needs to know in order to accomplish its purpose? (2) What subquestions must be answered before the single question can be answered? (3) Do we have sufficient information to answer the subquestions confidently? (4) What are the most reasonable answers to the subquestions? (5) Assuming that our answers to the subquestions are correct, what is the best solution to the problem?

A decision to use a particular agenda is based on certain characteristics of the task. If the task is difficult, the group may want a relatively complete agenda. If multiple solutions seem likely, the group may want to engage in some idea-generation technique. If high cooperation is needed to make a decision and carry it out, then the group should spend time in step 3 of the creative problem-solving sequence. If the group is not very familiar with the problem, then it might choose to map the problem carefully by step 1 of the single question sequence. If a high level of acceptance of a diversified group is needed, then step 2 of the ideal solution sequence might be important.

A leader can make the most efficient use of an agenda by publishing it in advance, tailoring it to the specific problem, allowing the members to modify the agenda, posting an abbreviated version of the agenda where all can see it, and using the agenda to help group members check the quality of their decision.

Brainstorming and nominal group technique were discussed as idea-generation techniques. Both are ways of getting group participation by withholding criticism while members are listing ideas. Brainstorming is a group technique in that members interact. Nominal group technique does not involve member interaction as the group generates ideas.

Buzz groups are used to gain input from all the members of large groups. Here the group is broken into subgroups of six members each and given six minutes to generate ideas. The leader of the large group gathers the ideas and presents them to the reassembled large group.

Quality circles are decision-making groups found in the workplace. They are composed of volunteers who deliberate about work problems and are led by a supervisor who acts as a facilitator.

Groups can make decisions through consensus, compromise, majority vote, decision by leader, or arbitration. Consensus means that all members find the decision acceptable.

Compromise involves giving up some of what members want in a solution so that the group can agree. Majority vote suggests that the decision is made on the basis of what most of the members want. Decision by the leader means that the leader listens to the group discussion and then forces the group to go along with the decision he or she favors or makes. Arbitration is a method of deciding by which a disinterested third party hears each position and makes a decision. Each of these methods of deciding has its implications, and must be carefully considered.

EXERCISES

1. Write a critique of your current group's decision making. Include a description and evaluation of:
   a. The group's organizing effort
   b. The adequacy of the information collected and shared
   c. The climate of the group
   d. Group conflict
   e. Group decision making
   f. Each member's contributions to the group

2. Begin by selecting a problem, as a class, for which any of the decision-making agendas presented in this chapter would be appropriate. Try to find a problem that interests as many people as possible. Now form four groups, with each group taking a different agenda—reflective thinking, creative problem solving, ideal solution, or single question. Have each group member prepare a discussion outline using the particular agenda. Bring these to class and discuss them in your groups. Then, as a group, construct a discussion outline that all members agree is reasonable. Finally, using this agenda, conduct the discussions in class with the remainder of the class serving as observers.

3. Observe a decision-making group in your community. Write down the sequence of steps the members appear to follow. Write a three-page critique of the effectiveness of their decision-making agenda.

4. In small groups, brainstorm with members to see how many problems you can discover related to student life at your college or university. Do you find the number of problems you are able to discover to be large? Are there problems in the group's list that you would not have thought of personally if the group had not participated in brainstorming? Now focus on the brainstorming process. Was it easy to avoid criticism of others' ideas? What are the problems associated with using this technique? How can a group overcome these problems?

5. Conduct a nominal group technique session in your class. Arrange the room so that each group is seated in a semicircle and facing a flip chart on the wall. If this is not possible, use the chalkboard to record your suggestions. One member of each group should be appointed to conduct the nominal group session for your group. Work on a problem your instructor assigns, or pick one of the topics discovered during the brainstorming session described in exercise 4 above. After the session, discuss how successful the group was at using nominal group technique. What problems did you encounter? How might a group avoid these? When is this technique likely to be most useful to a group?

6. Divide the class into buzz groups. Give each of these groups six minutes to generate suggestions for the question "What might be done to improve the college library?" Designate a member of your group as the buzz group spokesperson. Your instructor will act as the overall group chairperson. After the session, process the experience in your group. How effective was the buzz group technique? What problems did your group discover with using the technique? What might a group do about these problems? When is this technique especially useful?

7. Form small groups or use existing small groups to investigate and propose solutions to a problem. Each group is to select a campus issue to discuss in class. The group selects an issue, researches the issue, selects an agenda, and conducts a final decision-making session on the problem in class. Tape-record this final session.

NOTES

1. Victor H. Vroom and Arthur G. Jago, *The New Leadership: Managing Participation in Organizations* (Englewood Cliffs, N.J.: Prentice-Hall, 1988).

2. John Dewey, *How We Think* (Boston: D. C. Heath, 1910).

3. Ibid., 6.

4. Research suggests that the first step, establishing operating procedures and analysis of the problem, is related to group problem-solving effectiveness. See Randy Y. Hirokawa, "Group Communication and Problem-Solving Effectiveness II: An Exploratory Investigation of Procedural Functions," *Western Journal of Speech Communication* 47 (1983):59–74.

5. John K. Brilhart and Lurene M. Jochem, "Effects of Different Patterns on Outcomes of Problem-Solving Discussion," *Journal of Applied Psychology* 48 (1964):175–179.

6. John K. Brilhart, *Effective Group Discussion*, 4th ed. (Dubuque, Iowa: Wm. C. Brown, 1982), 202–203.

7. Ibid.

8. Ibid.

9. Carl E. Larson, "Forms of Analysis and Small Group Problem-Solving," *Speech Monographs* 36 (1969):453.

10. Ibid.

11. Randy Y. Hirokawa, "Group Communication and Decision-Making Performance: A Continued Test of the Functional Perspective" (Paper presented at the annual meeting of the Speech Communication Association, Boston, 1987).

12. Ibid. See also Randy Y. Hirokawa, "Discussion Procedures and Decision-Making Performance," *Human Communication Research* 12 (1985):203–224.

13. Brilhart, 205–206.

14. See David R. Seibold, "Making Meetings More Successful: Plans, Formats, and Procedures for Group Problem Solving," *The Journal of Business Communication* 16 (1979):3–20.

15. Alex F. Osborn, *Applied Imagination: Principles and Procedures of Creative Thinking* (New York: Scribner's, 1959), 300–301.

16. Ibid., 300–301.

17. S. Kanekar and M. E. Rosenbaum, "Group Performance on a Multiple-Solution Task as a Function of Time Available," *Psychonomic Science* 27 (1972):331–332.

18. André L. Delbecq, Andrew H. Van de Ven, and David H. Gustafson, *Group Techniques for Program Planning: A Guide to Nominal Group Techniques and Delphi Process* (Glenview, Ill.: Scott, Foresman, 1975), 7–16.

19. Susan Jarboe, "A Comparison of Input-Output, Process-Output, and Input-Process-Output Models of Small Group Problem-Solving Effectiveness," *Communication Monographs* 55 (1988):121–142.

20. Delbecq, 4.

21. J. Donald Phillips, "Report on Discussion 66," *Adult Education Journal* 7 (1948):181–182.

22. Randy Y. Hirokawa, "Improving Intra-Organizational Communication: A Lesson from Japanese Management," *Communication Quarterly* 30 (Winter 1982):35–40. This essay provides an interesting contrast between Japanese and American styles. It is excellent background for understanding why the concept of quality circles has been so successful in Japan.

23. Larry R. Smeltzer and Kittie W. Watson, "An Analysis of Communication Skills in Productivity Improvement Groups" (Paper presented at the annual meeting of the International Communication Association, Honolulu, 1985).

24. There is a demonstrable relationship between cohesiveness and quality decisions. But apparently a third factor must be present—the group must approach its decision making systematically and in a rational manner. See Randy Y. Hirokawa, "Consensus Group Decision Making, Quality of Decision, and Group Satisfaction: An Attempt to Sort 'Fact' from 'Fiction,' " *Central States Speech Journal* 33 (1982):407–415.

25. Anne Gero, "Conflict Avoidance in Consensual Decision Processes," *Small Group Behavior* 16 (1985):487–499.

26. Julia T. Wood, "Consensus and Its Alternatives: A Comparative Analysis of Voting, Negotiation and Consensus as Methods of Group Decision-Making." In Gerald M. Phillips and Julia T. Wood (eds.), *Emergent Issues in Human Decision-Making* (Carbondale, Ill.: Southern Illinois University Press, 1984).

RECOMMENDED READINGS

John E. Baird, Jr., *Quality Circles: Leader's Manual* (Prospect Heights, Ill.: Waveland Press, 1982).

Norman R. F. Maier, *Problem Solving and Creativity in Individuals and Groups* (Belmont, Calif.: Brooks/Cole, 1970).

Carl M. Moore, *Group Techniques for Idea Building* (Newbury Park, Calif.: Sage, 1987).

Alex F. Osborn, *Applied Imagination* (New York: Scribner's, 1957).

David R. Siebold, "Making Meetings More Successful: Plans, Formats, and Procedures for Group Problem-Solving," in Robert S. Cathcart and Larry A. Samovar, eds. *Small Group Communication: A Reader*, 5th ed. (Dubuque, Iowa: Wm. C. Brown, 1988), 209–224.

CHAPTER 4

Understanding Verbal and Nonverbal Messages

OBJECTIVES

After reading this chapter you should be able to:

Draw, label, and explain Richards's triangle of meaning.

Define the term *frame of reference,* and explain how a person's frame of reference can cause difficulty in small groups.

Separate denotative and connotative meaning.

Explain how perception, ambiguity, too much information, and too little information can influence accurate communication processing.

Avoid language that labels or connotates inferiority.

Explain the fundamental idea of a ladder of abstraction, and show how the abstracting process can create difficulty for decision-making groups.

Specify the functions of nonverbal messages and show how each of the four functions bears upon accuracy in group communication.

Recall the six nonverbal codes we present, and specify their uses.

Explain the three major categories of nonverbal problems.

Given the text materials, apply our suggestions for improving nonverbal communication to particular examples of communication.

Name and explain the components of the listening process, describing potential difficulties that might be encountered with each.

Specify the five strategies that can be employed to improve listening.

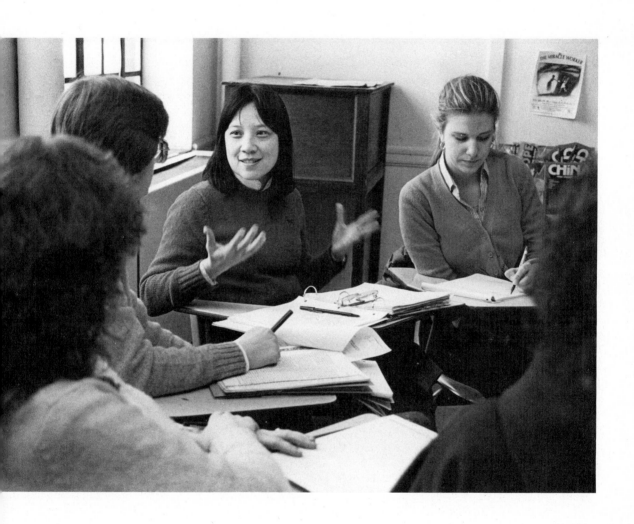

Think for a moment about a community action group trying to influence the city council to provide better lighting in a west side neighborhood. Perhaps you can imagine yourself as one of the members of such a group, drawn together from diverse backgrounds and not particularly well acquainted.

Such a group called itself the Maryknoll Neighborhood Association. It wanted to get funding included in the city's public works department budget to double the number of streetlights in the neighborhood. Jerry Lewis, the elected leader, suggested that participants draw up a list of recent security problems and gather a small group to go to the next council meeting to present their case. Further, he suggested that they arrive early and sit together. A number of those present spoke in favor of this plan until Sally Davis objected. She argued strongly against this idea. Instead she argued that two or three of them should visit each council member to plead the case. Others joined her in opposition and, as a result, no decision was reached.

A talk with Sally after the meeting revealed that her difficulty with Jerry's plan resulted from misunderstanding what he had in mind. She knew that the council had a reputation of not responding to large groups pressuring it to take action. She interpreted what Jerry said to mean this type of show of power. Jerry intended a small group who would present a petition and make a carefully documented presentation. But misunderstanding prevented any action.

Obviously, Jerry and Sally did not understand each other. Why did they have such a problem? What can they do to prevent it from happening next time? The answers to these questions are complex, but worth your time and effort. You will surely experience this common problem as a group member. You may also be one of the many people who feel frustrated and tense after such an experience. Knowing how to use language skillfully and effectively can help you to avoid some of these problems.

This chapter will help you understand verbal and nonverbal communication in groups. The first part of this chapter explores the nature of verbal messages. An understanding of how messages are created could have been helpful to Jerry and Sally. Next, some of the most common barriers to effective verbal communication are presented. The discussion of verbal communication concludes with some suggestions that will help you to improve your verbal skills in these areas.

The second part of the chapter begins with a discussion of the functions of nonverbal messages. Careful attention to group members' nonverbal behavior can often cure misunderstanding. If Jerry and Sally had been more aware, they might have explored differences before this talk turned to anger. They might have adjourned with agreement instead of failure.

After a description of the functions of nonverbal messages, problems related to them are raised. The ambiguity of nonverbal communication and the "unintentionality" of nonverbal communication factors that inhibit nonverbal message exchange are discussed. Finally, some ideas that will help you to improve your nonverbal communication skill are provided.

The third part of the chapter addresses listening. We begin by introducing the major components of the listening process. Since problems are associated with each of these components, we discuss those next. The chapter concludes with some recommendations about how to develop listening skills.

UNDERSTANDING VERBAL MESSAGES

Imagine yourself as a member of a group appointed to provide suggestions for dealing with a growing drug problem in your community. The group has five members—the owner of the local mercantile store; the production manager of a small cookie manufacturing plant (he is from France, and has been in this country only three years); a pastor of a church (it has a drug counseling program); the principal of a high school; and you (a representative from the college).

The Concept of Meaning

How do you know what words mean as group members exchange messages within their meetings? How do you know what a particular sentence means? How do you know what is meant by the phrase "drug problem"? You will not be surprised to learn that a number of theories attempt to answer this question. Whole books have been written on the subject.[1] One explanation was developed by I. A. Richards,[2] whose characterization of meaning is often referred to as the triangle of meaning. The diagram in Figure 4.1 shows how symbols, thoughts, and their referents are related.

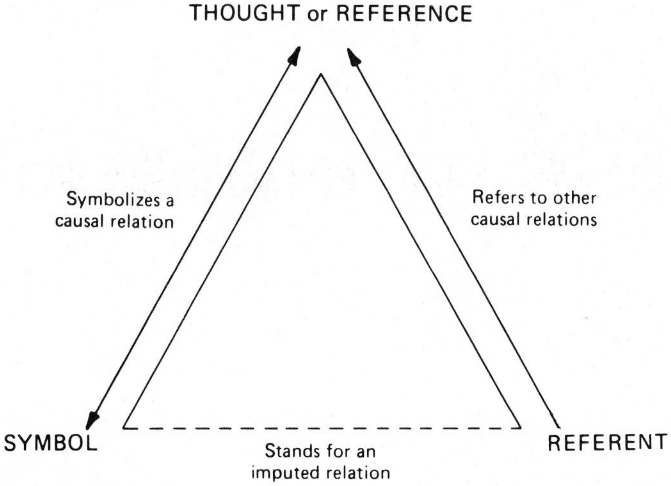

THOUGHT or REFERENCE

Symbolizes a
causal relation

Refers to other
causal relations

SYMBOL

Stands for an
imputed relation

REFERENT

FIGURE 4.1
The Triangle of Meaning

Figure "Thought or Reference" from *The Meaning of Meaning* by C. K. Ogden and I. A. Richards.
Reprinted by permission of Harcourt, Brace and Jovanovich, Inc.

One easy way to understand Richards's triangle is to think of it in terms of the drug problem your group is to consider. Suppose we turn back to the question "What is meant by the term 'drug problem'?" You might imagine the production manager saying, "A drug problem is a situation where a significant number of people in a community are abusing drugs." The pastor might say, "A drug problem is the emotional trauma a person and his or her family feels as the drug begins to control the person's life and relationships." The high school principal might say, "Meet me behind the football stadium tomorrow at four P.M. and I'll show you a drug problem."

Each of these represents a different kind of meaning for "drug problem." The first is a dictionary definition of the symbol. This is represented by the bottom left of Richards's triangle, the symbol. The second definition is a report of a member's thoughts about "drug problem," how he or she experiences the drug situation. This is represented by the upper point of the triangle. The third definition is an actual presentation of the drug problem, the referent. A *referent* is the object or event to which the symbol refers. The triangle's lower right corner represents this kind of definition.

At this point many students may ask, "So what?" The remaining markings on the triangle can help you to understand language and some of the common misconceptions related to its use. Look now at the part of the triangle that shows the symbol (word) and the referent (thing). Notice that this part is represented by a dotted line. The breaks in the line show that there is no direct connection between words and objects they represent. For example, if you said "drug problem" to any of these committee members, would they point to the same situation you had in mind? Some would; others would not. If you move the other way, perhaps you can see the problem. Suppose you took someone to the corner of Main and Spring at 9:00 P.M. Suppose further that you asked the person to tell you what he sees. He says, "This is the corner of Main and Spring with some people standing around." You are thinking "drug problem" because you see people smoking marijuana; he is thinking "geography." The same referent has produced different symbols. There is obviously some relatedness, but the relatedness is indirect.

Notice the solid line between the symbol and the thought (or referent) on the left side of the triangle. This line represents a causal relationship. Using symbols, "drug problem" does cause meaning in the head of the person hearing it (and in the head of the person using it). Moreover, having the idea or thought causes the person to produce the term in order to communicate or to think about the situation. Thus there is a two-way causal relationship between symbol and thought.

Now study the relationship of thought to referent. An arrow shows a one-way relationship, suggesting that an object or referent cannot appear merely by thinking about it. But we can be stimulated to think about an object by observing its presence.

There is a very important remaining relationship: the symbol-thought-referent relationship suggested by the solid part of the triangle. Meaning between a symbol and referent is achieved by means of the thought process. To say this another way, meaning— the relationship between symbol and referent—is created in the head of the person who is using the symbol. The committee investigating the drug problem may experience its first problem because of this phenomenon and never know it. But if you know how meaning is related to symbols and referents, you may be able to take some action to avoid the problem. The degree of difficulty your group will experience is related to the degree to which the members' frames of reference overlap. Let us turn to these topics.

Frame of Reference

The meaning you generate for a set of words depends on the experiences you have had with those words. This set of experiences is commonly called the *frame of reference.*

Because your experiences with words are unique—unlike those of any other human being—your frame of reference is always different from anyone else's. Your frame of reference for "drug problem" will include a variety of experiences with drug problems. Perhaps you recall experiences you have had. That idea carries you to the unique characteristics of drug use by college students. Suddenly other people's experiences with respect to drugs come into your mind. You begin to focus upon how people you know think about drug use. The frame of reference you bring to the discussion of this issue is individual and probably very complex.

The uniqueness and complexity of a person's frame of reference can be a source of difficulty in small group decision making. Imagine how difficult it would be to explain all the experiences that come together to make up your frame of reference. You would have to take a lot of time, and you would have to organize it carefully. You would need to go into considerable detail, since each person's frame of reference is unique. You would need to explain the ideas, feelings, and values related to each connected experience. Frankly, it is hard to imagine a group being willing to sit still long enough to gain this kind of understanding.

Of course, this illustration has been invented. But too often group members misunderstand one another, and they need to share their frames of reference. Since they cannot or will not sit still long enough to do so, they simply do not understand what others are saying. The fact that group members do not understand one another's frames of reference can obviously be a problem.

Overlap of Experience

Working together and communicating with one another may not be as hopeless as we have made it seem. People who live in the same culture, who experience the same settings, and who frequently share experiences soon develop an overlap of experience. This sharing of experiences enables group members to create similar meaning in their heads when they communicate.

Group members create meanings for words through the experiences they have had with those words. They expect other group members to have meanings similar to theirs because their experiences are similar. So an important task for your committee considering drug abuse is to discover what experiences its members have had with drug problems— and in particular with this drug problem. This sharing process represents the transactional nature of communication. Understanding does not come from a one-way flow of communication. It is the result of a transaction among the participants in the process.

This transactional sharing process serves two purposes. First, the group develops a group frame of reference. Members learn of one another's concerns. This helps them talk to one another and to understand how other members are unique. Thus, we see the second purpose of this talk—to uncover differences in the way members view situations and issues.

Of course, some aspects of the group members' experiences will not overlap. For example, the French member of your group will have had experiences of how French people deal with drug use and abuse that are unique to him. It is important to know about these unique ideas and experiences so that they can be taken into account as you talk and work together.

Denotative and Connotative Meaning

You already know what is meant by the words *denotative* and *connotative,* but we think it is useful to review these concepts in order to make a point about developing more substantial group frames of reference. Denotative meaning is the generally understood meaning of a word and is found in a dictionary. It is the objective description of what the word "means." Connotative meaning is a subjective meaning for a word based upon personal experience with the word. It involves the emotional and personal reactions a person had when the word was experienced in its various contexts.

Exploring the denotative and the connotative meanings of key concepts in a group discussion can be very helpful to a group. Knowing the denotative definitions of key words will often allow a group to understand specific problems more fully. On the other hand, the connotative definitions of terms give a group a sense of the harm people are experiencing as a result of some problem. Both understandings are important for a group.

Consider the drug problem and the committee again. The group might construct a denotative definition of the phrase "drug problem"—"a situation in which a significant number of people in a community are abusing drugs." A connotative definition would be quite different—for example, "the emotional trauma a person and his or her family feels as the drug begins to control the person's life and relationships." It seems clear that connotative meanings provide additional useful information—information about how members are experiencing a problem.

PROBLEMS WITH VERBAL COMMUNICATION

Both the nature of language and the way meaning is ascribed to language are potential problems for communicators in groups. But this is not where the difficulties end. Four additional difficulties seem to come up frequently in small groups that prevent accurate processing and understanding of others' messages. *Perception* is the process of becoming aware of people, objects, and events by taking in information through the senses. Sometimes perception is a problem. A group member focuses your attention on a message in ways that cause you to be misled. At other times, the *ambiguity* of our language creates difficulties. You use words in your group that are difficult to define because of their abstract quality. Or, perhaps the way people or things are labeled presents problems. And groups encounter two other problems. They sometimes gather so much information that the members experience information processing problems. Or the opposite can be true: The group has too little information to be effective.

Perceptual Difficulties

Perception is a process because it occurs in a step-by-step progression. We take in information. We organize that data. We interpret and evaluate what we have received. The process sounds simple, but it is not. Many of the perceptual problems members experience grow out of three basic characteristics of perception: (1) Perception is a subjective process. (2) People strive for stability in their perceptions. (3) People assume that what they perceive is meaningful.

Subjectivity When members observe their group interact, they are selective in what they choose to notice. Members often select what is important to them but omit what is important to the person who is speaking. They "tune in" to what they want to hear; they "tune out" what they do not want to hear. You can imagine how this selectivity can create problems in groups. Take this example. Suppose you are part of a department in an organization related to your profession. You and several other department members meet to discuss a schedule of training programs for employees in the department. Several ideas are discussed, and the group ends up with five programs. As group leader you summarize what you believe the group consensus to be. But Jean objects: "We had a program on career planning. We said we would do that instead of one on computer applications." Who is right here? It turns out that after additional discussion you are correct and Jean is wrong. She "tuned out" when the group said it would keep career planning in reserve as an alternative. She did not perceive the group's communication that enthusiastically endorsed the idea.

You can combat such an error in several ways. One is to say back to the other person what you think was said, but in your own words. In other contexts you also might check your perceptions with a friend who was present as well. Often these techniques will help you discover differences that can be talked about. Finally, in a group meeting you may need to resolve differences by going directly to the leader of the meeting. However perceptual bias is addressed, a group needs to learn a method for overcoming the potential difficulties that flow from selectivity in perception.

Stability Psychologically, we expect group members to behave consistently over time. We know from our past experience in the group how a particular individual behaves and acts. We know what is important to that person, and therefore we expect things not to change. Put another way, we expect stability.

In this context, then, stability is the same as predictability of behavior over time. We expect the president of the Kiwanis Club, who has regularly started meetings on time, to begin on time today. We expect a classmate who seems always to be late to walk in late today. We barely pay attention if our predictions are correct, but we notice if the president is late or the student gets to class ahead of time. And the trouble is that we tend to develop biases on the basis of our expectations. Especially if someone's behavior is not stable, we are likely to distrust that person. Moreover, we tend to anticipate one another, sometimes wrongly, because we expect stability of behavior. If you *think* John is going to take a particular stand on some issue in the group meeting, you are likely to *hear* that stand whether he takes it or not! You might even choose a wrong—and potentially harmful—strategy *before* John has a chance to speak!

You might find yourself expecting stability in groups and perhaps forcing biases. Beyond being aware of the bias, we think you ought to try actively to avoid it. Check out what you think a group member is saying—especially with those you know well. The group members you know well are the ones you are most likely to anticipate and therefore perceive inaccurately.

Meaningfulness   We often assume that the other member is making sense—that what is being said is meaningful, but sometimes this just is not the case. Nevertheless, we always seem to try to make logical sense out of what has been said. This is the principle of meaningfulness in action. You may have perceived things in what a group member said that are not even there—filled in the "holes" to make the message meaningful. Overcoming this perceptual problem is difficult, since you may not even know that you are filling in missing parts.

Ask questions when something is not clear. Make it your general policy to go over the conclusions informally with a friend after a group meeting. If you are leading a group, summarize your group's progress and conclusions frequently. All these suggestions will be helpful in avoiding perceptual problems.

Abstraction in Language Use

To understand the idea of abstraction, consider the various terms that could be used to describe the leader of the chamber of commerce. A member might say, "George conducts our meetings in an orderly fashion and with considerable skill and grace." The member could be more and more abstract. Perhaps she might just say, "George leads our group well." Or perhaps she says simply, "George leads." Each time the member picks language, she is choosing some level of abstraction. In this case, if the speaker moves from "George conducts our meeting in an orderly fashion and with considerable skill and grace" to "George leads," she moves farther away from identifying characteristics of George's leadership.

The general semanticist S. I. Hayakawa[3] suggested an "abstraction ladder" to help people visualize the process of abstracting. We could place the terms on such a ladder and they would look like the representation in Figure 4.2. The lower on the ladder, the easier it is to visualize the detail of the phenomena. The higher up on the ladder, the more general the description becomes.

But how does understanding abstraction help us in our group communication? Abstractions are generalizations that allow us to talk about the similarities among several

FIGURE 4.2
Abstraction Ladder

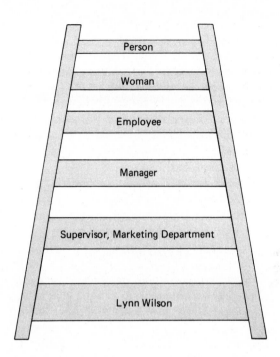

objects. We can say the words "man" or "woman" and classify people into one or the other category. This allows us to generalize about a group of similar people. But the higher on the ladder the abstraction, the more we must ignore the uniqueness that makes the objects of our attention different. This can obviously lead to serious group communication problems.

Dale G. Leathers[4] used confederates to introduce abstract language into the deliberations of laboratory discussion groups in order to study what would happen. Suppose in a discussion about how to improve members' participation, a member interjected the terms "relational deterioration," "tangential motives," "disparaging interaction," and others. This language use might be disruptive. Without definition and illustration, we are unlikely to know what the person using such terms actually means. The result may be frustration for the group. What Leathers found was that these abstract statements disrupted the discussion. The more abstract the statements, the more disruptive they were. Typically the discussants became confused. Sometimes they became tense. Some members withdrew from the discussion altogether. You can see from these reactions that ambiguous language can produce significant problems for small group discussions.

Labels and Language

The language we use in our talk about one another shapes the way we feel and think about other people and also the way that other people think about themselves and our relationship with them. The use of racist or sexist language in interactions in a group can seriously affect the relationships and spirit of cooperation that are so necessary for group productivity and satisfaction. Sexist and racist language usually defines relationships as superior or inferior, and that kind of definition is counterproductive.

We all have taken on the language we learned as we were growing up. So our use of language may seem somewhat automatic. It is possible to change the language you use to refer to others if you understand the damaging aspects of it and wish to change. Throughout this book, we have illustrated a style of writing that reflects our view of equality. We have switched to the sexually neutral plural (they), employed the he-or-she structure, and balanced our references to males, females, blacks, whites, old, and young in roles. We invite you to work on the labels you use in your talk if you believe you need to do so.

Too Much Information

An employee of a public accounting firm said after a recent group meeting: "For me there was just too much to remember. I tried to keep track, but there were so many things and some of them didn't pertain to me." We think that statement reflects a common problem called *information overload.* Undoubtedly everyone can experience information overload—especially when meeting with a large group of active, involved participants.

Information theorists have been studying this problem for quite some time. George A. Miller[5] has calculated the number of items of information an individual can effectively work with at one time. It turns out to be quite small. For most people it is seven, plus or minus two. To put this finding into a group context, if you have a group of seven, and if each member presents one idea, the members of the group are at or near capacity! Information overload can easily become a problem, because as items are added beyond the seven they may force earlier items out of the short-term memory before full processing can occur.

The group situation is especially difficult because usually a decision-making group will consider multiple ideas. Wise leaders encourage members to generate many ideas. But the group may experience overload. Consider the problem this group faces. A company that manufactures paper clips had decided that it would like to run a series of advertisements that would call attention to its company's name. It wanted the series to focus on imaginative uses for paper clips. Williams Advertising believed that the way to begin such a project was to gather a group of four or five people to generate ideas. Amazing as it sounds, the group gathered for this project generated twenty-three ideas. Narrowing these ideas to the five "best" was a considerable problem. It is difficult for a group to consider that many ideas. It suffered from information overload. The group created a communication problem that it must address. In the next section some strategies for dealing with information overload and the other problems presented so far will be described.

Too Little Information

It is always possible that a group is operating with too little information. This difficulty may result from two circumstances: The group members do not possess the needed information, or the group members do not realize the need to present information that they actually possess.

This information problem often has as its underlying root the failure to ask appropriate questions. It is the questioning process that guides in the collection of information for deliberations. So failure to have adequate information is probably a problem of not asking the right, or perhaps enough, questions. Perhaps the discussion question was not adequately focused or worded. Perhaps some question critical to analysis of the problem was not asked. We addressed the issue of posing discussion questions and research questions in Chapter 2.

Question asking can ensure that a group addresses the important issues in the discussion, has adequate information, and manages relationships effectively. Each of these functions of question asking is especially important to the effective processing of information in groups. We will take them up momentarily, but let's first examine what it means to ask a good question.

The good question   A good question has two characteristics: It is answerable and it is designed to meet a purpose. A question can be unanswerable for two reasons. It might be that there is no practical way of knowing the answer. For example, do you suppose the question "How many unmarried teen-age women in the city of Chicago became pregnant last year?" is answerable? It seems highly unlikely that all pregnancies in this category were ever recorded. Perhaps someone has a rough estimate, so that this question is answerable in some form.

Another kind of question that is unanswerable is the one that is too ambiguous. Suppose a group investigating a campus parking problem asked the question "How many students are late for their eight o'clock class?" On first glance, this seems to be an answerable question. But the question actually poses two additional questions: "Under what conditions?" and "On what days of the week?" Weather conditions and the day of the week will undoubtedly produce different answers. These need to be clarified in order for the question to be answerable.

A good question is also designed to meet a purpose. The overall purpose of a question is to seek either specific or general information. A question that seeks specific information produces a limited response. Such a question is referred to as *closed.* Once the response is given, the question is answered and there is no need for further response. Here are some questions of this type:

"How old was Nat when he first got into trouble?"

"Do we all agree with this solution?"

"To whom do we submit this report?"

A question that seeks general information is classified as *open-ended*. The purpose of such a question is to invite a variety of answers, encourage elaboration, or solicit a number of viewpoints. Exploration of causes of a problem, posing of solutions, and evaluation of ideas are times when you will want to ask the open-ended question. Here are some typical open-ended questions:

"What factors seem to have caused the decline in enrollment?"

"What are the goals we hope to achieve?"

"How can Mom, Dad, Bill, and Jean best share kitchen duty?"

The functions of questions   Questions are designed to serve particular functions during a small group decision-making discussion. We suggested above that these are (1) guiding the discussion to ensure that the important issues are effectively and efficiently discussed, (2) ensuring that adequate information is brought to bear on the discussion, and (3) maintaining a productive climate and interpersonal relationships.

GUIDING THE DISCUSSION   Questions that guide a discussion deal with group process. General questions that are useful in guiding group process make up the agendas presented in Chapter 3. These questions help orient and guide the group as it moves through the information-processing function. Questions are also asked that seek guidance and orientation. You can get a grasp of what guiding means if you think of these questions as seeking procedures or orientation. Here are some questions that seek procedures:

"How shall we attack this problem?"

"What agenda will we use to guide us in making our decision?"

"Do we move to solutions next?"

Questions that seek orientation are like these:

"What is our goal in this discussion?"

"Have we completed our work with criteria?"

"Has everybody said what he or she wanted to say about what might be causing this problem?"

ENSURING ADEQUATE INFORMATION   A group must have adequate information if it is to perform its task effectively. This information takes the form of fact, opinion, or value. We made the distinction between fact and opinion (inferences) in Chapter 2. Recall that a fact refers to a piece of information that can be verified or that has been repeatedly reported as true. Here are some questions that seek facts:

"How many incidents of vandalism were reported in the neighborhood?"

"Did the president say that she was aware of this spending problem?"

"Sally, what did you find out about eligibility requirements for this scholarship?"

Questions of opinion differ from those of fact as they ask for a conclusion, an inference, based on someone's observation and interpretation of what has or is or will be happening in the world. In the case of small group deliberations, these are questions about others' opinions, interpretations, and judgments about facts the group is processing. Examples of the kind of questions asked to seek opinion are these:

"Is there a need for additional secretarial help in the department?"

"Does this candidate meet the needs of our church?"

"What would be the effect of shifting the hours of operation from 8:00 until 5:00 to 7:00 until 4:00?"

A question about value calls for members to offer their judgment about the merit or worth of an idea. Asking for a value statement suggests that some comparison is being made to something else. Here are examples of questions asking for an assessment of value:

"Would it be more beneficial to add buses to shuttle people into the work site or to build additional parking spaces?"

"Would it be better to plan just two spectacular events for the year?"

"How well has the decision not to add a second family car served us?"

MAINTAINING A PRODUCTIVE CLIMATE AND RELATIONSHIPS Questions that ask members to consider climate and/or relationships can be important to the well-being of the group. The relationships we develop can have a significant effect on our willingness to work productively on the task. Tension can rise as signs of frustration, anger, boredom, or alienation are ignored. Showing concern about them and bringing them out so they can be dealt with are functions of the relationship question. Some examples of relationship-oriented questions are:

"Now that we have had a chance to get acquainted, does everyone feel like they know one another well enough to move on?"

"Mike, you seem a bit on the quiet side today. Is something wrong?"

"Is anybody else upset with the way we are working together today?"

There is a great deal of power in asking the right question at the right moment. Most of the time someone in the group will try to answer the question and the group's effort, as a whole, will benefit from it.

INCREASING VERBAL EFFECTIVENESS

Knowing the nature of language and how meaning is derived can help you avoid some of the more common communication difficulties. Problems of perceptual bias, language ambiguity, and information overload may all be treated easily by any group member who knows how. In this section some specific advice for handling these kinds of communication problems in groups is presented. The section is arranged according to the language you might use to verbalize the problems.

PROBLEM

You aren't sure that your group understands you. What can you do?

LANGUAGE AND/OR SUGGESTIONS

1. Recall the ladder of abstraction. Try to keep what you have to say as concrete as possible.

2. Include examples and illustrations of what you mean. (This is what a public speaker does to increase clarity.) For example, if you were talking about the drug problem, you might recount a specific case.

3. Watch for nonverbal cues. If you see that people seem puzzled or distracted, clarify or give an example. You might say, "I'm not sure I was clear. I'll try again."

4. Ask someone to summarize the progress the group has made and/or ideas that have been presented so far. Or ask someone to paraphrase so that you can see if people understand. You might say, "I presented several ideas and want to find out if I've been clear. John, would you mind feeding them back to me?"

5. You may be experiencing an organizational problem instead of an abstraction difficulty. In this case be sure to state one point at a time. Then be careful to organize what you have to say. You could follow this simple outline: (a) show the relationship of what you are saying to the remarks of the last speaker(s); (b) state the idea; (c) explain the idea; (d) develop the idea through examples or evidence; and (e) show that what you have said relates to the topic being discussed.

PROBLEM

You're confused. You're not clear about what has just been said by a group member or what has just happened.

LANGUAGE AND/OR SUGGESTIONS

1. Ask the speaker to give an example or illustration. You might say, "John, I'm having trouble understanding your point. Could you give me an example?"

2. Paraphrase what the person has said in less abstract terms. Say, "I want to make sure I've understood. Let me see if I understand."

3. Sometimes ambiguity is the problem when you do not understand the specific

task the group is undertaking at the moment. Ask the group to focus briefly on where it has been and where it is going. You could say, "I'm trying to put Jill's comments into the context of what we are doing and am having trouble. Could we take a moment to review?"

4. Ask a direct question. Say, "John, I want to be sure I've understood you. Do you mean . . . ?"

PROBLEM
You want to guard against any perceptual bias you may be experiencing with respect to what a member has just said.

LANGUAGE AND/OR SUGGESTIONS
1. Paraphrase the content back to the speaker and check to see if you are accurate.

2. Check your interpretation with a colleague from your group.

3. Take notes. Often this focuses your attention more and will help you to get more of the message.

4. Try to put yourself in the place of the person speaking. If you can empathize with the speaker you may "tune in" to what he is saying and thus avoid your personal bias. Imagine what the person was thinking and feeling as he experienced the event. Try to figure out how the speaker is connecting the ideas to what has already been said.

5. Paraphrase the content of the person's message; then try to formulate a good question. Often the question might relate to the significance of the issue. You might say, "How does this relate to [the previous issue or decision]?"

PROBLEM
The group is processing too many ideas—information overload is hampering your group's productivity.

LANGUAGE AND/OR SUGGESTIONS
1. Combine related issues. Channel capacity can be increased by placing items into a larger class. To illustrate, group the causes of a problem under two or three separate categories. "I see these causes as falling under three categories. [Name the categories.] Could we group them under each category, and then discuss the categories and causes in each?" (Be careful here that you do not become so abstract in the categories you use that you experience the abstraction problems we discussed earlier in this chapter.)

2. Try to eliminate solutions or ideas that do not seem relevant to the discussion. You might say, "We've been working so hard on generating ideas that we have made a long list. Are there any of these that we might be able to cross off in favor of others?"

3. See if you can combine and reformulate the ideas or solutions that seem relevant.[6] Perhaps the other group members can help in this process. You

might begin by pointing out the problems created by too many proposals, then talk about how the group can combine and reformulate.

Verbal communication and the problems related to its use have been considered to this point. Meanings are related to our personal experience, so any attempt to share an idea in a group may lead to misunderstanding. Small groups can improve understanding by members' defining terms both denotatively and connotatively.

Group communication is also affected by perceptual biases, ambiguity of language, and information overload. Each of these was discussed, and suggestions for coping with problems that might arise from each were offered.

UNDERSTANDING NONVERBAL MESSAGES

Most people find nonverbal communication to be an intriguing subject. Perhaps this fascination arises because an important part of the message is carried by nonverbal behavior. This seems reasonable when you consider that cues come from the group's physical setting, placement and seating of members, appearance and clothing, body movement and posture, eye contact and movement, facial expressions, and various vocal cues. These cues give the group members information about how other members perceive themselves and the message sender.[7]

Consider the impact of the arrangement of seats in a meeting of a college curriculum committee. It illustrates one aspect of nonverbal communication in groups. The committee is reconstituted each year, so nearly all of its members are new. It is traditional for this group to elect a chairperson at the first meeting. Prior to the meeting, one member, Bob, had decided that it would be an interesting experience to lead such a group. So he approached one of the members to seek nomination. This person told Bob that she and two other members had met and had decided to nominate Sue for the position of chairperson. Bob arrived at the meeting and noticed the seating arrangement pictured in Figure 4.3. What do you make of what you see?

Sue had taken a central place near the head of the table. Those who intended to nominate her sat together on one side of the table, and to her immediate right. On the other side of the table there was another block of three members, 6, 7, and 8. Members 1 and 9 sat away from other members of the group—apparent isolates. And no one sat next to the associate dean. Where would you sit if you wanted to assume a leadership role in this committee? If the placement and seating of people really do make a communicative difference, then observing the seating pattern could be very useful to you. Where people sit may provide information about the group's role structure and patterns of influence.

A person who wants to maximize his or her effectiveness for making leadership contributions would sit in a central location. In this case one of the central seats still available is to the immediate right of the associate dean. Here good eye contact can be maintained with most of the group. In addition, the seat next to the dean is nearly as

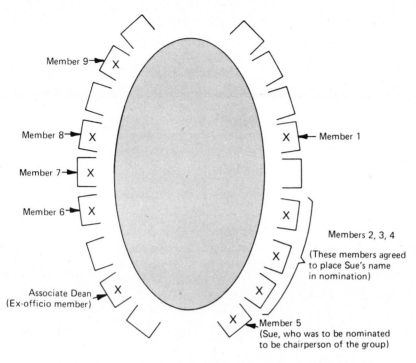

Where would you sit if you wanted to share in the leadership of this group?

FIGURE 4.3
Seating Arrangement of College Curriculum Committee

central as that taken by the person to be chosen leader. (Incidentally, Sue *was* chosen to lead the group.)

Other status and role considerations became apparent as the group met. It turned out that members 1 and 9 were in fact isolates—they communicated less than any of the other members, and they remained apart from the group. Members 6, 7, and 8 were acquaintances and therefore were sitting together. Because they were different from one another in attitudes and expertise, and because they rarely saw one another outside the meeting, they were active in the meetings but never acted in concert. Bob took the seat next to the dean. He tried to be an active member of the group and to influence it in productive directions.

This rather extended and personal example was presented to give you some appreciation of how important just one set of nonverbal messages may be in a small group. Of course, these work simultaneously with other nonverbal message systems and with language. What comes next is a discussion of how these nonverbal message systems function and how they interact with language. Some of the key pitfalls to watch out for are suggested, and some specific advice about how you can improve your own nonverbal behavior is given.

The Functions of Nonverbal Messages

The relationship between verbal and nonverbal messages is very complex. Although writers have identified at least six important relationships, these basic functions can be reduced to four: *reinforcement, modification, substitution,* and *regulation.* Try to keep in mind the example we gave of the seating arrangement of the college curriculum committee. This situation provides an illustration of these four functions.

A word of caution seems wise here. People do not use nonverbal systems very uniformly, so much of what you sense of members' nonverbal communication will be somewhat ambiguous to everyone, including the person generating it. These four categories, then, can describe how nonverbal signals function, but they cannot describe how a particular member uses particular cues for particular meanings or nuances. Where another's nonverbal messages are ambiguous, it is best to ask for a translation into words. Chapter 9 will suggest how to do that. For now, consider the four basic functions of nonverbal messages.

Reinforcement   Sometimes nonverbal messages reinforce the verbal message by *repeating* what the words say. The seating arrangement was described, and a picture of what it looked like was produced. You might describe the layout of a parking lot and also use your hands and arms to gesture in ways that will repeat the message. Repetition of this type introduces redundancy into the communication, which helps your listener to understand and remember your message.

Facial expressions, like gestures, can also serve as reinforcement. You often use facial expressions to *elaborate* on meaning as you try to describe feelings or emotions. For example, a person may—in recounting the frustration she experienced in trying to interview a reluctant expert for her group—tense the muscles of her nose, tighten the muscles of her arms, and gesture rigidly. Clearly understanding the other person's emotional state is a very important part of processing his or her message accurately. Since the face, posture, and gestures of the person often reinforce the expressed feeling, paying attention to these may yield a big payoff.

Nonverbal messages also reinforce the verbal by *accenting* important points. Certain words were emphasized as the seating arrangement of the college curriculum committee was discussed. Typesetters use italics for emphasis. We do essentially the same thing with our voices, faces, hands, arms, and bodies. Authors italicize to help the reader know what they think is important—they want to reinforce those parts of the message. Group members emphasize the important aspects of a message by raising volume, setting words off by pauses, and gesturing with their hands. These reveal the organization and key ideas of the message. You will be better able to understand the speakers' messages if you pay close attention to how they are reinforced nonverbally.

Modification   Suppose that Sue, curriculum committee chairperson nominee, sat in the central position she chose but avoided eye contact. Perhaps her face carried an expression of disinterest; maybe she even slouched in the chair. When asked if she would be willing to serve if elected, she shook her head from left to right and back and forth, saying, "Well . . . uh . . . I suppose I would serve if elected." Would you believe her verbal message? Her behavior would contradict her verbal message. Sometimes nonverbal behavior is purposeful; sometimes it just seems to slip in without the speaker's knowing it. But people generally believe nonverbal messages and thus modify what a person says. What is far more likely is that Sue's behavior would not have been as clear as we described it. Most nonverbal communication is very subtle and idiosyncratic. That is, the nonverbal cues are fleeting and very personal. Still, a group's success may be in jeopardy if members don't pay attention to the nonverbal component. Sue's subtle cues of disinterest could be overlooked. If they are, and the group elects her to do the important job of leading, the group could be buying trouble.

Substitution   If you knew that Sue had been approached about leading the curriculum committee and then you saw her take a chair at the head of the table, you might conclude that her behavior was a substitute for the words, "I'm interested and willing to be chairperson of this group." Consider some of the other ways in which group members communicate with one another nonverbally. They fidget in their chairs, stand up to indicate adjournment, look disinterested when they are not prepared, avoid eye contact to signal that they do not wish to speak, maintain eye contact to signal that they want a person to speak, and the like. All of these signs substitute for the verbal message, so all are important clues to what is going on in the group. A group will generally be more productive if the leadership pays close attention to them.

Regulation   Substitution and regulation are closely related. Group members regulate one another's behavior by substituting nonverbal messages for words. To illustrate, it is common for group leaders to use eye contact, head nods, and gestures to encourage and discourage contributions. Members who begin to talk at the same time may look to the designated leader for a cue as to who should continue. A leader may maintain eye contact and give head nods to cause a speaker to continue, or perhaps to cause a person to elaborate. On the other hand, these behaviors may be withheld to discourage a talkative member.

Members indicate their desire to talk through nonverbal signals, too, thus regulating the behavior of the entire group. One may lean forward and raise her hand slightly. Another may even open his mouth and make some nonverbal utterance—perhaps an "uh" sound. Still another may suddenly lean forward and begin speaking. Finally, members use hand gestures to slow down and speed up speakers. Do you ever find yourself making small upward motions in an oval pattern in an attempt to cause a very slow speaker to talk faster?

So there are many examples of the four functions of nonverbal messages. Members *reinforce* one another and their own statements with nonverbal messages. They *modify* their spoken words with nonverbal messages. They *substitute* nonverbal messages for spoken words, and they *regulate* one another nonverbally. Learning to do these things comes quite easily and naturally, since nonverbal messages are a part of each person's fluency. But, like the use of language, fluent use of nonverbal messages is rarely conscious behavior. And since our use of these codes tends to be idiosyncratic and very subtle, group members may be generating confusion as well as understanding. The next section will focus your attention on ways to use nonverbal message systems on purpose.

USING NONVERBAL CODES

There is much to know about nonverbal codes within the context of small group communication. We have described four functions that may be accomplished by any nonverbal code. But we want you to be able to *choose* nonverbal messages. Here we will present six different kinds of nonverbal codes and their uses: physical environments; appearance; gesture, posture, and movement; face and eye behavior; vocalics; and time. After reading this section you should be able to put what you have read to deliberate use in groups. If you do so, you will be able to make a contribution to your groups regardless of the contexts in which you find them.

Physical Environments

You already know that the place where you hold a conversation has an effect on the conversation. Consider the effect of moving a conversation with a group of colleagues from place to place. Suppose the conversation takes place in the company cafeteria. Now suppose it is being held in the back of a corporate conference room. Now imagine having it in the parking lot. Each time you change the environment you change the conversation. This principle of environmental effect holds for other groups, too. Environment affects a group, although many groups will attempt to get their tasks done regardless of the environment. They resist moving even though the environment may be affecting their task adversely.

One important environmental factor is the attractiveness and appearance of the meeting room. Abraham Maslow and Norbett Mintz[8] investigated the effect that different environments had on group members' attitudes toward the task and the emotional states evoked. Subjects rated a group of photographs in three settings: a room that looked like a janitor's closet (the ugly room), a professor's office (the average room), and a living room with nice furniture (the beautiful room). The subjects gave more positive ratings to the photographs, enjoyed the task more, and wanted to stay with the task longer when they worked in the beautiful room! In addition, the ugly room caused the group members to feel tired, irritated, and unpleasant.

What can be concluded from this study? It is pretty good evidence that the surroundings make an important difference to the ways people behave. Of course, few meetings are conducted in living-room-like surroundings. Still, it is possible to find a reasonably comfortable, well-illuminated (but not bright enough to cause eye tension) meeting place, and there is much that can be done to make any room more attractive. For example, chairs can be moved so that they are arranged comfortably. People meeting in a very large room may want their chairs closer than if they were in a smaller room. Of course, objectionable and distracting clutter can and should be removed. Groups do adapt, of course, so it is not necessary to worry about environmental characteristics that cannot be changed.

The seating preferences and arrangements that group members adopt affect both member participation and leadership emergence. A number of researchers have reported an interaction pattern when people are seated across from one another. Steinzor; Strodtbeck and Hook; and Hearn[9] have all found a strong tendency for communication to flow between members across the table more than between adjacent members. They also found that this effect can be negated if eye contact is blocked by some sort of table arrangement and by certain personality characteristics. For example, group members who are sensitive to rejection seem not to follow this pattern.[10]

The quality of interaction also seems to be affected by seating arrangement. Russo[11] presented diagrams of five different seating arrangements of six-member groups seated at a rectangular table with a single member at each end and the other four people seated two on each side. Figure 4.4 shows the arrangements he tested. Subjects were asked to guess whether the pairs were intimate/unacquainted, friendly/hostile, talkative/untalkative, and equal/unequal. What Russo found was that the greater the distance between the two people, the less acquainted, friendly, and talkative they were thought to be.[12]

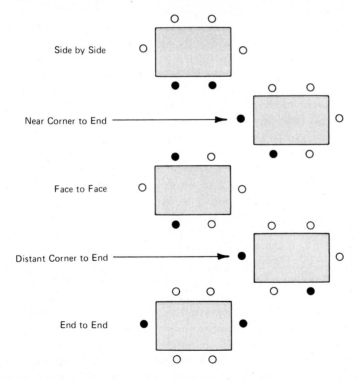

Blackened circles represent positions in the arrangements that were examined by Russo.

FIGURE 4.4
Seating Arrangements in Russo's Study

When you can do so without appearing to be manipulative, seat talkative members on the same side of a rectangular table with another person between them. The person in the middle may suffer at first, but only a little—and the group will benefit greatly.

If it is not possible to control the seating arrangement of too-talkative members, the flow of talk may still be controlled through eye contact, head nods, and so forth. Along these same lines, the fewer empty chairs at a meeting, the less interpersonal distance and the more the perception that the situation is friendly and intimate—and the greater the interaction.

The emergence of a person whom the group will accept as its leader is also affected by seating arrangement. When members identify their leader, the potential leaders generally are persons who interact with the group members easily. For this to happen, the person needs to maintain eye contact in order to recognize other members' needs and to regulate the flow of communication. L. T. Howells and S. W. Becker[13] reasoned that the group member who could control the communication most—the person who could maintain face-to-face eye contact—would most likely emerge as the person the group would consider its leader. They seated five-member groups at a rectangular table, two persons on one side and three on the other, to test this hypothesis. The members on the two-person side would have the opportunity to maintain eye contact with more members, so Howells and Becker thought they would be the most likely candidates for emergent leader. This is in fact what happened; from twenty groups studied, fourteen members from the two-seat side emerged as leaders. Only six from the three-seat side emerged as leaders.

If it is important to lead in a particular meeting, you can take a central position to maintain maximum eye contact with members. If you want to decrease your chance of being selected as leader—an entirely sensible choice for some very busy people—then reverse this advice. On the other hand, if you want to equalize the seating advantage among the members, choose a circle.

Appearance

It is commonly believed that you can learn a great deal about a person merely by observing his or her appearance. People do, in fact, make judgments about others on the basis of their appearance.[14] Individuals who are thought to be physically attractive are also seen as more personable, persuasive, interesting, confident, sociable, serious, and outgoing than individuals who are not perceived as physically attractive. So physical appearance can have an impact on your perception of group members, and can have an impact for you as a group member as well.

What do you make of this information if you are "sort of average"? Many people who are not beautiful are personable, confident, persuasive, sociable, serious, outgoing, and more! So it seems reasonable that physical attractiveness is not necessarily tied to physical beauty. Rather, it appears to be tied to cultural norms. You can keep physically fit and be well groomed. Most people can control their weight and make sure their clothes are clean and fresh.

With regard to dress, group members should generally adhere to the degree of formality called for in any particular context. If you are not familiar with the usual dress standard, ask someone who knows. Study the dress habits of those in your group or organization. Look for elements of dress these people share, and if it seems reasonable, follow their lead.

Keep in mind that dress is particularly important when you are meeting with the group for the first time. Factors such as task-relevant knowledge, rate of participation, and ability to do the task do not become more important than image until the group members become acquainted with you.[15]

Gesture, Posture, and Movement

Gesture and movement help to regulate the flow of communication in groups, so it is important for you to learn to let your body communicate. John E. Baird and A. Schubert[16] reported that leaders gave more positive head nods than nonleaders and that they gestured more. Certain nonverbal behavior controls or directs interaction among group members. Later Baird[17] demonstrated that this nonverbal participation is related to leadership emergence as well. Relatively high-status people tend to show more relaxed posture than lower-status group members. On the other hand, such behaviors as uncrossing arms and legs, unbuttoning a coat, and general relaxation usually signal openness and a feeling of equality.[18] A sense of how much a person feels like a part of the group as a whole can be gained by noticing the angle at which a member's shoulders and legs are turned to the group.[19] So using your body to communicate can have a very direct impact on the leadership you can contribute. Yet giving specific suggestions about how to gesture is not possible. It is good advice to say that you should follow your natural inclination to gesture or posture or move about. If you are able to do that comfortably, you will appear more at ease—and you will amplify and enrich what you are saying with nonverbal messages.

Face and Eye Behavior

Because facial cues are important indicators of a person's orientation, the face exerts a special influence. Dale Leathers reviewed the literature on facial expression:

1. The face communicates *evaluative judgments*—good and bad—through pleasant and unpleasant expressions that suggest whether the communicator sees the current object of his attention as good or bad.

2. The face communicates *interest or disinterest* in other people or in the surrounding environment.

3. The face communicates *intensity* and, hence, degree of involvement in the situation.

4. The face communicates the amount of *control* the individual has over his own expressions.

5. The face probably communicates the intellectual factor of *understanding* or lack of it.[20]

One group of researchers even found that smiles and head nods produce greater credibility.[21]

Eye contact usually produces less ambiguous messages than does facial expression. People make direct eye contact when they want to indicate they are open for communication, and when soliciting feedback after making a statement.[22] People use eye contact to decrease distance psychologically, and sometimes to show hostility.[23] Group members view eye contact as important. Judee K. Burgoon discovered that, when student groups were allowed to arrange their desks any way they wanted, they adopted a U pattern.[24] This allowed them to maintain eye contact with one another and with the instructor.

Constant eye contact makes other people nervous, because it can be a sign of confronting behavior. But keep in mind that in our culture the listener maintains more constant eye contact than the speaker. When you are listening to other group members, where is the focus of your attention? If it is not on the speaker, what do you think other members might conclude? Clearly, use of appropriate eye contact is an important leadership skill you might wish to cultivate.

Vocalics

Such characteristics as aptitudes and interests, personality traits, ethnic background, education level, anxiety, and other emotional states are judged by listening to other's voices. Some of these vocal factors are not easily controlled, but with effort you can control others. Careful attention to your articulation, rate of speech, and fluency may help you to produce the kind of image you wish to project.

Consider the stereotypes that people have about cues given off by the voice. The breathy female voice has a stereotype of sexy, pretty, and maybe not to be taken seriously. The stereotype of a male with a high voice can be equally problematic. Beyond these stereotypes, people who use choppy sentences may be viewed as not knowing what they want to say. You may not be aware of what you are communicating, but the impact of voice can be considerable. You might find that tape-recording yourself in a group meeting is quite informative. What do you think other group members might conclude from your vocal presentation of yourself?

Use of Time

Two aspects of time are important to a small group. First, inferences people draw from starting meetings on time or late are often important. Time may mean money to everyone at a meeting. The people at the meeting are probably taking time away from their work to attend—and at considerable cost to their organizations. Start at the designated time if you have control. If you are a member, arrange to be at the meeting place on time so that you do not delay the rest of the group. Your use of time may be more than a matter of courtesy—it may be a matter of money—and it may be a factor in the group's success.

Second, when a meeting drones on and on, people become uneasy and uncomfortable. People can maintain attention and a fairly high level of participation for only about one hour. Leadership in this regard means being sensitive to the group's needs. If the meeting is beginning to drag, you can suggest a short break or recess. Be sure that you specify the *length* of the break. If you are the group chairperson, be sure to begin the meeting promptly after the break.

Problems in Using Nonverbal Messages

It seems easy to see that the very nature of nonverbal messages sometimes presents problems in groups. Suppose you are a member of a group with one person who never says anything. Her silence certainly communicates—but what? Is that person shy? Is it that she has nothing to say? Is she preoccupied by some personal or emotional problem? Did she spend most of last night working on a term paper? Is she merely tired? We suspect that you cannot answer these questions. The woman's silence communicates, but it does not communicate very clearly.

Nonverbal messages are ambiguous   Ambiguity creates many problems for small group members. For instance, group members often must guess about what is going on. Misinterpreting others' nonverbal expressions can be just as damaging as misunderstanding what they say! People are unique. Their experiences are also unique. How they experience a particular context—such as a group meeting, for example—can readily change the meaning they get. A smile may be a greeting in one context and "I put one over on you" in another. Even subcultural differences can affect how we communicate without words. The amount of eye contact expected and the degree of personal closeness permitted vary from culture to culture and subculture to subculture within a single community, and cross-cultural groups may be in for some surprises.

For example, if you had a person from Thailand in your group, and if you crossed your legs so that the sole of your foot was pointing at him, he would be insulted!

Nonverbal messages are often unintentional   When group members read an unintentional cue as intentional and act on it, unnecessary interpersonal conflict can ensue. Suppose John, a member of your group, was concentrating on an idea that he was going to present and stared out the window as he thought. The staring behavior was probably unintentional, in that he did not intend it to create an impression. A conclusion of "disinterest" from this unintentional nonverbal behavior might lead you to the wrong conclusions about John. You might be very embarrassed if you chose to act on your interpretation of this unintentional behavior.

Nonverbal messages can inhibit communication   Sometimes a group member's nonverbal behavior inhibits communication. For example, consider the person who talks in a group while staring at the wall. Group members may suspect he would not notice their departure if they moved out of the room. By staring at the wall—by not adhering to the expected eye-contact behavior—this person seriously inhibits communication in his group. But eye contact is not the only kind of nonverbal behavior that might inhibit communication in groups. Sometimes group members attend meetings in inappropriate clothing, fidget in their seats, doodle on paper in front of them, and the like. These behaviors communicate about group members, even if unintentional. They also can be generally distracting to others.

Consider this nonverbal behavior observed in a planning session of a group of young adults who were developing a fund drive for a nonprofit organization. There were four men in business suits and two women, one in a conservative dress and the other in a tailored wool suit. Fifteen minutes late, the final member of the group, a woman named Stella, bounced into the room saying: "I'm so sorry I'm late . . ." No one heard the end of that sentence, we suspect. The woman was wearing blue jeans and a V-neck sweater. Of course, *she* was embarrassed to discover she had worn the wrong clothes. Stella left the meeting almost as soon as she got there.

So nonverbal messages can cause problems. You need to find ways you can address them.

INCREASING NONVERBAL EFFECTIVENESS

If you decide to improve your effectiveness in using nonverbal messages, you'll want to know, first, what needs improving. One way to identify areas for improvement is to try to isolate problems you have had in the past, then find ways of addressing them. In this section, some of the more common problems in nonverbal communication have been selected, along with some suggestions you might wish to try.

PROBLEM
You find that some members talk too much, others talk too little.

LANGUAGE AND/OR SUGGESTIONS
1. Try to regulate the talk patterns by eye contact and head nodding. Avoid eye contact with the talkers; increase your eye contact with those who are silent.

2. Examine the seating arrangement. Maybe the talkers are seated across from one another. In an ongoing group whose members value one another and the group's task, you may be able to approach the more active members and secure their agreement to sit in positions that will minimize the problem. Seat talkative members next to one another if possible. Seat less talkative members across from one another and in central positions. Be careful not to interpret the silent members' nonverbal behavior as a lack of interest. Bormann[25] found that these members were most often experiencing a high level of primary tension, even though they offered the excuse of being uninterested.

PROBLEM
You want to be more influential in a new group.

LANGUAGE AND/OR SUGGESTIONS

1. Sit at the end of a table if possible. If this is not possible, try to sit on a side where you can address and make eye contact with the majority of the group's members.

2. Make frequent eye contact with members and the group as a whole.

3. Pay close attention to the nonverbal cues. You can provide support, reinforce people, clarify, and the like when you are sensitive to the nonverbal cues others are presenting. These help you to provide both social and task leadership. (You will want to review Chapter 7, "Leading Group Meetings," carefully.)

PROBLEM

What can you do about the ambiguity problem in groups?

LANGUAGE AND/OR SUGGESTIONS

1. Check out your perceptions when you can comfortably do so. Use tentative language to let the other person know that you are checking out an inference. You might say either publicly or in private, "I noticed you were [are] staring out the window. You are usually with us. I wonder if there is some problem."

2. Realize, as Joseph DeVito has said, "Nonverbal behaviors are normally packaged."[26] What he means is that a nonverbal behavior is generally accompanied by other nonverbal behaviors that go along with and support the primary behavior. When you observe someone staring out the window, for example, study the facial expression, posture, and other cues that may help you understand what is happening.

3. Try to be aware of the context. Careful attention to the context is always important. Ask yourself, "How does this behavior relate to how the person has been contributing and to what others have been saying?"

PROBLEM

You think some members seem to feel excluded.

LANGUAGE AND/OR SUGGESTIONS

1. Make eye contact with these people.

2. Ask yourself, "Am I being sensitive to these members' feelings and viewpoints?" If you answer no or you aren't sure, then try to give more attention to these people.

PROBLEM

You are worried about giving off unintentional nonverbal cues in your group. What can you do?

LANGUAGE AND/OR SUGGESTIONS

1. Ask a friend (who might also be a member of your group) privately, "I've been

wondering how I'm coming off in the group. I want to do my best. How are you experiencing me as a group member?"

2. Self-awareness is the only other answer to this problem. Since you cannot easily observe some of your behaviors, try to be aware of what you are doing as you observe others. Often their reactions will give you a cue as to what you are doing.

PROBLEM

You think a member of the group is inhibiting communication by certain nonverbal behavior.

LANGUAGE AND/OR SUGGESTIONS

1. The behavior might be unintentional. If you think the behavior is unintentional and the member values the group, you may be able to approach the person privately. Be supportive. (Be sure to read the materials in Chapter 9 on being supportive.)

2. If the disruptive behavior seems to be intentional, then the group leader may need to talk with the person. A decision about who should talk to the person depends on who is most likely to be successful. Supportive communication principles should enhance the likelihood of success.

3. The group may need to discuss this problem. Do not take the leader and group member by surprise with such an issue. Check it out with them before the meeting. Be as supportive as possible.

We have presented options. You must decide which of them, if any, is best suited to you and to a particular group situation. Be flexible. Incorporate them into your own style as completely as you can. And *practice.* Learning a new way to communicate is much, much easier when you rehearse.

LISTENING

The processes involved in listening are much more complex than they first appear to be. The process is noisy and highly subjective. Beyond that, listening is a process that is composed of four component subprocesses, and each of the four can work independently to create errors in listening.

The Components of the Listening Process

The four components of the listening process are sensing, attending, understanding, and remembering. Let's examine each of these components more closely.

Sensing   Sensing is the act of receiving stimuli through the five senses. It is not necessarily a conscious act. For example, any sound wave that has sufficient intensity to reach the ear may be heard. You may ask, then, why you are unable to hear the ticking of the clock when you are working until it is called to your attention. We would answer that in fact you *could* hear the clock. The sound had sufficient intensity to reach your ear but was blocked by the second major element of the listening process.

Attending   You may not be selecting the particular stimulus—the ticking of the clock—to be part of your consciousness. We would say you were not attending. Theoretically, you are able to sense and attend to thousands of stimuli at a time, but you cannot attend to all the potential stimuli. Therefore you select those which are important to you and ignore the others.

Perhaps you failed to notice footsteps as someone entered the room because you were paying attention to a book you were reading. You filtered out the irrelevant. But if the footsteps had been those of your boss, who wandered in to talk with you, you would have filtered out an important sound. Filtering of this kind can also happen when you are listening to someone talk. You may filter out important pieces of information.

Understanding   The third component is understanding—interpreting and evaluating what comes in through the senses—in this case the ears. This step is so important that one writer has based his whole model of the listening process on it. Blaine Goss presents an information-processing model of listening in which he suggests this pattern: Signal Processing (understanding the segments and structures of what we hear) → Literal Processing (understanding the meaning and simple implications of what we hear) → Reflective Processing (understanding a deeper meaning through critical analysis and coming to appreciate what we hear).[27] Thus understanding is an important part of the listening process.

It does not matter if you can hear and attend if you cannot attribute meaning to what is heard. When you understand messages, you pick up meanings similar to those intended by the person speaking. You may understand even *more* than other people intend to communicate by observing nonverbal messages.

Remembering   Like attending, remembering is highly selective. To illustrate this idea to yourself, talk with someone about a movie you have both seen. You may discover that you have remembered the things most interesting and useful to you and have forgotten others. Your friend will have remembered what he or she found interesting. Comparing notes, you'll probably discover that you have remembered different details. You select not only what to attend to but what to remember. You can see how easy it is for a message you give to be understood and remembered as a considerably different message by another person.

Listening Problems

Each of the four components—sensing, attending, understanding, and remembering—gives rise to certain problems. We will discuss the problems before introducing techniques to overcome them. Our reason for organizing the material in this way is that the components are closely related to one another and sometimes problems overlap.

Problems with sensing   Two problems are related to sensing, physical impairment of the sensing mechanism and external noise. Obviously, not being able to sense adequately makes it hard for the listener—and a trip to a competent professional would be in order. Once the problem is solved, you can train yourself to take maximum advantage of your sensing ability.

The second problem is noise, or interference. Everyone who has attended movies can recall the experience of someone nearby talking or joking. The talk made it more difficult to hear accurately. But talking is not the only kind of noise; the sounds of people passing by or automobile or airplane sounds are other examples. Inadequate light may impair your sight and also be "noise." Temperature may be another.

For some people, both impairment of sense and unwanted noise affect the listening process at the same time. For example, a person with normal—stereophonic—hearing can select which ear to attend. If a source of unwanted noise is between that person and another, the listener can tune out the side with the noise and focus upon the side with greater fidelity. People with hearing in only one ear have to take in all sound-based information through that ear. They have no choice about how to use their hearing apparatus to suppress interference. A typewriter or a television set between a listener with one good ear and the source of speech can—and does—directly and strongly affect the communication process.

Problems with attending   Attending difficulties are more numerous than sensing problems. Five aspects of attention inhibit listening.

SELECTIVE PERCEPTION AND ATTENDING   People perceive and attend selectively. On the basis of past experience with situations and people, we select what we believe worth perceiving and attending. Because things are always changing, we nearly always need to adjust our sense of what to attend to.

POOR ATTENDING HABITS   Ralph Nichols and L. A. Stevens[28] cite three poor attending habits to which we want to call your attention. Some people learn to fake attention. They sit as if they are listening carefully but are in fact thinking about something else.

A second poor attending habit is to avoid difficult listening. In other words, people who do not expose themselves to difficult listening situations do not gain practice in attending to difficult material.

The third poor attending habit is to listen only for facts. This kind of attending may cause the listener to miss important cues about the message. Tone of voice and variations in the rate of speaking are two auditory factors that often reveal a great deal about the message. People who have trained themselves to listen for and jot down facts may miss these nonverbal cues and thereby misunderstand the message.

LISTENER ATTITUDES AND NEEDS THAT INTERFERE   Attitude will have a significant impact on how people attend to a message. For example, if you were forced by your company to attend a seminar, your attitude might get in your way as you tried to listen. Status can be a related problem. If you think it is inappropriate for group members to be offering you advice, you will pay less attention when they do. The same attitude-perception mechanism works when a person tries to listen to a co-worker who has a different perspective on how to do a job.

In addition, people attend to stimuli that satisfy their needs.[29] We often hear what we *think* was said because our needs and values cause us to ignore disconfirming stimuli.[30]

LOW INTENSITY OF THE MESSAGE   Some messages may be presented in such an unenthusiastic way that they are difficult to attend to. You may have discovered how difficult it is to listen when an instructor drones on and on. Nichols[31] suggests that deciding early in the listening task that you have some use for the material will help your ability to attend to it. Other techniques, such as active listening, discussed in the last section of this chapter, will also help.

UNACCUSTOMED LENGTH OF THE MESSAGE   Donald Campbell[32] found that the longer the message, the greater a person's loss of information. People have a natural tendency to shorten, simplify, and eliminate detail when listening to a long message. In addition, people tend to drop the middle of a long message.

Problems with understanding   Understanding and agreement are different concepts. Some people say they don't understand when actually they don't agree. Problems of understanding can be attributed to four sources.

DIFFERENT FIELDS OF EXPERIENCE   You know what words mean from your experience with them. Your past experience with the words we are writing here, with this context (you are reading, if not studying, this text), and with this content will all be relevant to your interpretation. For example, if you have read another author's definition and discussion of the concept "field of experience" and it differs from this one, you may have trouble understanding this passage.

INABILITY TO EMPATHIZE   Since people all have different fields of experience, then for almost every issue, the likely outcome of these differences is that people will hold different values. People are likely to disagree some of the time—maybe most of the time—if their orientations are very different. This tendency sometimes makes it difficult to see another person's way of looking at a situation. (Sometimes it is hard even to imagine another way of viewing a particular situation.) A frequent result is that people spend time mentally criticizing another person's view, constructing arguments to refute his or her ideas, and not listening carefully.

Empathizing is an activity in which participants attempt to put themselves in another's mental and situational framework. By its nature, empathy requires a more active mental commitment to what is being said. That is why empathizing creates greater understanding.

POOR USE OF FEEDBACK   People can create problems for themselves because they do not bother to get and give adequate feedback. Almost everyone has stopped at a service station to ask for directions to an unfamiliar location. What can you do to be sure you understand the directions? One technique is to repeat the directions back to the person and ask for correction of any errors.

MENTAL SETS   The fourth problem related to understanding is often alluded to by such terms as "closed-minded," "overly critical," and "polarized viewpoint." Mental sets such as these can cause listeners to assume that they know what is right and prevent them from understanding another's view. We are certainly not saying that you should not have opinions. You need to acknowledge, however, that others also think and have something to say. Unless you can momentarily put your opinions aside, you may not even hear what they are saying.

Problems with remembering   How long will you remember what you have heard? Tony Buzan[33] has suggested that you will forget 80 percent of the details in just twenty-four hours. The curve that Buzan plotted is based on data he collected with students who had memorized word lists (Figure 4.5). Buzan discovered that we are not 100 percent efficient at remembering, even when we have just completed a learning task. Notice the rise at the end of the task—the mind keeps working and making connections. Our remembering is more efficient for a short period after we've completed a learning task than it is *during* the task. Researchers have been aware of this forgetting curve for a century. Herman Ebbinghaus[34] did basic research with forgetting in 1885. Compare the Ebbinghaus curve with Buzan's. Notice that negative acceleration of the retention curve seems to be the general rule. The Ebbinghaus data are based on the number of nonsense syllables remembered. Buzan's data represent remembering real words. The Buzan curve is calculated with respect to the subject's ability to recall the memorized words. This difference in methodology is important for those studying memory. For us, the important principle is that both researchers reported the same relatively rapid drop in remembering.

Developing Listening Skills

Work hard at listening.   Becoming a better listener requires the *belief* that listening can be hard work. In this respect it is the same as other skills. It involves making an effort to get the main point, the information you need.

For example, suppose a member of your group seems to you to talk too much. "He has an opinion about everything," you say. This is so much the case that you have developed the habit of discounting his opinion. During one meeting he says: "I've found some important information on the problem. . . ."

Given your prior experience with this member and your attitude about the value

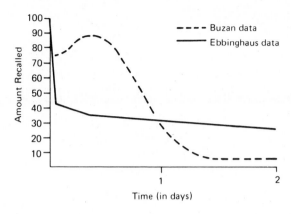

FIGURE 4.5
Forgetting Curves

Source: Adapted from *Use Both Sides of Your Brain* by Tony Buzan. Copyright 1983 by Tony Buzan. Reprinted by permission of the publisher, E. P. Dutton.

of his contributions, you may find it very hard work to stay with him and to get his point.

Paraphrase the content.   The technique of paraphrasing will help you to attend more carefully and to know if you understand. By paraphrasing the content, a technique also called active listening, you can say back to the speaker what you believe he or she is trying to say. Thus you are forced to concentrate on what is being said. Paraphrasing is not parroting but putting what you have heard into your own words. When you paraphrase, you'll know if you understand. You can continue if you do; you can be corrected if you don't.

You may argue that paraphrasing everything the other person says would drive anybody mad. You are right. Paraphrasing is a special technique that should be used when the information being given (1) is particularly important to you or the organization, (2) is complex or involves several steps, and (3) involves a problem and the person has come to you for help. You must also have the time to exert the needed effort. Routine talk and information sharing do not usually require this special attention. If you learn to use it properly, paraphrasing is a powerful listening technique that brings with it impressive benefits.

You may also argue that paraphrasing seems artificial. We think that the artificial sound of the talk will disappear if you practice its use. One reason paraphrasing sounds funny is that people use the same lead-in to active listening every time. Often they say something like, "What I hear you saying is . . ." This is a perfectly good lead-in, but if overused it causes the conversation to sound artificial. Learn a variety of ways of saying, "I want to feed back what you've said."

Check out your inferences.   Listening is more than just hearing what was said directly. It is often difficult for people to say directly what they are feeling, needing, or wanting. Thus it becomes a useful listening technique to verify your inferences when the other person is not being particularly clear. This skill requires a high degree of selectivity in responding to the other person's talk. Inferences about negative feeling, for example, ought to be carefully weighed before responding. In this regard, plan and practice saying,

"What I'm guessing you mean [feel, need, or want] is . . ." Otherwise the usefulness of the check-out technique will be limited by the sound of artificiality.

Remember that it is very hard for many people to communicate the feelings associated with the content of their talk. When there is an underlying feeling that is clearly evident, it is probably better to respond to it. Carl Rogers[35] suggests that responding to the obvious feeling facilitates the expression of related feelings and helps both the listener and the speaker to understand the surrounding feelings and assumptions, needs, or other thoughts. So when those feelings are an issue, we think it is a good idea to focus on them.

Empathize with the speaker.   Empathizing is a most useful listening technique—getting into another's frame of reference rather than "listening" to your own view. Those who teach transactional analysis, a psychological method of improving interpersonal relationships, suggest that it is important to adopt an attitude that the other person is okay.[36] Jack Gibb[37] suggests that one of the six characteristics of a supportive climate is empathy. Carl Rogers[38] tells us that accurate empathic understanding of his clients' private worlds is an essential part of the relationship.

Empathic listening involves suspending evaluation. Evaluative listening is a deliberate activity and is, therefore, different from empathic listening. Charles Kelly drew this distinction clearly in his comprehensive dissertation research on listening in an industrial setting:

> The difference between empathic listening and deliberative [evaluative] listening is primarily motivational. Both listeners seek the same objective: accurate understanding of communication from another. . . . The empathic listener lets his understanding of the speaker determine his modes of evaluation, which are automatic; the deliberative listener's understanding of the speaker is filtered through his predetermined modes of selective listening, and he actually spends less time as a communication receiver. The empathic listener is more apt to be a consistent listener, and is less prone to his own or other distractions.[39]

The deliberative listener pursues an evaluative orientation from the start. In contrast, the empathic listener tries to withhold evaluation at least long enough to understand the other person's view.

Work on remembering.   It is possible to prevent the sharp drop in the amount of content remembered after an exchange, but not to prevent some drop. Three important techniques aid memory: organization, repetition, and association.[40]

In his useful and well-written book *Use Both Sides of Your Brain,* Tony Buzan suggests ways to intervene in the forgetting process. Study his graph of the forgetting curve pictured in Figure 4.6. He suggests that you take notes during the listening activity, if possible. If it is not, then make some notes within about ten minutes of

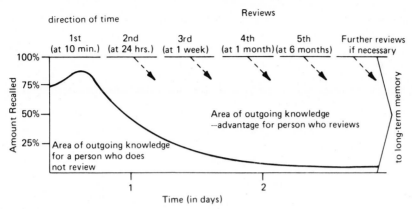

FIGURE 4.6
Spacing Organizing and Practice Sessions To Aid Memory

Source: Adapted from *Use Both Sides of Your Brain* by Tony Buzan. Copyright by Tony Buzan, 1983. Reprinted by permission of the publisher, E. P. Dutton.

listening. Afterward, reorganize the notes and add detail. Do this within about ten minutes of completing the listening. Buzan suggests both a review (repetition) and an organizing session. This may be enough for most listening activities.

If the content of your listening activity is something you need to remember over an extended period of time, you may want to practice recalling ideas. The practice session should be different from the first review session. Write down all that you can remember. Compare your writing with your own notes. Then relearn what you have forgotten. Space these practice sessions, as the figure suggests, at twenty-four hours, one week, one month, six months, and so on (if necessary). This kind of practice permits interruption of the forgetting curve.

As a further aid, the content of what you want to remember might be linked by association to some experience already familiar to you. This suggestion works, but you must use it correctly. The familiar experience must be sufficiently similar to what should be remembered. Rely on note taking for recollection of details, but on association to remember the broad concepts.

Some general principles of note taking seem to apply:

1. *Discover the speaker's organizational pattern if there is one.*

2. *Keep precise notes.* Note taking can get in the way of listening. Use either key words or key phrases. Later fill in enough detail to be sure of complete information recall.

3. *Develop a personal shorthand for common words and terms.*

4. *Review and rewrite your notes within about ten minutes of completing the listening activity.* Buzan contends that this takes advantage of the peak of remembering capability. Your mind continues to make associations and linkages for a short period after you complete the listening task.[41]

Try these memory techniques. They help to improve memory, and they will also help you to begin forming habits that will pay off as you move up into the management of an organization.

SUMMARY

This chapter was written to help you understand the effective use of verbal and nonverbal messages within group contexts. Interpreting verbal messages requires the application of your personal experience to the words being used by group members. Since each person is unique, accurate interpretation of meaning depends on similar experiences. When fields of experience do not overlap, we use words differently, and this causes many of our group communication problems. Groups can create a group frame of reference by sharing denotative and connotative definitions. Verbal communication is also affected by perceptual bias, ambiguity of language, and too much or too little information.

Nonverbal messages form an important part of the total group communication event. They serve to reinforce the verbal message through repetition, elaboration, and accenting. Sometimes they modify the words by contradiction. When this takes place, the nonverbal portion of the message is generally believed. Some nonverbal messages serve as substitutes for the verbal message, whereas others may regulate the flow of communication.

The physical environment of a group—the attractiveness and appearance of the meeting room—can cause the members to view the task more positively and thereby enjoy it and want to stay with it longer. Seating preferences and arrangements also affect groups.

Personal appearance, gesture, posture and movement, face and eye behavior, vocalics, and use of time also communicate in a group setting. Take care that you dress appropriately and keep physically fit and well groomed. Use of gesture, posture, and movement may help determine your influence and leadership emergence in the group. Positive head nods and greater gesticulation help people to emerge as leaders. Face and eye behavior convey evaluation, interest, intensity of involvement, amount of control, and probably understanding. Close attention to faces pays off. Additional information is often inferred from the voice. Attention to the voice may reveal the speaker's interest, personality, educational level, and emotional state. Finally, use of time is an important message system in groups. Starting meetings on time and regulating their length can help the efficiency of any group.

Nonverbal messages are ambiguous, can be unintentional, and do inhibit communication. You must depend on the context to interpret the meaning of the message. It is also helpful to remember that some of the nonverbal messages you observe may be unintentional and therefore misleading. Messages like improper clothing, fidgeting, and doodling can distract the listener and create problems for the group. Finally, specific strategies for coping with particular problems that flow from inaccurate nonverbal messages were suggested. Be sure as you decide about alternatives that you consider the situation and your own personal style.

Our discussion of listening began with a description of the four components of the listening process: sensing, attending, understanding, and remembering. Each of these presents a potential area of difficulty for a listener. If your sensing mechanisms are faulty, you will not receive the message. If you are distracted and do not attend, you will not know what is said. If you do not understand, you may assume one message when the speaker means another. If you cannot remember the message that you processed, your whole listening effort is wasted.

We discussed problems associated with each of these areas. Sensing problems may be related to actual defects in the mechanisms or to noise from the environment. Attending problems emerge from a greater range of difficulties. These include selective perception, poor attending habits, the listener's attitudes and needs, low-intensity messages, and messages that are too long. Difficulties related to understanding can be attributed to four sources: different fields of experience, inability to empathize, poor use of feedback, and various mental sets. Finally, as forgetting curves demonstrate, people forget much detail unless they themselves intervene in some way.

We concluded that important listening skills must be practiced if they are to be acquired. The five suggestions are:

1. *Work hard at listening.* Avoiding distractions is hard work.

2. *Paraphrase the content.* Active listening will force involvement.

3. *Check your inferences.* Checking will allow confirmation or denial.

4. *Empathize.* Empathy helps you understand the speaker's view.

5. *Work on remembering.* Note taking, association, and review help memory. Practice and understanding will bring improvement.

EXERCISES

1. Describe any problems your group has experienced with perceptual bias, ambiguity of language, labeling, too much information, and too little information. Identify any nonverbal problems that were experienced.

2. Make an audio tape of one of your group's problem-solving discussions. Analyze the verbal interaction of your group. Identify the major incidents of functional and dysfunctional language use. For the instances where language use was causing difficulties for your group, what steps would you suggest to help group members improve?

3. Write a short essay that describes your experience in groups where the following language problems affected the group's efficiency and productivity: frame of reference, overlap of experience, and denotative/connotative meaning. Be sure to give specific examples of each. Tell how language problems can affect the group.

4. Discuss in your group ways in which a group member might overcome perceptual problems, ambiguity of language, and information overload. Under what circumstances might these become serious problems for a group?

5. During a group discussion have one of the observers ask the group to "freeze." Then ask each observer to discuss the posture of one of the discussants. What does it seem to be saying about the member's relationship with the group? What does it say about the member's feelings about the group? After observers do this a few times, members and observers discuss the implications of the observations.

6. Ask groups to meet at two different locations while carrying out a class project. Then each member should write a two-page reaction paper in which the effects of the environments are compared and contrasted. The question this essay seeks to answer is "What difference did the environment make to your group climate and task productivity?"

7. Suppose you were in charge of plans for a decision-making meeting where you know two powerful and aggressive members will be in attendance. This is a five-member group. What steps might you take in arranging the environment to minimize this potential problem? Discuss your answer with classmates. How do their suggestions differ? Can the class agree on what might be the best plan?

NOTES

1. For example, Ragner Rommetviet, *On Message Structure: A Framework for the Study of Language and Communication* (New York: Wiley, 1974).

2. C. K. Ogden and I. A. Richards, *The Meaning of Meaning* (New York: Harcourt, Brace and Company, 1923), 11.

3. S. I. Hayakawa, *Language in Thought and Action* (New York: Harcourt Brace Jovanovich, 1964).

4. Dale G. Leathers, "Process Disruption and Measurement in Small Group Communication," *Quarterly Journal of Speech* 55 (1969):288–298.

5. George A. Miller, "The Magic Number Seven, Plus or Minus Two: Some Limits on Our Capacity for Processing Information," *Psychological Review* 63 (1965):81–97.

6. B. Aubrey Fisher, *Small Group Decision Making,* 2d ed. (New York: McGraw-Hill, 1980), 82–83; 149–154.

7. Dale G. Leathers, "The Informational Potential of the Nonverbal and Verbal Components of Feedback Responses," *The Southern Speech Communication Journal* 44 (1979):331–354.

8. Abraham H. Maslow and Norbett L. Mintz, "Effects of Esthetic Surroundings: 1. Initial Effects of Three Esthetic Conditions Upon Perceiving 'Energy' and 'Wellbeing' in Faces," *Journal of Psychology* 41 (1965):247–254.

9. B. Steinzor, "The Spatial Factor in Face-to-Face Discussion Groups," *Journal of Abnormal and Social Psychology* 45 (1950):552–555; F. L. Strodtbeck and L. H. Hook, "The Social Dimensions of a Twelve-Man Jury Table," *Sociometry* 24 (1961):397–415; G. Hearn, "Leadership and the Spatial Factor in Small Groups," *Journal of Abnormal and Social Psychology* 54 (1957):269–272.

10. Albert Mehrabian and S. G. Diamond, "Seating Arrangement and Conversation," *Sociometry* 34 (1971):281–289.

11. N. F. Russo, "Connotations of Seating Arrangements," *Cornell Journal of Social Relations* 2 (1967):37–44.

12. This finding has been further substantiated by J. J. Edney and M. J. Grundmann, "Friendship, Group Size, and Boundary Size: Small Group Spaces," *Small Group Behavior* 8 (1979):124–135.

13. L. T. Howells and S. W. Becker, "Seating Arrangement and Leadership Emergence," *Journal of Abnormal and Social Psychology* 64 (1962):148–150.

14. See Keith Gibbins, "Communication Aspects of Women's Clothes and Their Relation to Fashionability," *British Journal of Social and Clinical Psychology* 8 (1964):301–312; Ellen Berscheid and Elaine Walster, "Physical Attractiveness," in Leonard Berkowitz, ed., *Advances in Experimental Social Psychology* 7, (New York: Academic Press, 1974); C. L. Kleinke, *First Impressions: The Psychology of Encountering Others* (Englewood Cliffs, N.J.: Prentice-Hall, 1975).

15. See Marvin E. Shaw, *Group Dynamics: The Psychology of Small Group Behavior* (New York: McGraw-Hill, 1981), 319–320, for a more complete review of this research.

16. John E. Baird and A. Schubert, "Nonverbal Behavior and Leadership Emergence in Task-Oriented and Informal Group Discussion." (Paper presented at the International Communication Association Convention, New Orleans, 1974.)

17. John E. Baird, Jr., "Some Nonverbal Elements of Leadership Emergence," *The Southern Speech Communication Journal* 42 (1977): 352–361.

18. Gerald I. Nierenberg and H. H. Calero, *How to Read a Person Like a Book* (New York: Pocket Books, 1973), 46.

19. Stewart L. Tubbs, *A Systems Approach to Small Group Interaction* (New York: Random House, 1988), 203.

20. Dale G. Leathers, *Nonverbal Communication Systems* (Boston: Allyn and Bacon, 1976), 33–34.

21. W. Gill Woodall, Judee K. Burgoon, and Norman Markel, "The Effects of Facial-Head Cue Combinations on Interpersonal Evaluations," *Communication Quarterly* 28 (1980):47–55.

22. James McCroskey, Carl Larson, and Mark Knapp, *An Introduction to Interpersonal Communication* (Englewood Cliffs, N.J.: Prentice-Hall, 1971), 110–114.

23. Ralph V. Exline, "Explorations in the Process of Person Perception: Visual Interaction in Relation to Competition, Sex, and the Need for Affiliation," *Journal of Personality* 31 (1963):1–20.

24. Judee K. Burgoon, "Spatial Relationships in Small Groups," in Robert S. Cathcart and Larry A. Samovar, eds., *Small Group Communication: A Reader,* 5th ed. (Dubuque, Iowa: Wm. C. Brown, 1988), 360.

25. Ernest G. Bormann, *Discussion and Group Methods: Theory and Practice,* 2d ed. (New York: Harper & Row, 1975), 183.

26. Joseph A. DeVito, *The Interpersonal Communication Book* (New York: Harper & Row, 1983), 191–192.

27. Blaine Goss, "Listening as Information Processing," *Communication Quarterly,* 30 (Fall 1982):304–307.

28. Ralph Nichols and L. A. Stevens, *Are You Listening?* (New York: McGraw-Hill, 1957).

29. Lee Thayer, *Communication and Communication Systems* (Homewood, Ill.: Richard D. Irwin, 1968), 51–53.

30. Ibid., 53–54.

31. Ralph Nichols, "Listening is a 10-Part Skill," *Nation's Business*, 45 (1957): 56–60.

32. Donald Campbell, "Systematic Error on the Part of Human Links in Communication Systems," *Information and Control*, 1 (1958):334–369.

33. Tony Buzan, *Use Both Sides of Your Brain* (New York: Dutton, 1976), 49–50.

34. Herman Ebbinghaus, *Über das Gedächtnis: Untersuchungen der Experimentalen Psychologie* (Leipzig: Dancher und Humbolt, 1885). Interest in researching this phenomenon has begun to pick up in the last few years in relation to split-brain studies and their offshoots. In all the research we know about, the retention curves look about the same as the two we present.

35. Carl Rogers, "Releasing Expression," in *Counseling and Psychotherapy* (Boston: Houghton Mifflin, 1942).

36. Dorothy Jungeward, *Everybody Winds: Transactional Analysis Applied to Organizations* (Reading, Mass.: Addison-Wesley, 1974), 208–212.

37. Jack R. Gibb, "Defensive Communication," *Journal of Communication*, 11:3 (September 1961):141–148.

38. C. R. Rogers, "The Interpersonal Relationship: The Core of Guidance," *Harvard Educational Review*, 32 (Fall 1962):416–429.

39. Charles Kelly, "Empathic Listening," in Robert S. Cathcart and Larry A. Samovar, eds., *Small Group Communication: A Reader*, 2d ed. (Dubuque, Iowa: William C. Brown, 1984) 297.

40. James F. Deese, *The Psychology of Learning*, 2d ed. (New York: McGraw-Hill, 1958), 237–248.

41. Buzan, *Use Both Sides of Your Brain*, 55.

RECOMMENDED READINGS

Peter A. Anderson, "Nonverbal Communication in the Small Group," in Robert S. Cathcart and Larry A. Samovar, eds., *Small Group Communication: A Reader*, 5th ed. (Dubuque, Iowa: Wm C. Brown, 1988), 333–350.

John C. Condon, *Semantics and Communication*, 3d ed. (New York: Macmillan, 1985).

H. Lloyd Goodall, Jr., *Small Group Communication in the Organization* (Dubuque, Iowa: Wm. C. Brown, 1985), Chapter 3, "What You Should Know About Communication in the Small Group."

Andrew Wolvin and Carolyn Gwynn Coakley, *Listening*, 3d ed. (Dubuque, Iowa: Wm. C. Brown, 1988).

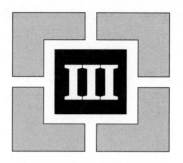

Participating in
Group Meetings

CHAPTER 5

Encouraging Group Development and Evolution

OBJECTIVES

After reading this chapter you should be able to:

Name and explain five motivations for belonging to groups; then specify how knowledge of these five motivations might be useful to a long-time group member.

Recall and explain Bales's, Fisher's, and Poole's explanations of group development.

Describe how knowledge of Bales's, Fisher's, and Poole's developmental explanations may be useful in encouraging a group's development.

Identify, define, compare, and contrast social tension, primary tension, and secondary tension; then explain how knowledge of social tension theory may be useful to an individual group member.

Describe Scheidel's and Crowell's notions of idea development in a problem-solving group, naming each stage in the process, and explaining the communication behavior to be found in each stage.

Specify how knowledge of the spiral model of idea development may be useful to a group member who wishes to encourage group development.

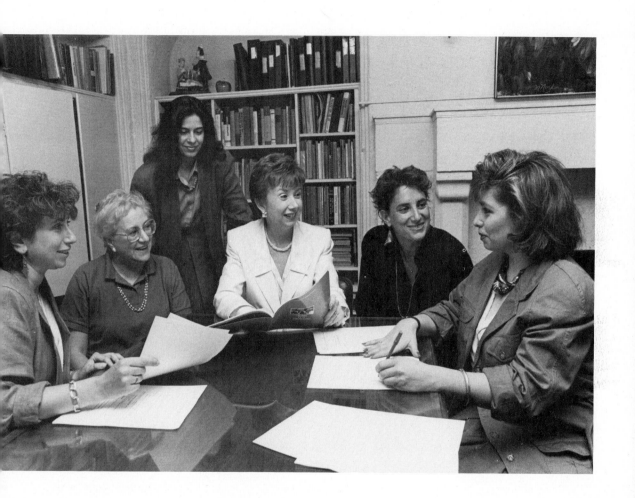

Suppose you are asked to serve on a committee to consider changes in general education requirements for all students at your college or university. You have some ideas about general education and are flattered to be asked. You agree to the appointment. The president selects an eight-member committee composed of five faculty and three students. You are one of the student members. The first meeting is next week. You begin to think about what the meetings will be like. Can you imagine what will happen? Would you be able to make a sequential list? Stop—and we hope you actually will—and try to make such a list. How many items do you have?

How did you do at crystal-ball gazing? Perhaps you were able to make some pretty good predictions. Yet you may have been frustrated in your attempt. Or perhaps you realized the difficulty of this task and did not try it. We think your ability to operate productively in groups rests in your ability to wrestle with some of these questions. Some generalizations about groups come from scholars who have investigated these issues. Their work will help facilitate the development and evolution of groups.

Motivations for volunteering to participate in groups is the first topic of this chapter. You will not always be able to know why people belong to your group, but when you do you can help them to be more productive by giving attention to their needs. Next, phases of group development are considered. Then, the topics of task development, social tension, and idea development are addressed. Each of these group processes happens with some regularity in its sequence. Knowing these sequences can help you to understand and make predictions about your group. Also, the "how to" question is addressed. How do you make use of this information to facilitate your group's development? Finally, practical suggestions for putting what you have learned into practice are offered.

MOTIVATIONS FOR MEMBER PARTICIPATION IN GROUPS

Examine your motives for being a member of a particular group. Do you have a group in mind? If not, stop for a moment and pick one. Now think both of yourself and the other members of the group. A good question to ask yourself is, "What things do members of the group receive that keep them in the group?" See how many different motivations you can list on a piece of paper.

Now check your list against the one presented below. See how you did. Perhaps our words are a little more "academic sounding," but see if your ideas match these. People are motivated to belong to groups because of (1) attraction to others in the group, (2) attraction to the group's activities, (3) attraction to the group's goals, (4) attraction to being affiliated with the group, and (5) attraction to needs outside the group. We will take up each of these ideas, with illustrations of each and suggestions for group development. The motives for belonging that a person brings to a group affect the development potential and direction of the group. These motives can be used to develop other members' motivation to participate. And, in doing so, the development of the group as a decision-making team is affected. The subsequent sections will examine these motives and demonstrate their potential for use in developing groups.

Attraction to Others in the Group

Ask any group of people to describe why they are attracted to one another and you are likely to get a variety of answers. You can gain an appreciation of the complexity of this issue by considering someone you know in a group, to whom you are attracted. Now take a moment to think of several of the reasons you like to be with that person.

Do you find the person physically attractive?

Do you have similar interests?

Do you have attitudes and values that seem to match reasonably closely?

Do your important values match closely?

Do you see yourselves as having similar personality characteristics?

Are you of similar economic status, race, and so forth?

Do you see the person as having abilities similar to yours?

Count the number of times you said yes to the questions asked. You are likely to have several yeses, because attraction is a complex issue. People are attracted to groups for a variety of reasons. Pete Wells belongs to the Rotary because the members he knows represent an image he admires. Al Smith belongs to a study group at his church because several of its members are interested in tennis. Sally Williams belongs to a group investigating computer needs in her department because she enjoys the people who volunteered to work in the group. Motivations for being part of a group are varied, and not always related to the task of the group.

Attraction is related to pleasing physical characteristics, similarities in attitude, belief, personality, race, economic status, and perceived ability of the other person. Perhaps the strongest of these—and the most often studied—is perceived similarity of attitude. Theodore Newcomb[1] conducted the classic study in this area when he invited a group of students to live in a house rent free if they would participate in an experiment. His experiment demonstrated the strength of similarity. He asked seventeen men to live in the same house for two years. After they occupied the house, he gave them a series of tests to measure attitudes and values. He also checked the room assignments and likings of group members. He discovered that liking was based on proximity—how close to one another in the house they were physically situated. Later, when he retested the interpersonal attractions, he found a shift. Now those who perceived themselves to be similar in attitudes had developed attractions. Newcomb concluded that people initially got to know those closest to them. Then, as they were able to know others in the house, they were attracted to those who were similar. Keep in mind when you look at why members are attracted to groups that similarity is a good starting place.

Attraction is also related to personality similarity. Byrne, Griffitt, and Stefaniak,[2] for example, had 151 subjects respond to items on a scale that would measure personality characteristics. Then they examined a stranger's responses that agreed with their choices—25 percent, 50 percent, or 80 percent of the time. Next the subjects rated the stranger's attractiveness. The more the stranger agreed, the more the person was liked by the subjects.

The details of these two studies are presented for two reasons. First, it is useful for you to have an appreciation of how researchers approach and examine issues such as these. Second, the kind of evidence that supports these generalizations is important. There is also support to show that attraction is related to economic similarity,[3] race,[4] and similarity of ability.[5] The findings related to similarity of ability are interesting. Initially people were attracted to those who had previously been successful at a given task. However, when they had the opportunity to shift from their initial choices, in time unsuccessful people chose unsuccessful partners.

Attraction to Group Activities

Sometimes people belong to a group because they enjoy some aspect of the task that members do.[6] But this is not always the same thing as valuing the goal of the group. For example, imagine an athletic woman joining the sorority softball team to participate in its athletic program but not really embracing its primary goal of socializing. Some people belong to a civic group in order to socialize with its members rather than to work toward achievement of its goals. You can imagine how important it could be to realize that particular members are not especially interested in the group's goal. If you try to motivate such people by emphasizing commitment to the group's goal, your success is likely to be minimal. On the other hand, you may be able to link achievement of their needs to the group goal and be successful. For example, a sorority might show how other athletes are attracted to groups with strong social programs. This may give the woman who joined to participate in athletics a reason to support the social program, too.

Attraction to Group Goal

Perhaps the most important reason for a member to belong to a group from the standpoint of group development is attraction to the goal. Sometimes it is difficult to separate this kind of attraction from valuing the group's activities. We showed you how it is possible to value certain activities and not be attracted to the group's goal. It is important that you be able to spot this situation when it happens.

Attraction to the goal contributes more to a group than mere achievement of particular ends. Members who are committed to the goal may work hard on being able to get along. They may even be able to put aside differences and hostilities because they value goal achievement. Sherif and Sherif[7] vividly demonstrated this aspect of goal achievement in their famous boys' camp experiment. They created hostility between two groups of boys through various manipulations. For example, they invited both groups to a party in which half of the refreshments were badly damaged. They invited one group earlier than the other so that they had opportunity to serve themselves the undamaged portion of the food. This they did; the other group became predictably angry. Next they tried to manage the conflict by creating a goal to which they thought both groups would be attracted. They arranged a baseball game in which their camp would play a neighboring camp. The embracing of this attractive goal served to ease much of the hostility and created a new group loyalty.

Attraction to Being Affiliated with the Group

Groups allow people to interact and thereby fulfill a need to affiliate with others. You undoubtedly know of people who do not really care about the task of the group, are not really interested in the group's goals, and may even not wish to get involved with the members on a personal level, but who attend some of the group meetings. You might suspect that affiliation with the group per se is rewarding—and it is. These people like to be able to say that they are members. Perhaps they believe that belonging to these groups gives them some sort of prestige. The aim of their attendance at a few meetings is to keep themselves in good standing so they can say that they belong.

Need for affiliation when it is a member's sole attraction to the group may present a difficult problem for the leader of a task group. How do you interest the person in the group's goals? If you cannot do this, then the member's presence may be disruptive. Your group can suffer significantly if you have several of these members. Imagine a PTA member who attends an occasional meeting. This person is uninformed. He or she may want to discuss an ongoing issue, but the effort is more disrupting than helpful. The next section of this chapter presents some specific suggestions for making productive members out of people who have this type of need.

Attraction to Needs Outside the Group

Finally, it is clear that some people belong to groups for reasons that may have nothing to do with the group's task, goals, members, and so forth. Perhaps you know of a fellow student who has joined groups in order to bolster her or his employment résumé. Some people belong to religious groups not because they are particularly attracted to the religious activities, but because it is the socially acceptable thing to do. Sometimes businesspeople belong to civic organizations because they think it will be good for business.

You can imagine the problems it might create for your group if you have members who are pursuing goals primarily outside the group. They may be totally unreliable, may attend only rarely, and can even be disruptive when they do attend, as they have not taken enough interest to know what is happening.

Encouraging Group Development: Motivation through Meeting Needs

People perceive their membership as satisfying some need, and this can serve as an important source of motivation for those providing leadership.

The problem for members and leaders who wish to develop their group is finding out what the motivations of various members might be. If you find that you have a number of people who are motivated by a particular need (say affiliation), you might try to get them to value the group members more. Perhaps you invite them to one of the group's social functions. This may promote cohesiveness and may also develop their commitment to members and the group, thereby enhancing productivity.

Sometimes it is the activities of the group that interest the member, with goal achievement being of little concern. Of course, if the group's activities are only task related, this is not a problem. One method of using this attraction to motivate is to link the activities to goal attainment. For example, if the person's primary motivation is to participate in your group's philanthropic effort, you might be sure that you devote some time in each of your meetings to this issue. You might emphasize how important you think this activity is and tell the person how much you appreciate his or her contributions in this area. You would also want to show how accomplishment of this philanthropic activity is related to the overall task.

Still others may belong to your group to try to fulfill their need for affiliation with others. These people may not care much about the group's goals or task or even the particular attributes of its members. We pointed out what a difficult problem this can be. It may be impossible to generate commitment to the group task. If this is a chronic problem that is in fact disrupting the group, you may need to make the problem an agenda item. The group's members need to affirm their commitment to the tasks and goal. The group might decide, for instance, that regular attendance and work on the task are necessary for continued membership in the group. If these people enjoy the affiliation with the group members enough, they may be motivated to embrace and work on the task in order to meet that need.

Finally, some members may belong to a group for a goal that is outside the group's purpose. They may wish to receive the benefits that outsiders might attribute to them because of their membership in the group. If the members are not genuinely interested in the task and in this case may not even particularly value the members, then your group may have to make membership contingent upon maintaining a particular level of involvement. This is hard to do, but it is one of the more practical solutions to this kind of motivational problem.

PHASES IN GROUP DEVELOPMENT

Suppose for a moment that you think the career for you is in medicine. Maybe you decide to specialize in pediatrics. Part of your task would be to guide children in their development. So you would be involved with parents, too. You would watch for normal developmental processes and alert parents to what normal expectations might be. You would use your knowledge of how children develop to know how a child is doing and to help you spot difficulties. Sometimes you might encourage parents to refrain from certain behaviors that may hinder normal development. On the other hand, you might encourage them to do things that would help develop motor skills.

Groups also develop in rather predictable ways, though most people are unaware of that process. But if you understand the process of group development you will be able to make more meaningful contributions to the groups and organizations to which you belong.

Group Development

One of the most interesting findings about group development is that task groups are thought to pass through phases in evolutionary and decision development. Understanding this phase development is particularly important to you because, as Marshall Scott Poole put it, the research suggests "a logically ideal format for decision making" that "may well be the simplest effective path a decision-making group could follow."[8] Although there have been many studies of this phenomenon, here we will present three. These three, taken together, will give you a firm understanding of group development. The first, from the research of Robert F. Bales, focuses on the evolutionary development of a group. The second, from the work of B. Aubrey Fisher, addresses a second key aspect of group development—decision development. The third, from research by Marshall Scott Poole, rounds out the discussion by helping us understand what happens when the Fisher model doesn't fit a particular group.

Robert F. Bales   Bales was the first scholar to attempt controlled study of the group development process. He identified two predominant concerns in groups.[9] These concerns, socioemotional and task, are evidenced in interactions about interpersonal relationships and accomplishment of the task. Bales found that issues related to one or the other of these predominate at particular times. As a group is forming, for example, the issue of who the members are and how they will relate interpersonally is foremost. This does not mean, of course, that task concerns will not be addressed as well, but that the socioemotional, relationship-related interaction predominates. As these interpersonal issues are settled and the group matures, task-related issues become more prominent. Now the group can focus its attention on production and thereby achieve maximum effectiveness in its decision making. So we find socioemotional and task phases as a group interacts over a period of time.

Issues of relationship and task cycle back and forth as the situation of the group changes. Thus we might expect each new meeting of an ongoing group to begin with relational talk being prominent as members become reacquainted. Then, the group might move on to a period in which task issues are central as it devotes more attention to accomplishing its task. We might also expect that when a group takes in new members or changes in some other way—perhaps the status of a member changes—the group might move to a period in which relationship talk predominates.

B. Aubrey Fisher   A scholar in the field of communication studies, Fisher has focused on the task dimension of decision making. Fisher[10] analyzed the content of audio tapes of ten interacting groups, using a category system that excluded their social dimensions. His focus was on the process whereby members' preliminary ideas are transformed into consensus decisions. Thus he was interested in the number of favorable, unfavorable, or ambiguous opinions offered; the evidence presented; the support given to opinion; modifications offered; attempts to clarify; and agreement or disagreement with others' opinions. You can tell by the kinds of behaviors he identified that his concern was definitely with contributions related to the emergence of a decision. From this work, Fisher identified four phases that seem to occur consistently: orientation, conflict, emergence, and reinforcement.

The *orientation* phase is characterized by members' spending most of their time agreeing with each other, clarifying, and giving information. They often present ambiguously worded suggestions and tentative statements. For example, a member might say, "I think the problem might be that Nat is bored with the job." Another member might say, "That certainly might be part of it. But outside factors may also be a problem here." Notice the tentative language. There is very little disagreement. They are testing the group and feeling their way, as they do not yet know what to expect. Usually members of a new group do not know one another well and therefore are unwilling to risk assertive behavior. You would not be likely to hear, "This is the way it is and we should accept it as being that way." Fisher suggests that this behavior serves "to avoid disrupting the developing social climate."[11]

Opinions about the decision are in the process of formulation, even in this first phase. For example, the member agreement above serves as a base for the future. Here any tentative agreements have an impact on what is to follow. Often these preliminary opinions change in the other phases to opinions favoring the decision proposal, as the process evolves with increasing intensity. Yet this agreement process is often hard to recognize during the first phase, when ideas are expressed ambiguously and voicing of agreement is in a tentative form.

The orientation phase, then, is centered around behavior that allows the group to get acquainted, clarify the task, and suggest tentative ideas and attitudes. People are testing the group to find out where they stand and how they will be received. They avoid assertive behavior that might lead to disagreements and conflict.

Members eventually come to understand the group and task. They have made up their minds by this second phase and now are willing to express their opinions more assertively. Here a favorable proposal is frequently followed by the expression of an unfavorable attitude. John might say, "I think the department's production is falling off because there are so many people sick." Mary might reply, "John, there is no evidence to support that. In fact, we've had people out before and kept production up. Remember . . ." Through this process the key decision proposals become evident. This phase is termed *conflict* because members feel free to enter into arguments with one another. Notice that Mary freely disagrees with John. They bring out evidence to support their positions and may even engage in debate with each other.

Polarization of attitudes can take place as a decision proposal emerges. So groups often find themselves divided into two coalitions—one favoring each side of the proposal. The opposition here is genuine. Those members who do not participate in the debate at this point are considered deviates. The normative behavior in this phase is "dissent, controversy, social conflict, and innovative deviance."[12]

Two events characterize the *emergence* phase: dissipation of conflict and argument, and a return to ambiguity of comments. We can expect more tentative language again. Words like "might," "perhaps," and "seems" begin to reappear. If you were counting the statements of dissent, of unfavorable opinions, you would find fewer than in the previous phase. Coalitions weaken as the statements that opposed the emergent decision become more ambiguous. You find less positive reinforcement of others' unfavorable attitudes. Perhaps John says to Mary, "I guess I can see your point. That's a good way to look at it." In addition, members expressing these ideas drop the presentation of the supporting evidence and reasoning that previously bolstered them.

There is a return of the ambiguity of the initial orientation phase, but it serves a different purpose here. Members are modifying their dissent. This represents a process of changing their stand on the issue. You can understand how unlikely it is that persons who have been in opposition will make an immediate about-face and favor the decision. Opposition is now expressed through ambiguity rather than direct opposition, but attitudes are being modified. As we observe more ambiguous comments from the coalition against, we will also see an increase of favorable opinions toward the decision proposal. The polarization of the conflict phase dissipates.

During the emergence phase many of the group members seemed to favor the decision, but consensus was not achieved. Consensus is achieved during this final, or *reinforcement*, phase. Evidence is still being offered in favor of the decision, but now it serves a different purpose. Here the evidence reinforces the decision that the group has made. John might say, "I see that Mary's idea is right. I remember some data we collected about a year ago that supports this interpretation."

Fisher says, "Members constantly and consistently express opinions favorable to the proposals and positively reinforce one another's favorable opinions with expressions of agreement and additional social support."[13] You might hear, "I'm so glad we were able to finish this today. I thought it would take two meetings. We really worked hard."

The dissent that characterized the conflict phase—and to some extent the emergence phase—is nearly nonexistent here. Very few negative attitudes toward the proposal are observed and almost no social conflict is present. This lack of conflict serves a function in the group—it reinforces the unity of opinion that has developed among the group members. There are other signs of this growing unity. The ambiguous comments of the emergence phase have lessened considerably. Tension is replaced by jovial, loud, boisterous, laughing behaviors. The group process in this phase has as its outcome the building of commitment to the group decision.

In summary, Aubrey Fisher has discovered that groups go through four phases in the process of making decisions. They orient themselves, engage in conflict, modify the opposition to allow the emergence of a decision, and finally reinforce the emerging decision in order to achieve consensus. Fisher attempted to observe this developmental process free from the social dimension of the group. The success of his attempt to divorce the social dimension is questionable. Some scholars believe that it is possible to divide considerations like that, but the social and task dimensions are so intimately related that complete separation is impossible.

Marshall Scott Poole   Sometimes we observe a group in which these traditional phase models don't fit. Marshall Scott Poole developed a model that explains what is happening when the traditional model doesn't fit. His model, a multiple sequence model, provides an explanation that will help you understand what is going on when this developmental process occurs.[14] The keys to understanding this exceptional case phenomenon are the concepts of activity tracks and breakpoints. Poole reasons that there are three basic activity tracks in groups: task-process activities, relational activities, and topic activities. These ideas should not be new to you, as we have introduced each of them before. Task-process activities have to do with the decision-making process. Relational activities focus on social processes. Topic activities are represented by different areas of content. Table 5.1 presents a classification for task and relational activities. Topic activities, of course, will depend on the issue being discussed.

When these activities develop together and at roughly the same speed, we have the recognizable phase development that was presented when we discussed Bales's and Fisher's ideas. In the orientation phase, a group may orient itself toward the decision-making process, and toward one another socially, discussing topics suitable to orienting. On the other hand, the group may get oriented toward the decision-making process and be ready to move on, but still work on issues of relational orientation. Thus the group

TABLE 5.1   Classifications for Task-Process and Relational Activities

Task-Process Activities	*Relational Activities*
Problem Activity: 1. Problem analysis	*Work-Focused Relationships:* 1. Focused work (no criticism; extended idea development and analysis) 2. Critical work (idea development through criticism and repartee)
Executive Activity 2a. Orientation 2b. Reflection on process	
Solution Activity: 3a. Establishment of solution guidelines 3b. Solution design 3c. Solution evaluation 3d. Solution confirmation and selection	*Conflict:* 3a. Opposition 3b. Resolution-accommodation 3c. Resolution-avoidance/smoothing 3d. Resolution-integration (bargaining/ consensus building/problem solving)
	Integration: 4. Integration
	Ambiguous Relationships: 5. Expression of ambiguity

Source: Marshall Scott Poole, "Decision Development in Small Groups, III: A Multiple Sequence Model of Group Decision Development," *Communication Monographs* 50 (1983):327. Reprinted by permission of the Speech Communication Association.

may move on to the conflict phase with respect to the decision-making process, but still be in the orientation phase relationally.

Group activities are divided by breakpoints. These represent transitions in the development process. When a breakpoint interrupts all three activity tracks at the same time, the group is following traditional phase development. Poole identifies three types of breakpoints. The *normal breakpoint,* the most common, occurs when a group moves from one topic to the next or from one activity to the next or to plan a task. The *delay* is a breakpoint that occurs when a group doubles back to repeat the same analysis or activity. The group is in a holding pattern until it moves to its next activity. The final breakpoint, the *disruption,* can be of two types. One type has its roots in *major disagreement* or *conflict.* The issue is such that it requires the group to redirect its activity toward the conflict and maybe even reorient itself. The other type of disagreement has its root in *group failure.* Here the group discovers that its effort is not going to be sufficient to meet the task goals. This too requires that the group analyze the problem and take some corrective action.

Fitting Together the Models of Group Development

The Bales model of development helps us understand the formation process in a group. Members must probably feel a need to "know" whom they are working with before they will be able to achieve maximum productivity. So a newly formed group will spend some time working on relationships before it moves to a phase when task issues predominate. If the group is ongoing, it will likely return to issues of relationship at the beginning of each meeting.

Fisher's research provides conclusions about how a general pattern of decision making develops. This pattern will repeat itself each time the group moves to a new topic of deliberation. So we might expect to see a series of spirals, each spiral representing the group approaching a new topic. Here is a summary of the important conclusions from Fisher's research:

1. Most groups go through some kind of orientation. They need time to discover who is in the group and what the group is all about.

2. Next, groups generally experience conflict. The intensity of the conflict may vary with the task, but differences in members come out. This conflict may involve ideas, personal relationships, and/or authority and influence among members.

3. Successful groups solve their differences and manage the conflict. They move to a period in which polarization and argument begin to diminish. Roles and norms seem to stabilize during this period. Unsuccessful groups eventually dissolve.

4. Groups that are successful enter a more productive period. The portion of their energy that has been devoted to group concerns can now be focused on the task.

5. Finally, groups go through some kind of leave-taking stage. This may be particularly evident in long-term groups, but probably takes place in most groups. Often successful groups feel good about their effort and take time to congratulate one another.

Marshall Scott Poole presents a refinement of these ideas to account for the circumstance when the activities in a group are not in synchrony. When this happens, he suggests that group development can be looked at through its three major activities: task process, relationships, and topics. In this case, movement from activity to activity within a track is defined by breakpoints.

Encouraging Group Development: Application of Task-Group Development Theory

Imagine yourself faced with a group experience and armed with this information about how decisions emerge. What will you do with the information? What kind of applications can you make? There are important applications, so take time to read carefully how you might use the information.

Consider that researchers from different backgrounds have discovered the same phases in task groups.[15] They used different terminology, but an analysis of their conclusions led us to the four steps.

These broad phases seem to develop naturally in many groups, although the specific content of each phase may differ somewhat from group to group. No one took these groups aside and taught them to move through these phases. The phases are functional because most groups seem to sense particular needs at different times in their group process and behave in ways to fulfill them. Thus it seems reasonable to assume that these communication behaviors are in part serving some important function for the group.

What if you do not observe these phases in your group? The breakpoints for different group activities may not be aligned. The phases may be moving at different rates for different group activities. But perhaps a phase has been skipped altogether. You might ask if the need for going through a phase is present. For example, do the members of your group know one another so well and understand the problem so well that they do not need to go through an orientation phase? If your answer is yes, then your group has probably been able to skip this phase. If the answer is no, you may need to exert some leadership. You might say, "I'd like to go back for a minute and make sure I understand our task. Let me try to say what I think we are trying to do."

But why do groups skip phases if they actually perform important functions? Two answers to this question are frequently mentioned. First, some appointed leaders guide their groups away from these functions. For example, the manager who led a task force to investigate absenteeism at a shipbuilding company began by saying, "What should we do about our attendance problem?" Through this question this leader bypassed the orientation phase. Instead the leader might have recognized the need for orientation. He might have said, "Let's focus on the problem for a minute. Could someone describe it in his own words?" Second, some group members assume that others in the group are sharing their understanding of the task and are as familiar with the task as they are. These people, too, may urge the group to bypass certain phases.

The problem for you is to decide if a real need is being ignored if your group bypasses a phase. But consider the possible outcomes of bypassing each of the four phases.

Phase 1   The orientation phase allows members to understand the task and one another's frame of reference. If a group skips this stage, it may move directly to conflict. The intensity of the conflict may be increased by the fact that members do not understand one another or the positions of members on the issue. Here are some key suggestions and/or questions the leader might pose to help a group in this stage:

> Introduce one another.
>
> Ask members to tell how they are associated with the project and their experience with it.
>
> Ask someone to verbalize the task.
>
> Make sure members understand the task.

Phase 2   The conflict stage serves the function of testing ideas on the road to the emergence of consensus. When a group skips this step, it may not have looked critically at the issues. This may produce an inferior decision because of superficial discussion. Here are some suggestions for helping a group through its conflict stage:

> Conflict is generally useful, so be patient in dealing with it.
>
> Clarify members' positions.
>
> Pose a middle ground.
>
> Pose alternatives that might be acceptable.
>
> Compliment members who are managing their conflict well.

Phase 3   The emergence phase serves the purpose of producing a decision, healing the wounds of conflict, and generating consensus. Some members may not be able to accept the decision if the group does not emerge from the conflict stage. Relationships may be damaged and polarization may remain if emergence does not take place. Here are some things you can do to help your group:

> Compliment the group on its progress.
>
> Verbalize consensus when you hear it.
>
> Compliment members on their ability to work through their disagreements.

Phase 4   The reinforcement phase calls attention to the good work a group has done and generates satisfaction for the group. Omission of this phase has implications for carrying out decisions. When the group must either advocate a solution to someone in authority for it to be carried out, or when members must do so themselves, omission of this step may cause them to have less commitment and vigor. The leader and members of a group might reinforce the group's decision by:

Complimenting the group on its effort.

Visualizing the implications of the decision.

Decision-emergence phase theory can help you anticipate what might happen next in your group. Sometimes members try to resist the conflict phase, for instance. They seem to believe that there is something wrong with their group if conflict arises. Decision-emergence theory alerts us to expect this; it tells us that groups naturally experience conflict and work through it. Thus if you understand phase theory and the fact that phases serve functions, you will realize that conflict serves an important and productive function for your group.

Understanding phase theory can help you to discover that your group has become stalled. We all have had experiences with groups being stuck in a particular phase. Often groups find themselves bogged down in the conflict stage. If you have experienced this problem, you will want to move your group out of conflict when possible. You will find some of the techniques presented in Chapter 10, "Managing Conflict in the Group," helpful in this effort.

Since groups do move through decision-emergence phases, it is important for you to know what these are. You can facilitate your group's development if you are able to identify the phases. You can (1) discover if your group has skipped a phase, (2) anticipate the group's movement through the phases, and (3) know when your group has become stalled in a phase. Discovering, anticipating, and knowing these things can allow you to provide the leadership necessary to facilitate group development and evolution.

Also, keep in mind that for some groups these phases are cyclic. Long-term groups that take on new members and new problems will recycle back to the orientation phase as they encounter these changes. If you are a member of a long-term decision-making group, you should expect such behavior. This expectation will help you to understand your group better.

But how can we identify a group that might not conform to the traditional phase model? Poole suggests that "there will be even, coordinated development among the three activity types for groups with (1) high consensus, (2) mutual or dominant involvement types, and (3) low- to intermediate-difficulty tasks.[16] A *high-consensus* group is one whose members have little difficulty agreeing with one another. A group whose members are *mutually involved* is one in which members are more or less equal relationally, even though differences may exist in the actual status of members. On the other hand, a group that is characterized by *dominant involvement* is one in which one or more members dominate and the other members depend on them for leadership, evaluation, and morale. In other words, the dominance pattern is "okay" with those being dominated.

Low to intermediate task difficulty results when a group's goal is relatively clear, the relationship between the causes and solutions to the problem is relatively clear, and the coordination of the group's activities is relatively uncomplicated.

Once you identify where the traditional phase pattern does not apply, you can follow through the developmental process by separating the three activity areas and then identifying breakpoints in each. Then analyze the development by asking yourself if the important functions of each phase are being performed within each of the activity areas. For example, can you identify the breakpoints that divide the three activity areas into phases? If you cannot do this, then probably one or more of the phases have been omitted from the activity area. Does the omission of a phase have an impact on the group? For example, if the orientation phase has been omitted from the relational activity track, what impact does that have? This is the kind of analysis you can do using Poole's model.

Social Tension

Social tension is the uneasiness that group members feel when they are uncertain about members' relationships. It is a factor in groups that exhibit a phaselike pattern. This kind of tension can be graphed in relation to time and a threshold of tolerance. That is, if we could measure the amount of tension being generated in a group as it meets over time, we might characterize this flow as graphically pictured in Figure 5.1. Notice that a tension level is represented by the dashed line. This line is labeled "threshold of tolerance" because tension levels above it cause the group discomfort. If the level remains too high too long, the group's productivity can suffer. Ernest G. Borman[17] distinguished between two types of social tension: primary and secondary. The difference between these two is one of source rather than level of tension.

Primary tension is a normal occurrence when people come together to work with one another for the first time. You experience it often on the first day of class because you are not acquainted with the professor and class members. Freshmen are often assigned roommates whom they do not know. The initial meeting is generally filled with primary tension. These meetings are usually characterized by long periods of silence, discussion of light topics, and tentative statements. Groups, too, experience these social inhibitions. Meeting for the first time—the fact that there is no history—means that members will not have generated expectations about how they will be received and how they are expected to act. Ongoing groups that do not meet for an extended time may even reexperience this primary tension when they gather for a meeting.

Primary tension in groups is evidenced by a particular kind of interaction. Members are usually very polite and, therefore, the intensity of the talk is very low. Sighing and yawning might be observed, as if members are bored or tired. People often speak softly and try not to offend one another. Frequently you will notice long pauses as members seem not to know what to say to one another.

Primary tension is nothing to be overly anxious about. It cannot be avoided. Just be aware that people who meet for the first time will not be as productive as they might be until they discover who is in the group and what they are like. You can also give

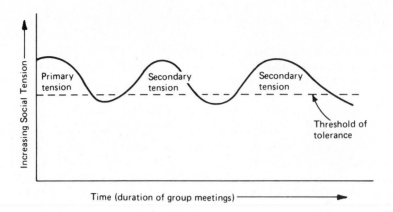

Display of Primary and Secondary Tension in a Hypothetical Group

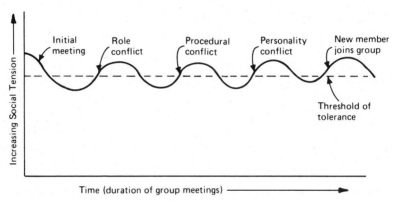

FIGURE 5.1
Phaselike Structure of Social Tension

each person a warm, friendly welcome. Beyond this, primary tension is often broken when someone in the group is able to introduce some humor. Perhaps you can do this. Then people will begin to laugh and perhaps feel more at ease.

Secondary tension is something to be expected in a group also. It is different from primary tension in that it occurs later in the meeting. It is related to topics different from getting acquainted. Members are often struggling to discover what roles they will play, to define their status in the group, to secure esteem and rewards. They may experience conflict over perceptions and personalities. These differences produce tension. Consider that groups are likely to have members who have very different ideas about goals, what is important and valuable, what solution might fit the problem, who should fulfill what role in the group, and doing one's part and being absent or tardy. You can undoubtedly add several more situations you have personally experienced when your groups have experienced differences. So the potential is present for significant tension in groups. Thus secondary tension is a serious problem for most groups. Figure 5.1 illustrates social tension in a group.

Frequently secondary tension is marked by a departure from the group's normal routine. There may be an outburst from some member. Often the interchanges are antagonistic and hostile. Thus secondary tension is marked by loudness. Two or more members may even try to talk at the same time—gone is the politeness that marks primary tension. Generally the group's interaction is monopolized by two or three members talking while others observe. Long pauses may be evident as members who are arguing try to gather their thoughts. Extreme secondary tension is unpleasant for the group and may even damage the group if it is not brought under control. Every group must develop means for dealing with secondary tension. Some general ideas about addressing this situation are suggested in the next section, which pursues the issue of encouraging group development.

Encouraging Group Development: Application of Social Tension Theory

You can make use of the ideas we have presented by providing leadership as needed. Suppose you expect primary tension in your group because it has not met for quite some time. You can allow some time for the group to get reacquainted. You may assure people that it is important to understand one another and the task before you move ahead to suggestions. This kind of assurance and reassurance can be helpful to the group. Recall that we said that primary tension is often broken by the introduction of humor. You may also be able to do this for the group.

The idea of managing social tension presents some problems. One of the difficulties you will face is knowing when there is too much tension. Healthy groups experience a level of tension that is within their range of tolerance. This keeps them alert, helps hold them together, and keeps them active. Healthy groups also experience tension that is above their tolerance level. This tension can overpower the group's task effort and depress its productivity. These groups reduce tension and then move on with the task. But how do we know how much tension is too much? Though many groups function with fairly high tension levels, it is impossible to make any definitive statement. Too much tension can be measured by a group's inability to function in the task area and to maintain a satisfying social climate. There is no absolute that can be applied to all groups equally.

Another problem in managing social tension is related to reduction techniques. What works for one group may be absolutely unsuccessful for another. Group members must monitor the situation and make decisions and take actions to manage it. Keep this in mind as some of the methods found successful for managing tension are discussed.

One role that develops in groups to manage social tension is that of the *tension releaser*. Often this is a person or persons who can make light of the situation. Phil Johnson, a member of a management group at a bank, was good at this. One day, when two people who were locked in an argument finally agreed, he joked, "Wow! I'm so glad you guys settled that. I was about to break out the squirt guns so you could have at it." Sometimes, however, this kind of carefree joking behavior can be quite unsuccessful in groups that are addressing certain kinds of problems. For example, persons experiencing a personality conflict may not find it easy to laugh at themselves or the situation. They are likely to resent the person and intervention of this type. Likewise, a serious dispute over the leadership role may not be appropriately met with humor. Members may find a person insensitive if he or she tries to approach this tension with humor.

An alternative to humor is *mediation*. This often works better than humor when members are experiencing some form of interpersonal conflict. A person who is respected by both parties can often provide leadership here. This intervention may take place either within or outside the group's regular meeting. The manager of a sales force for an office supply company resolved a disagreement over sales technique this way. "Joe, Jean, I see that you both are really involved in this issue—and I can tell you are dead serious about it. Maybe I can help. Would you consider this different position?" The techniques that might be used in this case are many. This topic is of such importance that it requires a detailed and careful treatment. Thus Chapter 10 has been devoted to the issue of conflict management. We will not take the space to repeat ourselves here.

Another successful tension-relieving technique is *scapegoating*. Sometimes this may produce negative results, but groups frequently use it to relieve tension. Most often the scapegoat is an outsider. In the world of work it is often a boss; in the classroom situation it is generally the instructor. These groups blame the person for their frustration and may even take that person on as the "enemy." A group of men found their funds for social activities depleted. Instead of placing the blame on themselves, the president released the tension related to the situation through a long speech about dues they had to pay to "national." This may be rather unpleasant for the scapegoat and thus can backfire and produce negative results.

Finally, a most successful technique for reducing tension is *confronting* it directly. This is probably the most difficult solution for groups. Most of us do not like the painful period of confrontation, but the outcome is often worth the effort. When a problem is such that it needs direct confrontation, it is generally too important to be ignored. One such real-life experience may convince you of the value of this type of confrontation.

A large paper-manufacturing firm holds an annual weekend retreat for its mid-level managers. Their leader poses management problems and the group is responsible for addressing them in a discussion format. During a recent retreat, a manager, Sue, produced considerable tension by always addressing the discussion first and by rattling off a solution from a management course she was taking at the local university. This was unnerving to other members of the group, and because of her rapid-fire delivery they were unable to understand most of what she was trying to say. She also usurped their opportunities to talk and make contributions. In addition, she would interrupt everybody, including the instructor. On the second day of the retreat, two of the class members decided to confront her.

> DON: Sue, we have been talking about this retreat and we want to talk with you about something.

SUE: What do you mean?

DON: We feel like we are not getting as much out of the retreat as we should. I feel this way and others say so, too. Usually, when John Smith throws out a discussion question you answer it immediately. But you not only answer it, you rattle off all the solutions from your class—and so fast.

SALLY: I agree. I feel like I'm not getting what I came for. I don't get a chance to talk.

DON: We appreciate that you have done your homework. And you certainly deserve a chance to talk. But we'd like to have our own chance, too.

Nearly every member had something to say. They did so in a direct but supportive manner. The result was a complete about-face. With the leader's help, the group was able to state specific behaviors that the problem member could change. She was willing and able to do so.

Confrontation will not always have such a positive effect. But avoiding problems does not mean they will go away. Usually they will remain, and their presence will cause destructive levels of tension. Keep in mind that the important thing for a group to do is to confront the problem overtly and as supportively as possible.

In summary, Bormann suggests that primary tension is related to the acquaintance process. Secondary tension results from perceptual problems, procedural disagreements, role development, and personality differences. Some methods for dealing with this conflict are humor, mediation, scapegoating, and confronting. Successful groups experience tension and manage it when it moves beyond their tolerance level.

Idea Development

Thomas M. Scheidel and Laura Crowell[18] found that idea development does not conform to a straight line. Instead, groups seem to develop a spiral of *anchoring* and *reach-testing* behaviors. We will address these ideas shortly. But first consider the underlying basis for this work.

Scheidel and Crowell attempted to describe idea development in terms of communication patterns rather than in terms of the task and social dimensions. Thus their work was limited to one aspect of group development—idea development—and does not give the broad picture as do the ideas we discussed with you above.

Scheidel and Crowell studied five trained discussion groups that carried out two-hour discussions in which the task was to evaluate a local newspaper. They tape-recorded the discussion and then evaluated the content for type of contribution. These investigators were interested in the amount of initiation, extension, modification, synthesis, confirmation, clarifying, or substantiation of ideas.

All of these behaviors can be seen in the development of an idea. Follow, for example, the development of this idea in a city council meeting:

INITIATION: "We ought to have an ordinance that will regulate businesses that come to town to sell their goods on a transient basis."

EXTENSION: "Yes. And the ordinance should cover door-to-door salespeople and those that rent temporary space."

MODIFICATION: "But it should be limited to people who come to town and sell. Not the kids who are selling for clubs or the farmer setting up a roadside stand."

SYNTHESIS: "So we ought to have an ordinance that regulates businesses that set up temporary sales locations but not temporary business by local people."

CONFIRMATION: "Yes. That is what we need."

CLARIFICATION: "I want to make sure I got this straight. You mean those people who come to town and set up in motels and the traveling salesperson. I know these people. They can be real rip-offs."

SUBSTANTIATION: "Yes. Last year we had seventy-five complaints to the chamber of commerce about inferior merchandise they sold. And they were no longer here to answer questions about the things they sold."

Scheidel and Crowell were also concerned about how people tested ideas. Assume for a moment that you are Tom Scheidel or Laura Crowell. What kind of pattern would you expect to discover in a decision-making discussion group? Start with your own experience. Does somebody introduce an idea that is then discussed and tested by the group? Does a member voice disagreement that then causes the group to test and modify the idea? Does the group spend considerable time refining an idea before it goes on to the next? Would you expect some sort of linking behavior—like the speaker who creates a transition to link ideas to one another? What comes next will be more meaningful to you if you stop here and try to answer these questions. Take your pencil and jot the answers, yes or no, in the margin if you like. Now read on.

If you are operating on the assumption that ideas in decision-making groups develop in a step-by-step line, then you may have answered yes to most of these questions. Scheidel and Crowell assumed that a linear model would include a sequence that looks something like Figure 5.2. This chain of events would reoccur for each decision made by a group.

However, a typical sequence of response did not follow this linear pattern. In fact, these kinds of statements accounted for only about 22 percent of the total comments. Further, most of the comments with respect to what others said were quite positive. A fourth of the comments were statements of agreement. Another fourth of the contributions

Initiation - - - - ► Extension - - - - ► Modification - - - - ► Synthesis

FIGURE 5.2
A Linear Model of Idea Development

were devoted to rephrasing (clarifying) and providing evidence to support (substantiating). Not much extension, modification, or synthesis was observed at all.

Scheidel and Crowell observed what they called a reach-test cycle. This pattern involved (1) the suggestion of an idea, (2) agreement by others, (3) presentation of examples to clarify the idea, and (4) affirmation that the information confirms the original assertion. Consider an interaction from a sorority meeting that illustrates this pattern. The group is considering what to do for a spring event:

1. "Let's make our spring social a beach party."

2. "That sounds like a good idea."
   "Yes. I think so, too."
   "Let's do it."

3. "We could go early—say nine a.m. Spend some time on the beach. Then go to a few of the entertainment spots while it's hot. Then back to the beach by three."

4. "Yes. Good idea."

This reach-test motion of the group is sometimes followed by a member negatively criticizing the idea. Scheidel and Crowell found, as pointed out above, that disagreement was rare. But when it happened it almost never took place immediately after the new idea was suggested. This decision point then serves as an anchor point of agreement. If the new idea has been rejected, then the group moves back to its previous anchor point. If the reach-tested idea is approved, a new anchor point is established. Then a new preliminary idea is presented for the group to reach-test. This process looks like the illustration in Figure 5.3. Notice that the process is not represented as linear at all. It involves cumulative and progressive movement in which the group introduces, confirms, clarifies, and substantiates ideas. When ideas are rejected, the group backtracks to the agreed-upon position and reconfirms its decision.[19]

This spiral pattern is the likely explanation for what many have thought to be an inefficiency of group decision-making process. The linear model assumes not much backtracking—obviously a straight line is the shortest distance between two points. Thus those who observe groups and discover that they are not moving in a straight line label groups as inefficient. It is not appropriate to describe the spiral movement as

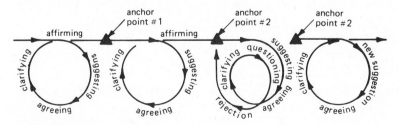

FIGURE 5.3
The Spiral Model of Idea Development

inefficient. Efficiency is related to more than doing a job quickly. For example, you would be unlikely to call a mechanic efficient who fixed your car quickly, but didn't do it carefully and correctly. If the spiral motion serves a purpose—suppose, for example, it helps the group to develop more commitment to its decision—then it may be the most efficient way to achieve a desirable end. It is quite possible that the spiraling has this effect, as much of it is devoted to voiced agreement. This type of agreement is especially necessary when it is important to achieve acceptance of a decision by most or all of the group's members.

Data that support this interpretation of the reach-test process were provided by a follow-up study on feedback in group decision making. Scheidel and Crowell[20] focused on the occurrence of feedback loops of the reach-test variety—an interaction pattern in which one person initiated a comment that was responded to by another person and then was reacted to by the initiator. Thirty-five percent of the interaction consisted of these patterns. It is amazing that there were so many of these special kinds of feedback loops. The most frequently observed feedback response was the statement of agreement (34 percent). An agreement-type feedback consists of a receiver making a comment to the source of the idea that shows agreement or asks for further clarification. The loop is completed by the source speaking again. Thus what we observe from the receiver is a reinforcing comment. This response seems to be encouraging to the original speaker, as he or she often speaks again.

A speaker in a service group might say, "I think our spring project should be to raise money to buy camping gear for the boys' home." Another member might respond, "That's a wonderful idea. We ought to do that." The first speaker would then continue, "We could sell doughnuts at the shopping mall on a couple of Saturday mornings." Thus the anchoring and reach-testing processes seem to serve the purpose of encouraging the group members and developing the acceptance necessary for commitment to the outcome of the group's task.

But what happens to ideas that are not reinforced? Suppose a person disagrees or presents negative modification of the idea. Dennis S. Gouran and John E. Baird, Jr.,[21] observed that group members have a tendency to change the subject shortly after the topic draws disagreement. Groups move to a new topic two to four comments later. So groups that do not find that they have an anchor of agreement drop the idea and pick up a new reach-test cycle in search of agreement.

Encouraging Group Development: Application of the Spiral Model of Idea Development

The spiral model seems to account for the apparent inefficiency of groups. This spiral movement may seem to be inefficient, but it seems to perform an important function for the group. Knowing that this type of movement is normal may help you to be more patient with your group. Remember that it is the process by which groups build consensus and commitment to their decisions.

This reach-test model may also suggest to us that there is a natural tendency in groups to avoid conflict. Recall that a fourth of the comments about others' ideas were statements of agreement. Another fourth were remarks that either clarified or substantiated. Only very rarely did a member disagree with an idea. This seems to suggest a need for members to foster an attitude that conflict is useful and can be handled in a manner that is supportive of members and the group. Members may need to make a special effort to analyze one another's ideas critically.

SUMMARY

Understanding the reasons members have for being part of a particular group is important. People belong to groups because of (1) interpersonal attraction, (2) attraction to the group's activities, (3) attraction to the group's goals, (4) valuing group affiliation, and (5) fulfillment of needs outside the group. Attraction is related to pleasing physical characteristics, similarity in attitude, belief, personality, race, and economic status, as well as to perceived ability of the other person. The reasons people belong to groups are related to needs that can be reinforced in order to develop commitment to the group and its goals.

Groups, like people, move through phases. Evidence was presented from three researchers, Robert F. Bales, B. Aubrey Fisher and Marshall Scott Poole. Their work suggests that groups move through four stages as they undertake their task: (1) orientation, (2) conflict, (3) emergence, and (4) reinforcement. Poole suggested three activity areas—task, relationship, and topic. Each may follow this phase cycle at different paces. We pointed out that these phases seem to serve certain needs and that when they are skipped, problems may result. The orientation phase allows members to understand the task and one another. The conflict stage serves the function of testing ideas on the way to emergence of consensus. The emergence phase serves to produce a decision, heal the wounds of conflict, and generate consensus. The reinforcement phase helps members to believe that they have done good work and generates satisfaction and commitment. The ability to identify these phases will allow a person to discover if the group has skipped a phase, anticipate the group's movement through the phase, and know if the group has become stalled in a phase.

Social tension in groups is both beneficial and harmful. A group needs a certain amount of tension to help hold it together and keep it active. Too much tension can be more than a group is able to tolerate and may destroy the group. Tensions experienced as a group is forming are called primary tensions. These are due to uneasiness among the members and uncertainty about the task. Other tensions develop as the group is working out roles and norms. These might be over leadership, and perceptions about procedure, personalities, and values. This tension level exhibits a phaselike structure in the healthy group. Groups manage tension through tension releasers, mediation, scapegoating, and direct confrontation. The important thing is that groups manage tension so as to keep it at a level that allows them to be productive.

Idea development is thought to follow a spiral structure. This pattern of development was first described by Thomas M. Scheidel and Laura Crowell. A reach-test cycle consists of four parts: the suggestion of an idea, agreement to the idea by others, presentation of examples to clarify the idea, and affirmation that the information confirms the original assertion. Groups move from an anchor point, a point of decision, to the next idea. Rejection of the idea means that the group moves back to its last anchor point and suggests a new idea to be reach-tested. This confirming pattern represented by the four-part cycle probably serves to reinforce the group's commitment to its decision. Leaders should realize that this function is taking place and not be unduly concerned about the apparent inefficiency it creates.

EXERCISES

1. Describe and analyze the development of your group. Also, describe and analyze the forces that attract you to and repel you from the individual group members and the group as a whole.

2. Consider why you joined at least three groups of which you are now a member. List the reasons you found each group attractive. How do these compare with the reasons for joining groups that were presented in this chapter? What motivational problems might have been generated by your reasons for joining the groups? Now compare one of these experiences with the experience you had when you considered joining a group but did not do so. What factors caused you to feel unattracted to this group? What might have been done to increase your attraction for this group? Write a three-page paper that compares and contrasts your personal experience with attraction and repulsion. Or, with the members of a small group, compile a list of factors that promote attraction and foster repulsion for a potential member of a group.

3. How often do group goals and individual goals match? Consider your experience with this issue. Make at least a page of notes that answer the following questions for you: What group stands out as one in which your goals and its goals were the most alike? What group stands out as one in which your goals and its goals were most different? Describe your attraction to each of these groups. Describe your participation in each of these groups. How did it differ in each group? Bring your worksheet to class and compare your answers with answers of the members of a small group. Is your experience like theirs? Is there a typical experience? What motivational factors are presented to the group when individual and group goals differ? What can be done when this happens?

4. Consider this question as a class. If you could pick members for a decision-making group, what characteristics would you want in order to create an ideal group? Give reasons for your choices. Try to construct an ideal five-member group.

5. Obtain an audio tape of a fifteen-minute discussion conducted by a group whose members are meeting for the first time, and without an appointed leader. In a small group, analyze the interaction. See if you can identify phases through which the group passed. Did the group follow the phases that Fisher suggests decision-making groups go through? If not, why do you think they did not follow the phase theory? If not, did the fact that the group skipped a phase, or perhaps moved through phases in a different order than Fisher suggested, make any difference in how the group did at decision making? Now identify at least two sequential decisions, one following the other. Did these decisions evolve as Scheidel and Crowell suggest they do? If not, how did they evolve, and how do you account for the difference between the way they evolved and the way Scheidel and Crowell suggested decisions evolve?

6. Analyze one of your group meetings for primary and secondary tension. At the end of an in-class group meeting, your instructor may allow time for you to address these questions: Was there any primary tension in your group? If so, describe the outward signs of the tension. How was the tension broken? If not, speculate as to why there was no apparent primary tension. Now see if you can identify at least two instances of secondary tension. What was the source of this tension? How did this tension manifest itself in group behaviors? How was the tension released? What are some other ways a group might deal with secondary tension? Suppose the tension was not released. Speculate as to how this might affect your group.

NOTES

1. Theodore M. Newcomb, *The Acquaintance Process* (New York: Holt, 1961).

2. D. Byrne, W. Griffitt, and D. Stefaniak, "Attraction and Similarity of Personality Character-istics," *Journal of Personality and Social Psychology* 5 (1967):82–90.

3. D. Byrne, J. L. Clore, Jr., and P. Worchel, "Effect of Economic Similarity-Dissimilarity on Interpersonal Attraction," *Journal of Personality and Social Psychology* 4 (1966):220–224.

4. Marvin E. Shaw, "Changes in Sociometric Choices Following Forced Integration of an Elementary School," *Journal of Social Issues* 29 (1973):143–158.

5. Marvin E. Shaw and J. C. Gilchrist, "Repetitive Task Failure and Sociometric Choice," *Journal of Abnormal and Social Psychology* 50 (1955):29–32.

6. M. Sherif and C. W. Sherif, *Groups in Harmony and Tension* (New York: Harper & Row, 1953).

7. Ibid.

8. Marshall Scott Poole, "Decision Development in Small Groups I: A Comparison of Two Models," *Communication Monographs* 50 (1981):20. Poole argues also that certain factors like conflict may interrupt the logically ideal format.

9. Robert F. Bales, *Interaction Process Analysis* (Reading, Mass.: Addison-Wesley, 1950).

10. B. Aubrey Fisher, "Decision Emergence: Phases in Group Decision Making," *Speech Monographs* 37 (1970):53–66.

11. B. Aubrey Fisher, *Small Group Decision Making*, 2d ed. (New York: McGraw-Hill, 1980), 145.

12. Ibid., 147.

13. Ibid., 149.

14. Marshall Scott Poole, "Decision Development in Small Groups, III: A Multiple Sequence Model of Group Decision Development," *Communication Monographs* 50 (1983):321–341.

15. Two research reports support the notion that there are recognizable phases in groups. See R. B. Caple, "The Sequential Stages of Group Development," *Small Group Behavior* 9 (1978):470–476; M. A. Bell, "Phases in Group Problem Solving," *Small Group Behavior* 13 (1982):475–495.

16. Poole, 339.

17. Ernest G. Bormann, *Discussion and Group Methods: Theory and Practice*, 2d ed. (New York: Harper & Row, 1975), 181–182.

18. Thomas M. Scheidel and Laura Crowell, "Idea Development in Small Group Discussion," *Quarterly Journal of Speech* 50 (1964):140–145.

19. Randy Hirokawa found that the need to cycle back to further investigate was a characteristic of effective groups. That is, a member will decide that some detail has been ignored and cause the group to cycle back for further exploration. See Randy Y. Hirokawa, "Why Informed Groups Make Faulty Decisions," *Small Group Behavior* 18 (1987):3–29.

20. Thomas M. Scheidel and Laura Crowell, "Feedback in Small Group Communication," *Quarterly Journal of Speech* 52 (1966):273–278.

21. Dennis S. Gouran and John E. Baird, Jr., "An Analysis of Distributional and Sequential Structure in Problem-Solving and Informal Group Discussion," *Speech Monographs* 39 (1972):16–22.

RECOMMENDED READINGS

B. Aubrey Fisher, "Decision Emergence: Phases in Group Decision Making," *Speech Monographs* 39 (1972):53–66.

Randy Y. Hirokawa, "Group Communication and Problem-Solving Effectiveness" *Human Communication Research* 9 (1983):291–305.

Marshall Scott Poole, "Decision Development in Small Groups III: A Multiple Sequence Model of Group Development," *Communication Monographs* 50 (1983):321–341.

Susan B. Shimanoff, "Group Interaction via Communication Rules," in Robert S. Cathcart and Larry A. Samovar, eds. *Small Group Communication: A Reader*, 5th ed. (Dubuque, Iowa: Wm. C. Brown, 1988).

CHAPTER 6

Roles and Role Emergence

OBJECTIVES

After reading this chapter you should be able to:

Explain the concept of role as it relates to participation in small groups.

Identify what is meant by role stability, including its impact on the functioning of a small group.

Differentiate between formal and informal roles.

Describe a model of role emergence that includes the concept of group reinforcement.

Suggest what is meant by role conflict, and speculate about some typical outcomes of this type of conflict.

List and describe the roles that fall under each of these categories: group task roles, group maintenance roles, and self-centered roles.

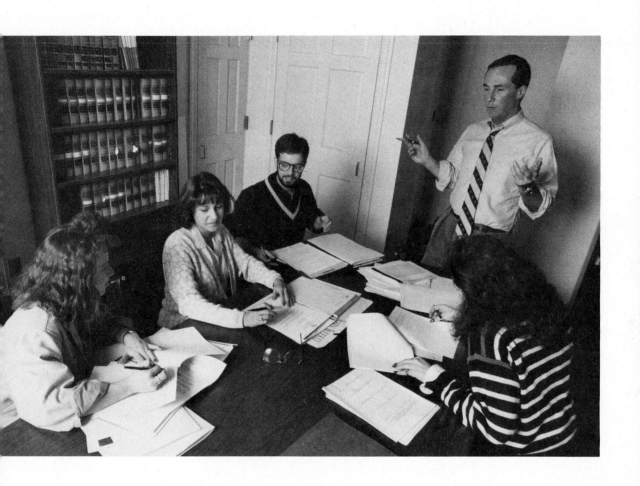

The program committee for the Parent Teacher Association met to plan activities for its six meetings for the year. The committee had five members, including the president and secretary of the organization. The group had spent a little time just chatting and getting acquainted when Dan McDonald, the program committee chair, interrupted.

DAN: I think we are all here and have had time to say hello. Let's get started. We will have six meetings this year. Five of them will include a program we plan; one will be a program put on by the students in the school. What ideas do you have for our programs?

GROUP: (Silence.)

MIKE: (Finally, after a short silence.) I've been having trouble dealing with my son's behavior. How about someone to talk about managing behavior problems?

DAN: Okay. Let's put that one down as a possibility. What's another idea?

GROUP: (More silence, with Judy finally speaking.)

JUDY: I think that handling homework is worth some good advice from an expert. Homework time at my house is awful. I'll bet others think that's a problem. How about you, George?

GEORGE: Well, Judy, I haven't noticed much difficulty with homework at my house. My children generally finish their homework by the time I get home from work. But if it's a problem for you, let's get someone to come and give advice.

ELIZABETH: Homework is certainly a problem, but I'm more concerned with all the trash on television. I'm worried about the violence and sex that my kids are exposed to on TV. I try to keep them from watching that stuff, but somehow when I'm not close by they tune it in. I'd like to have someone come and talk about this problem.

ROBERT: I'd like to backtrack on all of this, Dan, if I may. I think these are interesting ideas. But I think we need to understand more about what we're trying to accomplish in our programs. I'd like to have us talk about what programs were offered last year and how they were received, and then get back to suggesting ideas.

DAN: We could do that. What do others think about starting again?

GROUP: (Silence.)

DAN: Mary, do you have a suggestion about what we should do?

Think for a moment about the people in this short interaction among members of the PTA program committee. You probably formed ideas in your head about each of these group members. Your vision of these people would probably allow you to make predictions about their behavior in the future. The set of behaviors exhibited by each member is the beginning of a role definition for that person. Role is a concept that is central to understanding small group interaction. Role determines the structure of a group and its outcomes. The roles that are developing in this program committee may allow it to plan a year of exciting programs. On the other hand, the roles may lead to extended conflict, lack of agreement, and programs that will not serve the organization well. Role development may or may not allow the group to achieve its full potential.

We begin our discussion of role by explaining the concept. Next we suggest a model of how the roles in a group develop over time. This will lead us to two ideas related to the developmental process: role conflict and role strain. We will suggest how a group might address these role difficulties. Finally, we will present a scheme for thinking about roles as task roles, maintenance roles, or self-centered roles.

THE CONCEPT OF ROLE

Your first contact with the word *role* was probably in connection with an actor who assumed the role of a certain character in a play. You also assume certain roles in everyday life. You are a student, a daughter or son, a friend. Perhaps you are a worker within an organization. You learn how to play these roles through interaction with others. American culture tells us what roles ought to be.

In a sense, a small group is a culture. It, too, has a set of roles that reflect its members' views of the group's needs and the preferences of its individual members. A *role* is the set of behaviors displayed by an individual in relation to the expectations of the rest of the group members. A role is something that evolves out of the trial-and-error process—the members of a group teaching individuals which behaviors are appropriate and which are not by rewarding and punishing trials. If the individual cares about his or her membership in the group, then to that extent the group has power to mold the individual's role. Group members can reinforce certain behaviors and extinguish others, and by this process bring an individual into line with what the group needs or wishes from him or her. Sometimes a particular set of behaviors follows a pattern that can be described by a single term. *Leader* is an example of a term used to describe a particular set of related behaviors. These related behaviors taken together are called a role.

On the other hand, an individual must agree to play a particular role. When the individual agrees to play the role and the group positively reinforces performance of the role, *role stability* emerges. The person will generally continue to play the role on a regular basis.

The concept of role can be more fully understood by differentiating between formal and informal roles within a group. A *formal role* is assigned by the organization or group. It usually includes some title, such as president, vice-president, secretary, or chairperson. The assignment of this type of role may or may not be determined by a person's expertise or talent. For example, a man may be appointed to chair a group and not perform as we might imagine a chairperson should. A formal role, then, identifies a position and a set of behaviors that a person may or may not fulfill. The definition of this role remains roughly the same regardless of the person within it.

An *informal role* is regulated, often very subtly, between the group and the person who fulfills the role. The emphasis is on function rather than position. Thus a person may provide leadership functions and therefore fulfill a leadership role without the formal designation.

The formal role structure in an ongoing group, usually constituted by the organization itself, operates in addition to the informal role structure determined by the group. A network of informal roles is highly idiosyncratic to any particular group. And because of people's idiosyncrasies, the number of roles that can emerge in a group is considerable. With the exception of the role of leader, no role seems to be present in all groups.

Here we will present the process through which an informal role emerges, address the issue of role conflict, and then describe several of the usual roles found in decision-making groups. Keep in mind as we present these materials that we are discussing informal roles rather than formal roles or positions.

ROLE EMERGENCE IN SMALL GROUPS

Imagine yourself in your first job. You have been working for your employer for approximately a year. You open the morning mail and find an interoffice memo that appoints you to a committee to review dress standards for the organization. If you can, imagine yourself in the first meeting of this group. What will you do? What roles might you play? Will you lead? Will you be an important source of information? Will you be the person to challenge the group's ideas? Will you help other members to feel that they are part of the group? Perhaps you have served some of these roles for groups in the past. If so, you may do so again. The question of what role you will play in this group may be answered by considering how roles emerge in decision-making groups.

Ernest G. Bormann[1] provides a model of how roles emerged in groups he studied at the University of Minnesota. He presents a stimulus-response model that points to role emergence as a function of reinforcement through the group's interaction over time. Figure 6.1 displays the basic model. The schematic shows the options for the emergence of one role for a particular member. At a particular time, T_1, a member performs a given role behavior. A member or several members either give ambiguous feedback or encourage or discourage the member with regard to this role behavior. At another time, T_2, presumably the next opportunity the person has to perform the role behavior, the person behaves on the basis of the group's reinforcement or lack of it. If the group members have given ambiguous cues, the member will generally try the role behavior again. He or she does so until a clear signal is received from the group. If the group approves, the member will try the behavior again—this time with greater confidence. If disapproval is shown, the member is likely to quit trying to perform the role behavior. In cases where the particular role is important to the group, other members may attempt to provide it. This stimulus-response model operates for each role that emerges.

To show how a role might emerge through group interaction—and how powerful a group's ability to control the behavior of one of its members might be—suppose that

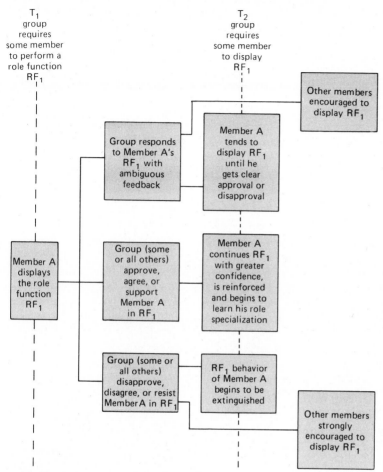

FIGURE 6.1
Bormann's Model of Role Emergence by Ernest G. Bormann.

Figure from *Discussion and Group Methods: Theory and Practice,* copyright © 1969, 1975 by E. G. Bormann. Reprinted by permission of Harper & Row, Publishers, Inc.

you join some on-campus group. You might imagine yourself in any of a variety of contexts—member of the student newspaper staff; member of a special-interest club in relation to your major department; member of the executive committee in a social fraternity or sorority; member of an ad hoc committee of the student government association; member of a subgroup in a course you're taking; student representative on some faculty committee. Let's suppose you join an ad hoc committee of the student government association. Interested and excited, you approach the first meeting very well prepared to discuss the topic, which, say, is selection of the entertainers the student government will support and bring to the campus in the coming year. Because the bottom line is a very large sum—$150,000—you have given a good deal of thought to the variety of speakers and entertainers you think would be appropriate. You have asked many of your friends to mention their interests. You have spent two nights walking the floors of the dormitory in which you live conducting a survey to discover what those students would prefer. You have even contacted one of the New York booking agencies to ask about the fees charged by several of the name entertainers you have identified. So you've come to the group prepared.

The chairperson opens the meeting with a little speech about getting the most for the money and then asks if anyone has any suggestions. You wait quietly for an opening. After several of the members—all of whom have been members of the committee before—have had a chance to speak, you discover that they have not really put much thought into their proposals. No one appears to know how much money would be required, or if the individuals named would be available. No one seems to have asked around to get representation from a cross-section of the student body.

So you begin to make your presentation. You say something like: "Hmm, uh. I did a little thinking about this before the meeting. I went around the dorm and asked one hundred and twenty people to mention entertainers they would like to bring to the campus if money were no object. I was surprised how easily their responses could be classified into categories. I'd be happy to say more, if you would be interested in hearing about it." You stop.

"Really?" "Wow! You did that?" "That's fantastic!" "Let's hear it." These responses seem to reflect the group's attitudes generally. People are interested. They are excited. They are reinforcing your behavior. They are telling you that they like what you have done and that they value you and your help. They are teaching you the behaviors that will become your role in their network. In this case your role might be termed information provider.

"Yeah. Uh. There were really four categories. One was rock music. One was country and western. One was serious lecture. One was classical and jazz music."

You are about to develop these categories further when one of the members says: "We tried classical and jazz last year. No one came to the concerts. We spent about a fourth of our budget to entertain about one hundred people."

Another member says: "That's that. No classical and jazz." A discussion on the categories follows, and the group finally eliminates classical, but not jazz, and agrees to try to get Grover Washington to come to the campus. In discussing your categories, the group has cemented your role of information provider in the group to some extent. You have provided leadership that members have valued. They have reinforced your behavior. Thus, by communication, you and they have had a most fundamental impact upon the group.

The process of role development can be quite subtle. Often a member may not be specifically aware of the group's reinforcement pattern or even of the group's particular expectations for a role. Awareness usually comes *after* the role behaviors have been performed and the expectations have been developed.[2]

The particular role a person plays will vary from group to group. Your own experience probably suggests this. If you think of the various groups to which you belong, you are likely to discover that you play different roles in each. This is because each member of a group develops a pattern of behaviors that takes into account personal abilities and willingness to play the role, *and* group approval. Thus roles are negotiated between an individual and the group's members.

ROLE CONFLICT

Joseph McGrath describes several role pressures that can result in problems for group members.[3] Two of these problems that can occur as a member attempts to carry out a role are role conflict and role strain. *Role conflict* results when a person tries to play two or more roles—generally in different groups—that are contradictory to each other. *Role strain* comes from not being able to perform a role. Of these problems, role conflict is likely to be more frequent, because members do not generally attempt to play roles for which they feel ill equipped.

Role conflict is most likely to occur when a person must take a role outside the group that is especially important. Suppose for example, that a prominent member of the community—say, the president of a local business—is appointed to a commission to study teen-age delinquency. This president has had considerable experience with young people whom her company has employed over the past five years. She has come to believe that companies cannot afford to spend resources on irresponsible or delinquent youths. Now she finds herself appointed to a committee that is charged with finding ways of employing these people. Although the president of a local firm can render a valuable service in this position, the woman in this example is unable to fulfill the role. Her role as president of her company conflicts with the role of group member. She cannot seriously entertain the idea of integrating these juveniles into the business community.

What usually happens in a case like this is that a person will enact the role of greatest personal importance.[4] In the case of the president of the local company, she will probably try to block any programs that try to integrate the juveniles of her community into local businesses.

Occasionally a group member might experience role strain. This happens most often when a member is appointed or elected to fulfill a role but is not equipped to do so. Sometimes the person finds that he or she has accepted the role because no one else will. Consider, for example, the person who is elected to chair a group without any experience at all in such a task. He or she might accept reluctantly because no other person will step forward and take the role.

An additional example is provided by the person who is asked to collect information and bring it back to the group but who has no particular access to the information or data-gathering skill. Role strain resulting from this kind of situation—one in which the person fills a role reluctantly—can affect both the social and task dimensions of the group. The person resents the imposition, so the climate breaks down. If the person does a poor job of carrying out the role, the task suffers.

Being alert to the potentials of role conflict and role strain is an important part of your functioning in a group. You can avoid role conflict in part through careful selection of participants. But when conflict has not been successfully avoided, a group may have to deal with the situation directly. (Some of the methods we suggest in Chapter 10, "Managing Conflict in the Group," will be helpful in coping with this situation.) Role strain can be minimized if group members are careful not to force a particular role on a reluctant person. Careful attention to the verbal and nonverbal cues a member gives off when a particular role is being suggested will aid in avoiding this difficulty.

FUNCTIONAL ROLES IN SMALL GROUPS

It may be that the most common question asked by those who want to do their best in group meetings is: "What do I do during meetings to make the best contribution I can?" In one form or another, that question has been asked for many generations. One of the most useful responses appeared in an essay written by Kenneth D. Benne and Paul Sheats.[5] These scholars studied the role behaviors that occurred in small groups engaged in problem-solving discussion. They divided those behaviors into three categories, which correspond to the three primary matters that every discussion group must confront—matters related to goal achievement, matters related to group identity, and matters related to the needs of individual members. Every behavior in a group falls into one or more of these three categories.

Group Task Roles

In the first category, Benne and Sheats identified certain role behaviors that helped groups to achieve their goals, whatever those goals were. What behaviors help a group to accomplish its tasks? Someone tries to give the group some semblance of order, and undoubtedly someone will criticize and evaluate suggestions, and someone else will summarize what has been said. Typically, if the group believes its work to be important, someone will keep some kind of record of its work. All these behaviors are what Benne and Sheats called *group task roles*. In all, they identified and described thirteen such role behaviors in the first category. Table 6.1 presents the kinds of roles Benne and Sheats had in mind. We will describe and give examples of each so that you can understand the typical behaviors of someone who is fulfilling each role.

TABLE 6.1   Group Task Roles

1. Initiator-contributor	8. Diagnostician
2. Information seeker	9. Orienter-summarizer
3. Information giver	10. Energizer
4. Opinion seeker	11. Procedural assistant
5. Opinion giver	12. Secretary-recorder
6. Elaborator-clarifier	13. Evaluator-critic
7. Coordinator	

1. Initiator-contributor   As the name suggests, this person initiates ideas and suggestions. The initiator-contributor comes up with new ideas and lines of discussion. You might hear, "How about taking a different approach to this chore. Suppose we . . ." If the contribution is related to an idea already being discussed, the role player will present a new or novel idea related to it. This person is the creative thinker in a group. He or she might begin, "You know there is another way of looking at this that we might want to consider." This function is performed by the designated leader when he or she introduces an issue for discussion.

2. Information seeker   Asking questions that seek information is an important function for all members of the group to perform. But a group may not have any formal procedure to ensure idea generation. And group members may also be reluctant to provide the needed information. So the group must rely on certain members to sense the need for more information and actively seek it.

   The information seeker asks for evidence that will allow judgment of the factual adequacy of ideas. This person might ask, "Does anyone have any data to support this idea?" The role player might, instead, ask for information or facts relevant to understanding the problem. Or perhaps this person will suggest that more information is needed before a decision can be reached. Perhaps the person might say, "I'd like to know more about what happened when they tried a play similar to this a couple of years ago. Let's find out and meet tomorrow to make a decision."

3. Information giver   The role of information giver is generally shared by many group members. It is obvious that the quality of a decision is related to the quality and quantity of information a group has to use. The information giver offers facts that are relevant to the group's task. The person who is playing this role well has the research skills, analytical ability, and knowledge to provide accurate and concise data when needed. As part of the information given, you may hear the source of the information. The information giver might say, "I asked Dr. Jones, a specialist in this kind of thing. He said . . ."

4. Opinion seeker   Opinions differ from information in that they are inferences or conclusions, whereas information is the observed data. The opinion seeker role is important because groups need members to offer conclusions about the facts they are processing. And, on the emotional side, members need to know how the others feel about the issues. If you were playing this role, you might say, "Does anyone else have an idea on this? Can someone clear up what this means?"

5. Opinion giver   The opinion giver offers analysis of the information being presented. This means that the person states beliefs or opinions about suggestions being made. Perhaps you might hear, "I think we ought to go with the second plan. It fits the conditions we face in the Concord plant best." The opinion giver might also indicate what the group's attitude should be: "We ought to take a hard line on absenteeism. If people miss work too frequently, we ought to let them go."

6. Elaborator-clarifier   Group members are not always clear about their ideas when they are processing information in groups. The person filling this role tests ideas and suggestions by elaborating on what is being said. The person may also test understanding by asking questions. For example, you might hear, "Do you mean that George actually said that he knew about the situation? I thought that that was your guess about what was going on." The elaborator-clarifier may also offer rationales for the group to consider. Perhaps a member will say, "I think we can tell Sue that we recommend this idea because . . ." Finally, this person might try to help the group visualize how an idea or suggestion would work if it were adopted by the group.

7. Coordinator   The coordinator tries to draw connections between what different members have said. This person might draw together information, opinions, and ideas or check relationships among information, opinions, and ideas. For example, a coordinator might say, "John's opinion squares pretty well with the research that Mary reported. Why don't we take that idea and see if . . ."

8. Diagnostician   The diagnostician analyzes and identifies task-related problems. This person also poses issues related to the problem being discussed and, in doing so, may redirect the group. Typically, a person in this role might comment, "But I think you are missing the main point. The problem is that we can't afford to have unsafe . . ."

9. Orienter-summarizer   When the group moves too far off the task, the orienter-summarizer senses the appropriate time to bring members back. You might hear, "This discussion of . . . has been fun. Let's get back to where we were a few minutes ago." Or the orienter may ask a question about where the group is headed to allow members to see that they have digressed: "I'm not sure where we are headed on this issue. What is the point?"

   This person also keeps the group oriented by helping members understand where they have been and what conclusions they have reached. This is accomplished by providing timely summaries as the group moves through the information processing. The summary may be followed by a question to check out the accuracy of the summary provided: "Is that what we've been saying?"

10. Energizer   A member energizes the group when he or she raises the level of enthusiasm for its work. This is often accomplished by "upbeat" nonverbal behavior. Enthusiasm is generated by having one or more people in the group with an optimistic outlook. The energizer may also recognize the need for someone to challenge the group. You might hear, "Come on, folks. We're almost finished. I know we can be through in a few minutes if we work at it."

11. Procedural assistant   The procedural assistant may take on a variety of tasks. He or she may organize such routine tasks as making seating arrangements, obtaining equipment, and handing out pertinent papers. This is an important role because it fulfills functions that assist the leader in making sure that the group has what it needs and that meetings run smoothly. When the role is performed by several people, it can help to build a sense that members care about the group and about unity. The fact that members are willing to pitch in spontaneously is one sign of a healthy, cohesive group.

12. Secretary-recorder   In many groups some person is assigned to take minutes of a meeting, serving as the "group memory." Obviously, keeping track of what is going on as a group is processing information requires skill and an ability to pay attention. This role presents a potential problem for the group, because the recording activity can limit other kinds of participation for some individuals. If the person doing the recording is also expected to provide certain data and expertise in information processing, then this individual needs to be a person who can record and participate otherwise. Be sure to appoint someone who can do both.

13. Evaluator-critic   The person fulfilling the evaluator role is referred to as the "critical thinker." This is an important role because the quality of a group's decision is a function of how carefully and critically it evaluates ideas. The person in this role analyzes or causes the group to analyze its accomplishments according to some set of standards without causing members to feel threatened. You might hear an evaluator-critic say, "Look, we said that we had only four hundred dollars to spend. What is being proposed will cost at least six hundred dollars. That's a fifty percent override."

This person also monitors the decision-making process to see that concensus has been reached. He or she may say, "What I hear people saying is that we must solve the attrition problem. Is that our first priority?"

Several of these task roles are critical to the group's effectiveness: initiator-contributor, information seeker, information giver, opinion seeker, opinion giver, and evaluator-critic. Group members must initiate ideas and provide information and informed opinion. It is also crucial for some members to seek information and opinions if what is being offered is not sufficient to produce high-quality analysis and decisions. Finally, effective analysis depends on members' being willing to think critically—and cause the group to think critically—about the ideas and information being presented.

Group Building and Maintenance Roles

Group life includes moments of success and moments of failure. When times are bad, group members need to focus upon their relationships. Sometimes damaging conflict must be managed. At other times individual members develop problems that adversely influence the group. For example, when a task force is called, each person has been asked to meet because of his or her personal expertise. If an individual suddenly stops making contributions to the group, the group loses the benefit of that person's input. Sometimes the tension levels in a group get so high that something must be done to break the tension. All of these concerns and others are in the social, or relationship, dimension of group communication. When they occur, the role behaviors Benne and

Sheats described as maintenance roles are needed. Table 6.2 lists the eight roles included in this category.

1. Supporter-encourager The person or persons in this role offer warmth, solidarity, and recognition to the group's members. Support may take the form of praise, agreement, or signs of acceptance. A supporter-encourager might say, "I really like that idea, John." Or perhaps you might hear, "Priscilla's suggestion is attractive to me. Could we discuss it further?" This person-to-person encouragement is a valuable motivator and builder of cohesiveness. When offered by a high-status member, perhaps the group's leader, it can have even greater effect. All members want to know that they and their work are appreciated.

2. Harmonizer A harmonizer is the person who helps a group manage conflict. He or she works to reconcile disagreements, mediate differences, and reduce tension. The harmonizer is likely to be well acquainted with the conflict management techniques presented in Chapter 8.

The person acting as harmonizer may also take on the role of tension releaser. Tensions are reduced by giving members the opportunity to explore their differences. Here are comments typical of a person in this role: "I don't think you two are as far apart as you think. Henry, are you saying . . . ? Benson, you seem to be saying . . . ? Is that what you mean?"

3. Tension releaser The tension releaser's goal is to relax group members. This may be accomplished by poking fun at a situation so that members laugh at the situation. It may even require a diversion—perhaps a joke that is totally unrelated to the particular task at the moment.

The tension releaser must be sensitive to the social demands of the group. Jokes that may be funny to an all-female audience may not be funny at all in a mixed group. Making light of some issues can obviously be in poor taste. When not played appropriately, the role may be viewed, instead, as the self-centered, playboy/playgirl role (discussed below).

4. Compromiser This person offers to compromise when it is clearly necessary for group progress. "Looks like our solution is halfway between you and me, John. Can we look at the middle ground?" is a comment typical of the compromiser.

The nature of the group decision-making process often requires compromise if the group is to reach its goal satisfactorily. Thus, in the task dimension, many of the group's

TABLE 6.2 Group Building and Maintenance Roles

1. Supporter-encourager	5. Gatekeeper
2. Harmonizer	6. Feeling expresser
3. Tension releaser	7. Standard setter
4. Compromiser	8. Follower

members must often play the compromiser role. Compromise will be necessary for some in the relationship dimension as well.

5. Gatekeeper   The person fulfilling the gatekeeper role tries to keep communication channels open. One responsibility is to manage tactfully the time allotted to each speaker. If some members seem to be monopolizing the interaction, the gatekeeper might ask, "Does anyone else have an opinion on this issue?"

   This person is also skillful at drawing silent members into the discussion. The gatekeeper is careful to notice quiet people early in the session and to ask for their input. You might hear, "Susan hasn't had the chance to say anything about this yet. Susan, I know you have been studying the problem. What do you think about . . . ?"

6. Feeling expresser   The feeling expresser monitors the feelings, moods, and relationships in the group. The person articulates these group feelings, as well as his or her own, when doing so is appropriate. You might hear, "Don't we all need a break right now? I'm frustrated and confused and maybe we all are. I'd like to take a break so we can come back fresh and ready to tackle this again."

7. Standard setter   This role requires the person in it to suggest standards for the group to achieve. Recall from Chapter 1 that standards related to group process are called norms. The standard setter may challenge unproductive norms or unproductive group behavior. For example, when a member is continually late for meetings, the standard setter might say, "John, we had to wait for you again. The delay means we won't get finished today. What happened?"

   Or the standard setter may be primarily concerned with setting criteria. You might hear, "In my view, this decision doesn't measure up to our best. We really haven't set any criteria, much less tried to apply them."

8. Follower   The follower goes along with the movement of the group. He or she listens attentively, accepting the ideas of others. Here is a typical comment from a person in the follower role: "I agree. Yes, I see what you mean. If that's what the group wants, I'll go along." In productive groups, members will usually not take on this role as their sole contribution.

Several of these building and maintenance roles are especially important to creating and maintaining an effective group. Cohesiveness is generally recognized as important for productivity; thus the supporter-encourager performs a needed function for a group. Conflict that is not managed effectively in a group can destroy its effectiveness. The harmonizer works toward this end. Tension levels can rise about the group's threshold for tolerance. The group needs a member to recognize when tension has been too high for too long, and to release it. Also, group members who are thinking critically about problems will undoubtedly have differing thoughts about what to do. Here the role of compromiser is crucial. Finally, a group must have standards—standards for behaving and for deciding—that enable it to be effective. Someone in the group must take the responsibility to help the group set and maintain standards. Thus five maintenance roles for groups are critical: supporter-encourager, harmonizer, tension releaser, compromiser, and standard setter.

Self-Centered Roles

Benne and Sheats described eight additional roles that they believed were usually counterproductive. These roles are *self-centered roles*, and they focus on solving individual problems. We do not mean to suggest that each of these role behaviors is always counter to the best interests of the group. We do mean to suggest that self-centered roles usually inhibit group success. But our point is really that analysis of the role behaviors occurring in a group will usually suggest the reasons for a group's being successful or not. Table 6.3 displays the categories of self-centered roles.

1. Blocker   The blocker prevents progress toward the group's goals by frequently raising objections, rejecting others' ideas, or taking a negative stand on issues. Issues that the group has already considered and decided may be reintroduced by the blocker. Blocking techniques are numerous. Some we've encountered are emotional outbursts, filibustering, going on and on with procedural objections, and examining a solution or idea word by word to make sure each is exactly right. One blocker we know, whose presence was needed for the group to operate, declared, "Wait a minute! That's not right! That idea is absurd. If you take that position, I simply can't continue to work with this group."

2. Aggressor   Some self-serving members struggle for status by trying to defeat one another. Their goal is to enhance themselves by lowering the status of others in the group. An aggressor was heard to exclaim in a loud voice, "Wow, that's really swell! You turkeys have botched things again. Your constant bickering is responsible for this mess. Let me tell you how you ought to do this."

3. Deserter   The deserter withdraws from the group's deliberation in some way. The person may act indifferent, aloof, and stiffly formal. Or the deserter might talk off the subject or engage in some sort of side conversation to avoid the issue. The person may merely sit in the group and daydream. A deserter may say to himself or herself, "Ho-hum. There's nothing in this discussion for me." But to the group the deserter says, "I guess I really don't care what you choose in this case. But on this other matter . . ."

4. Dominator   The dominator continually takes more than a fair share of the group's

TABLE 6.3   Self-Centered Roles

1. Blocker	5. Recognition seeker
2. Aggressor	6. Confessor
3. Deserter	7. Playboy/playgirl-clown
4. Dominator	8. Special-interest pleader

time. All members may dominate at some time or another, but this is not what the dominator role means. This person is a frequent monopolizer and may even interrupt and take the floor from others. The dominator might break in with, "Bill, you're just off base here. What we should do is this. First, . . ."

5. Recognition seeker   The recognition seeker attempts to call attention to himself or herself in an exaggerated manner: "I think . . . . Don't you think I'm right? [Don't you think I'm wonderful?]!" The role is played by boasting about present and past accomplishments, relating irrelevant personal experiences, and sometimes attempting to gain sympathy. Here is a typical comment: "You guys wouldn't believe the bad day I had yesterday! It started when I woke up and went on and on. Let me tell you what happened."

6. Confessor   The confessor role is played when a person presents his or her personal difficulties and feelings related to them in a task group. These are not task-related issues; they are personal matters that are unrelated to the task. The confessor is using the group for therapy. Generally the group cares about the person, so members turn their attention to helping. You might hear a confessor comment, "This is not exactly on the topic, but I'm experiencing a problem with a woman named Mary in my department. Yesterday, Mary and I had a fight about . . ."

7. Playboy/playgirl–clown   Some people love to be the clown in the group. Humor can be an important part of many group interactions, as it helps the group relax and attend to the task. Yet when the humor, horseplay, or cynicism is inappropriate, it can distract from the group's productivity. Members of the group may become caught up in the clowning and for the moment enjoy it. But later they may regret it, since the task remains incomplete. If members can play around without seriously damaging their productivity, then clowning serves a valuable purpose. When a person continually distracts the group from its task, the role becomes self-serving. Most of us can recall a typical lead-in from the clown: "Did you hear the one about the . . ."

8. Special-interest pleader   A member who speaks on behalf of an outside group, rather than the group of which he or she is a part, is pleading a special interest. When one group was deciding to whom it would award a contract, one member pleaded his special interest: "My friend Alan runs a company that makes this product. How about using his company? We might as well spend our money with people we know." The comment was a straightforward interest plea. No data were given to suggest that the firm offered advantages over others. The argument was merely on the basis of rewarding "a friend."

As you can see from studying these role behaviors, they often overlap. Indeed, there are as many roles as there are people in groups, and even during the course of a single discussion, each person will contribute a variety of appropriate role behaviors. Identifying the potential role behaviors will allow you to do two things. First, it will allow you to understand what is happening in a group while it is happening, and in case something is causing the group to be unsuccessful, you can intervene. Second, the analysis of group role behaviors should suggest ways of behaving that will help you achieve your own goals—and will help the groups to which you belong achieve their goals as well.

Ultimately, you are responsible for your own behavior in all groups you join. In a sense, as a member of the groups, you are responsible for their success or failure. What you do to encourage the group to set and achieve appropriate goals is a mark of your worth to the group. What you do to encourage the group to become more cohesive and a better team, and to establish a climate of trust in which communication can work well, is also a mark of your worth to the group. Together, these two categories of behaviors constitute important aspects of group leadership, the topic of Chapter 7. And leadership is not confined to those individuals who have been designated to lead groups. Each member of each group can contribute leadership. Each member should do so.

SUMMARY

In a sense, a small group is a culture and it, too, has a set of roles that reflect its members' views of the group's needs and the talents and preferences of its individual members. A role can be defined as a set of behaviors that an individual member displays in relation to the expectations of the rest of the group members. A member may take on a formal role that is assigned by the organization or group. This role usually has a title such as president, vice-president, or secretary. On the other hand, the person may take on an informal role. This type of role is characterized by behaviors that fulfill a function for the group. Such a function might be information provider, tension releaser, recorder, or leader.

Roles emerge through a trial-and-error process that has been described by Ernest Bormann. This stimulus-response model suggests that members attempt roles and the group either reinforces or discourages the role behavior. Over a period of time, depending on the group's reaction, the member continues or discontinues the playing of the role.

Two problems that can occur as a member attempts to carry out a role are role conflict and role strain. Role conflict results from a person's trying to play two or more roles—generally in different groups—that are contradictory to each other. Role strain comes from not being able to perform a role. Of the two problems, role conflict is likely to be the more frequent, because members do not generally attempt to play roles for which they feel ill equipped. These problems can be addressed by selecting participants carefully and not forcing a role on a reluctant group member.

Roles represent a wide variety of behaviors. There are those that are task centered, in that they help the group achieve its goal. Other roles are maintenance oriented. These are the roles that help care for a group and its members rather than the task. Finally, there are roles that are self-centered. These roles focus on achieving the aims of individual group members and, therefore, often detract from task accomplishment and group maintenance.

EXERCISES

1. Describe and analyze the functional roles of the members of your group.

2. Think of a group with which you felt particularly frustrated. What roles did the various members play? Can you account for your frustration through an examination of the participation of the other members? What might be done if you encounter a similar situation in the future? Answer these questions in a two-page analysis.

3. Role-play a problem-solving discussion, perhaps a case study given to your group by your instructor. Assign two of the self-centered roles to two of the members. Attempt to complete this discussion within twenty to twenty-five minutes. Following the discussion of the case study, conduct an analysis of the group interaction. What effect did the disruptive role playing have on the group's decision making? What leadership behaviors did members employ to attempt to overcome these difficulties? How successful were they? If they were, why were they? If they were not, why were they not? What might have been done that was not done?

4. Consider at least four groups in which you have held membership within the past two years. Describe your role or roles in each group. Make a list of these roles and then compare them with those of other members of the class in a small group. What do you discover? Do people perform a variety of roles? Do they, instead, play similar roles in the groups to which they belong? Does the role depend on the type of group? Does it depend on the commitment the member has to the group?

5. Observe a group with one or more of your classmates. Independently, list the functional roles each member serves. Compare your findings with those of others who are observing the same discussion. Do you agree on the roles being played by each member? If not, how do you account for your disagreement? Now divide the behaviors among task, maintenance, and self-centered roles. Were the important roles played? What role functions might have improved the decision making if members had fulfilled them?

NOTES

1. Ernest G. Bormann, *Discussion and Group Methods: Theory and Practice*, 2d ed. (New York: Harper & Row, 1975), 292–308.

2. B. Aubrey Fisher, *Small Group Decision Making*, 2d ed. (New York: McGraw-Hill, 1980), 169–170.

3. Joseph E. McGrath, *Groups: Interaction and Performance* (Englewood Cliffs, N.J.: Prentice-Hall, 1984).

4. Marvin E. Shaw, *Group Dynamics: The Psychology of Small Group Behavior*, 3d ed. (New York: McGraw-Hill, 1980), 278.

5. Kenneth Benne and Paul Sheats, "Functional Roles of Group Members," *Journal of Social Issues* 4 (1948):41–49.

RECOMMENDED READINGS

Kenneth Benne and Paul Sheats, "Functional Roles of Group Members," *Journal of Social Issues* 4 (1948):41–49.

Ernest G. Bormann, *Discussion and Group Methods: Theory and Practice,* 2d ed. (New York: Harper & Row, 1975), Chapters 8 and 9.

CHAPTER 7

Leading Group Meetings

OBJECTIVES

After reading this chapter you should be able to:

Define and differentiate between *leader* and *leadership.*

Define and differentiate between *designated leader* and *emergent leader.*

Explain the characteristic features of each of the following ways of looking at leadership, and suggest the utility that each perspective offers to group members: (1) the trait perspective, (2) the style perspective, (3) the functional perspective, (4) the situational perspective, and (5) the contingency perspective.

Specify and explain the characteristics of an effective group leader.

Recall the five major areas of responsibility that a successful group leader will attempt to manage, and specify how he or she might go about that attempt at management.

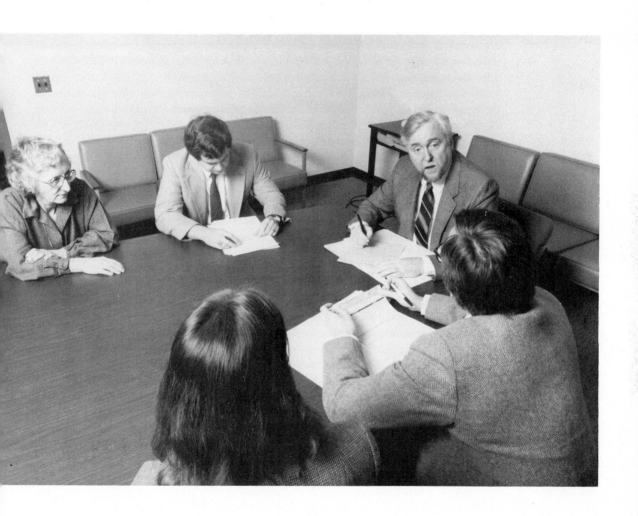

A management group of a local department store met in the company training room—one of those required affairs all individuals have to attend now and again. Poor leadership can be blamed at least in part for the way this meeting went. The time chosen for the meeting was poor, coming as it did in the middle of a very busy week just prior to a holiday. Moreover, the meeting was held at 1:00—just after lunch, and just before a 2:00 change of shift. Several department managers were concerned about the length of the meeting—they had to check in employees at 2:00. A good leader carefully selects an appropriate time.

The meeting included fifteen people from a variety of departments, and some department managers. Some of these people were not needed for this meeting and had no role in it. The agenda for the meeting was, ostensibly, to gather input on two questions: (1) What problems might develop from changing store hours? (2) If they were changed, what might the best hours be?

There was a hidden agenda, too. Indeed, there were at least two of them. One of the high-ranking managers was opposed to the proposals, but more than that, he appeared to be pushing for another manager who favored the change. This manager clearly wanted to teach the lower-ranking manager a lesson or two—perhaps well intended, and perhaps motivated by some animosity generated over a period of time and a history of conflict with the other manager. A wise leader would probably have specified a clear agenda, taking the needs of members into account, and would have done so well in advance of the meeting. Thus the leader might reduce the likelihood of private agendas being introduced. This store manager did not do so.

The meeting lasted more than an hour, and it concluded with the store manager receiving plenty of input. But it resulted in a set of unanticipated offshoots. The manager who was opposed came away from the meeting feeling more hostile than he had before. One of the other members of this group was from his department. The meeting brought out a soreness in their relationships, too. The management team had sustained a deep fracture, mostly as a result of the store manager's inability to lead and manage conflict in this group.

Many of these problems could have been avoided altogether if the leadership of this group had been more carefully planned and if the goals and the objectives of the meeting had been more carefully thought through. As the meeting progressed, more skillful leadership could have managed the conflict—could have brought out, or buried, if necessary, the hidden agendas and made clear that they were inappropriate. Something could have been done about the relationship issues that occurred. But none of this leadership was provided.

For a variety of reasons, the evolution of group phases, group norms, and group roles is not easy to observe in work situations. But we can examine student groups very closely, and we can ask our students lots of questions. At the same time, one advantage of working in an urban university is that the student population tends to be somewhat older than average. People take an hour or so from their workday to pursue a college education. As a method of research, we ask these individuals to tape-record their meetings, and to respond in notebooks to questions about what went on in their meetings and how they felt and what they thought. We make use of these reports throughout this chapter to draw inferences and examples that apply generally and relate them to the relevant research.

To illustrate the kinds of questions we asked students to consider, think of an uncomfortable, unprofitable group experience you have had recently. Did the faults have anything to do with leadership? Did the group have a leader? If it had a leader, can you describe him or her? For instance, did the leader move the group along in its task? Did the leader manage any conflict that arose? Or perhaps your group had no leader at all. Maybe several people were providing leadership. Did they move the group in the same direction? Or did they try to move the group in different directions? One or more of these questions probably reveal a problem or problems that account for the group's ineffectiveness.

You can also learn much by considering good groups that have effective leaders. So think, too, of the good groups you've experienced that have had effective leaders. What have they taught you?

This chapter begins by making a distinction between leadership and leaders. Next, we consider several perspectives on leadership. Then we show how ideas of each of these perspectives come together with research on leadership to suggest characteristics of effective leaders. The chapter concludes with concrete suggestions for improving your leadership skill.

LEADERSHIP AND LEADERS

One of the earliest decisions for any group is "Who will lead?" Sometimes the question is answered by someone in authority appointing a leader. For other groups, the group itself decides who will lead. This is a crucial question, for without adequate leadership both the quality of the group experience and the product of the group are in doubt.

A student chapter of the Public Relations Council of Alabama faced the leadership question and found the answer was not an easy one. In fact, the process the students went through took place over several meetings and was quite traumatic. Most of the group meetings had been largely social, with guest speakers. The members felt no need to single out any specific person as task leader. Then, in their fifth meeting, they decided to take on the task of producing a brochure about services offered by the American Cancer Society. This decision called for task leadership—a role that had not yet developed.

Two group members, Linda and Jeff, saw themselves as capable leaders, and both wanted very much to have the opportunity to lead. A struggle ensued. Sometimes Linda would be in control and some members accepted her. Then Jeff would get the floor and try to move the group in his direction. One group member in particular would follow. Then Linda would reverse the process. It took several meetings for Linda to emerge as the accepted leader of the group—and the competition was keen.

The group's answer to the question of who would lead detracted considerably from members' ability to accomplish the task. They were devoting so much energy to the leadership question that their productivity suffered.

Do not assume that this group did not have any social or task leader until members were able to select someone. Sometimes people wrongly draw this conclusion. The confusion lies in the difference between leader and leadership. *Leadership* is an influence process. *Leader* is a position within the group or perhaps a person who occupies that position. A leader may be formally designated or may evolve informally from the interactions of group members. Marvin Shaw defined leadership as "an influence process which is directed toward goal achievement."[1] Notice that this definition takes into account all kinds of leadership. For example, Linda might influence her group to socialize when it ought to work on the task. Her influence would qualify as leadership, but not in the desired direction. Again, a group member—say Marc—might influence another to leave the group's meeting early. This, too, would be leadership by Shaw's definition, although it would be leadership toward Marc's personal goal, and counterproductive to the group. Shaw's definition might be modified to take into account problems created by situations like these. Insert the word "group" before "goal" in the definition so that it reads: "Leadership is an influence process which is directed toward group goal achievement."

This definition of leadership omits specific reference to a leader. The term *leader* refers to a particular person who either is appointed to lead the group or emerges from the group membership. A person who is appointed to lead a group is generally referred to as a *designated leader* because someone in authority has appointed him or her to be responsible for directing the group. A department head provides a good example. So do the leaders of most groups whose members are named by some responsible person.

When leaders are appointed, an interesting phenomenon may occur. This problem is often illustrated in classroom discussion groups in which the leader is designated. Perhaps this leader has never led any group—and furthermore doesn't ever intend to do so. Maybe the group senses this, too. This person may be leader in name only—not accepted by the group as its leader or willing to try to carry out the role. (Recall that a role can't be fulfilled if a group is unwilling to allow it.) In such a case, a person might decide to do something to help the group move toward its goal. The group may accept the lead. When this happens, the person is called an *emergent leader.* Sometimes it is possible for a group to have both a designated leader and an emergent leader. The leadership responsibilities are divided. The designated leader may call the meetings and provide the agenda. The emergent leader influences the members in their effort to carry out the task.

Occasionally a group will reject its designated leader, but no one person will make influence attempts of sufficient quantity or quality to emerge as the task leader. In these situations the duties that might fall to an emergent leader are shared among several members of the group. For some groups this shared leadership can prove to be quite satisfactory. One member might fulfill the leadership task of managing conflict. Another person might summarize group progress. Still another member might encourage reticent members to participate. The leadership is shared with the designated leader, who convenes the meeting and circulates the agenda.

At times a member other than the designated leader might wish to lead, and the group might perceive this person as capable and even more desirable than the designated leader. This could set the stage for a leadership struggle, especially if the designated leader is not willing to share leadership and if the group is unwilling to follow the designated leader. A great deal of group energy might be consumed by such a role struggle—taking the group away from its specified task.

So if a group is meeting for a specified and short period of time—say one meeting—it is generally wise to have a designated leader who is well respected by the group and capable of supplying most of the necessary leadership.

PERSPECTIVES ON LEADER BEHAVIOR

The definition of leadership presented here embodies the key ideas about leadership. But there are a number of ways to look at leadership historically. Each of these perspectives allows us to discover something useful, but different, about leadership. So we are not advocating one particular view of leadership. Instead, we believe that you can learn useful things from each view. When these perspectives are taken together, a group of characteristics and behaviors emerge that can help you become a more effective leader. You will find these ideas grouped under the headings "Characteristics of the Effective Leader" and "Improving Your Leadership Skills." These descriptions are amplified with additional comments and suggestions.

The first approach—the *trait* perspective—is characterized by the question, "What personal traits would set a leader apart from others in a group?" The second perspective relates to leader *style*. People interested in this approach would ask the question "What particular patterns of behaviors can be observed in various kinds of leaders?" A third way of viewing leadership focuses on the *functions* a leader performs. This approach is characterized by questions like "What might a leader do to manage task and social aspects of the group?" The fourth perspective—the *situation* perspective—is characterized by such questions as "What kind of leadership is called for by a particular circumstance?" A final approach combines some of the others. It is often referred to as the *contingency* perspective. People who are trying to understand leadership from this view ask, "Given this task, what kind of leadership will be most effective?" Each of these perspectives is addressed in turn. The hope is that you will see the utility in each, and that they will inform your participation and leadership in groups.

We'd like to give you the opportunity to gain a sense of what leadership style you might pursue when faced with leadership responsibility. Table 7.1 is a questionnaire that will help you discover your situational style. Before you continue, take a moment to decide what action you might take in each of the twelve leadership situations. Then continue by reading about the different perspectives on leadership. After completing the reading, you will want to evaluate your responses to the twelve situations by using the coding scheme found in Figure 7.3 at the end of the chapter.

Trait Perspective

The term "born leader" is used to describe a person who is believed to possess the characteristics needed to be a successful leader. This view supposes that certain individuals

TABLE 7.1 Leader Adaptability and Style Inventory (LASI)

Situation	*Alternative Actions*
1. Your subordinates are not responding lately to your friendly conversation and obvious concern for their welfare. Their performance is in a tailspin.	A. Emphasize the use of uniform procedures and the necessity for task accomplishment. B. Make yourself available for discussion but don't push. C. Talk with subordinates and then set goals. D. Intentionally do not intervene.
2. The observable performance of your group is increasing. You have been making sure that all members are aware of their roles and standards.	A. Engage in friendly interaction, but continue to make sure that all members are aware of their roles and standards. B. Take no definite action. C. Do what you can to make the group feel important and involved. D. Emphasize the importance of deadlines and tasks.
3. Members of your group are unable to solve a problem themselves. You have normally left them alone. Group performance and interpersonal relations have been good.	A. Involve the group and together engage in problem solving. B. Let the group work it out. C. Act quickly and firmly to correct and redirect. D. Encourage group to work on problem and be available for discussion.
4. You are considering a major change. Your subordinates have a fine record of accomplishment. They respect the need for change.	A. Allow group involvement in developing the change, but don't push. B. Announce changes and then implement with close supervision. C. Allow group to formulate its own direction. D. Incorporate group recommendations, but you direct the change.
5. The performance of your group has been dropping during the last few months. Members have been unconcerned with meeting objectives. Redefining roles has helped in the past. They have continually needed reminding to have their tasks done on time.	A. Allow group to formulate its own direction. B. Incorporate group recommendations, but see that objectives are met. C. Redefine goals and supervise carefully. D. Allow group involvement in setting goals, but don't push.
6. You stepped into an efficiently run situation. The previous administrator ran a	A. Do what you can to make group feel important and involved.

TABLE 7.1   Leader Adaptability and Style Inventory (LASI) *(Con't)*

Situation	Alternative Actions
tight ship. You want to maintain a productive situation, but would like to begin humanizing the environment.	B. Emphasize the importance of deadlines and tasks. C. Intentionally do not intervene. D. Get group involved in decision making, but see that objectives are met.
7. You are considering major changes in your organizational structure. Members of the group have made suggestions about needed change. The group has demonstrated flexibility in its day-to-day operations.	A. Define the change and supervise carefully. B. Acquire group's approval on the change and allow members to organize the implementation. C. Be willing to make changes as recommended, but maintain control of implementation. D. Avoid confrontation; leave things alone.
8. Group performance and interpersonal relations are good. You feel somewhat unsure about your lack of direction of the group.	A. Leave the group alone. B. Discuss the situation with the group and then initiate necessary changes. C. Take steps to direct subordinates toward working in a well-defined manner. D. Be careful of hurting boss-subordinate relations by being too directive.
9. Your superior has appointed you to head a task force that is far overdue in making requested recommendations for change. The group is not clear on its goals. Attendance at sessions has been poor. Their meetings have turned into social gatherings. Potentially they have the talent necessary to help.	A. Let the group work it out. B. Incorporate group recommendations, but see that objectives are met. C. Redefine goals and supervise carefully. D. Allow group involvement in setting goals, but don't push.
10. Your subordinates, usually able to take responsibility, are not responding to your recent redefining of standards.	A. Allow group involvement in redefining standards, but don't push. B. Redefine standards and supervise carefully. C. Avoid confrontation by not applying pressure. D. Incorporate group recommendations, but see that new standards are met.
11. You have been promoted to a new position. The previous supervisor was unin-	A. Take steps to direct subordinates toward working in a well-defined manner.

TABLE 7.1   Leader Adaptability and Style Inventory (LASI) (Con't)

Situation	Alternative Actions
volved in the affairs of the group. The group has adequately handled its tasks and direction. Group interrelations are good.	B. Involve subordinates in decision making and reinforce good contributions. C. Discuss past performance with group, and then you examine the need for new practices. D. Continue to leave group alone.
12. Recent information indicates some internal difficulties among subordinates. The group has a remarkable record of accomplishment. Members have effectively maintained long-range goals. They have worked in harmony for the past year. All are well qualified for the task.	A. Try out your solution with subordinates and examine the need for new practices. B. Allow group members to work it out themselves. C. Act quickly and firmly to correct and redirect. D. Make yourself available for discussion, but be careful of hurting boss-subordinate relations.

Paul Hersey and Kenneth H. Blanchard, "LASI." Copyright © 1974, *Training and Development Journal*, American Society for Training and Development. Reprinted with permission. All rights reserved.

inherit unique leader characteristics that allow them to be successful. The trait perspective expands this idea. It assumes that leaders have certain personal characteristics that set them apart from nonleaders.

The trait perspective is illustrated by the recent experience of a nominating committee at a local church. A name was proposed for a leadership position. The suggestion was met by: "I don't think Ron would work out. I've known his family for years. They are not leaders. They don't have what it takes."

Imagine how important this perspective might be in the context of an industrial organization. A corporation could identify people who have the leadership traits that are desirable and then put those people into positions of power. The corporation could save thousands of dollars by selecting only supervisor-trainees who ranked high in specific traits. Moreover, management could measure the skill levels of existing supervisors and use these as the criteria for promotion—or even for continuing in a position. But does this approach, which seems to make sense, actually work? Several research reports suggest that it does not.

An essay by R. D. Mann[2] is instructive. He reviewed 125 leadership studies trying to link personality traits to performance in small groups. He was able to locate 750 findings about personality traits, but there was no consistency among the traits cited by the researchers. Some traits listed as important by one researcher were found to be insignificant by others.

Barbara P. Guyer[3] compared traits of discussion leaders, student evaluations of those leaders, and the grades assigned to the leaders by their instructors. She wasn't able to find a statistically significant relationship among the variables she studied. She concluded that "attention to personality traits . . . would have been of limited value in the selection of discussion leaders."

Style Perspective

Russ, a bright, ambitious, and capable management trainee, decided that in order to be successful he would have to work at learning to lead groups. In spite of his ambition, he was a little reserved, which caused him to take a back seat when it came to assuming leadership. But Russ had decided that he must overcome this problem—and now was the time to do it. He reasoned that he ought to study carefully the most effective leader-manager he could find. He figured this would allow him to learn firsthand what the most effective leadership style was.

So Russ modeled his own leadership style after the leader he perceived as being the most effective. This person's approach was to keep firm control. About six months later Russ was assigned the task of leading a group that was reviewing the company's dress policy. He led this group in accordance with the philosophy he decided was best. He believed that people need to be controlled—that productivity is best produced by careful, close control and a "take charge" attitude. He favored a style that embodied these philosophies.

On the other hand, he could have adopted a different style. If he believed that people need to be involved in the decision-making process and that people appreciate procedural help, then he probably would have adopted a style of leadership accordingly.

He could even have come to believe in a third philosophy. If he thought that attempts to guide groups were likely to lead to negative consequences and if he felt uncomfortable trying to influence people, he might have been likely to adopt a style that let people operate on their own.

These particular styles of leadership have been labeled *autocratic, democratic,* and *laissez faire.* Each style has its merits and will be discussed briefly, although there really is not much to be said about laissez-faire leadership.

Letting a group lead itself, if no one steps forward to provide leadership, might mean a disaster. If someone does lead, then that can be described as some kind of leadership style. For this reason laissez-faire leadership is not of particular concern. This leadership style encompasses the art of knowing when to stand back and let group members take charge. When the group has the talent, and does not really need the help of its designated leader, this may be an appropriate strategy. For example, some groups whose goal is learning do best if the teacher-leader allows participants to take charge of the activity.

Autocratic and democratic leadership styles have received a great deal of attention from scholars and researchers. Yet it is wise to look at this research from the perspective in which it was conducted. Most of the research compared "pure" examples of each style. But there is a vast middle ground in which leadership actually occurs outside the laboratory where it is being studied. You are unlikely to find a purely democratic or a purely autocratic leader. Keep this idea in mind as differences in these styles are discussed.

Much of the interest in the study of leadership styles began with Ralph K. White and Ronald Lippitt,[4] who studied groups of boys as they responded to the various leadership styles. Democratic leaders allowed participation in policy decisions. The boys were free to select alternatives and to work with whomever they chose. Autocratic leaders determined all policy, dictated techniques, and usually dictated work partners. Style accounted for clear differences in behavior. Boys who experienced autocratic leadership demonstrated thirty times more hostility and eight times more aggression than did boys who experienced democratic leadership. They also did more scapegoating, and their work was judged to be qualitatively inferior to the work of democratically led groups. We must be careful in making judgments about these data, however. The information was collected at a summer camp; thus it may be tied to the situation. Also, it involves the behavior of boys, which may not parallel that of adults at all. Sargent and Miller[5] found that autocratic leaders tended to rush through the question-and-answer process. Democratic leaders, on the other hand, attempted to encourage participation. Rosenfeld and Pax[6] discovered that autocratic leaders made fewer attempts to encourage members to participate, gave more negative reactions, and asked fewer questions.

Some researchers have examined the amount of structure a leader brings to bear on a task. William E. Jurma[7] has labeled this behavior *leadership-structuring style.* Someone who is a highly structuring leader will pay attention to group interaction procedures, help set goals, and stress equality. You might imagine a structuring leader spending time with the group doing the following: (1) setting goals and steps leading to their attainment; (2) clarifying task alternatives; (3) urging self-direction among members; (4) volunteering task-related information; and (5) urging members to treat one another with equality.

Contrary to what you might expect, participants who were low in task orientation were more satisfied than highly task-oriented participants when led by a highly structuring leader. Moreover, members of structured groups rated their tasks as more interesting, valuable, and important than those who participated in low-structured groups.

A group of people representing a countywide literacy council was called together to discuss program ideas. This group was led by a man named Lewis. He thought he understood what it takes to be a good leader—he had been enrolled in an advanced small groups class. Using a structuring style, he didn't realize that members of his group were following him but resenting him personally. The situation was such that they perceived themselves as peers. Thus the members appreciated the structure but believed that Lewis's autocratic leadership style was inappropriate for the situation—because they were all volunteers.

Perhaps members who are task oriented do not depend as much on the leader as do non-task-oriented participants. If this is the case, then it might explain Jurma's findings. But, beyond this inference, as a leader you need to be aware of two important principles. The first is that if you are confronted by a group of participants who are not task oriented, it would be wise to pursue a structuring style. (Jurma also discovered that discussions led by highly structuring leaders were judged by independent raters as being of higher quality than discussions led by nonstructuring leaders.) The second is that, in general, a democratic structuring style *produces higher satisfaction and better task performance* than do the nonstructuring and/or autocratic styles.

Functional Perspective

Recall Russ, the management trainee mentioned earlier in this chapter. Perhaps you thought it unwise of him to select a single effective leader and emulate that person's style. You might have suggested instead that he observe several leaders and ask what functions these effective leaders perform for their groups. He could make a list and then concentrate on learning how to provide these important services. This new approach would illustrate the functional perspective.

The functional view of leadership is represented by the question "What might a leader do to manage a group successfully?" Asking such a question invites long lists of leadership behaviors. Such lists can be both helpful and confusing. A person might discover from such lists some things to do when leading. Lists also can provide guidance in developing various leadership skills. But if the number of items on the list is great, it may be more confusing than helpful. One way to cope with this problem is to divide leadership into functional categories: task, procedural, and social.

Task leadership functions facilitate group processing and thinking about the task, such as generating ideas and information, processing that information, thinking critically about decisions, and clarifying ideas. These functions help the group to process information. Often we think about and work with the task and think that we are being productive. Productivity here is highly dependent on quality of thought. Securing the appropriate information and carefully processing it is the key. A skillful leader will help the group to be more productive in this area by helping the group analyze and decide about the task systematically.

Procedural leadership functions guide a group, or help the group members to work together smoothly and efficiently. A procedurally aware leader focuses on setting an agenda, regulating participation, summarizing group progress, and verbalizing consensus. These functions make a difference for most groups, but are difficult for many leaders to fulfill. Since they do not pertain directly to the discussion of the task, they are often overlooked. The skillful leader will realize the need for such guidance and will be careful to provide it.

Social leadership functions encourage and promote aspects of the social dimension. You may recall from Chapter 1 that this social dimension is critical to a group's success. Social leadership may sometimes cause a group to be diverted from its task. Although social leadership may serve an important purpose for the group, it is not directly task related. Robert Bales[8] was the first to demonstrate that the task and social-emotional leadership functions were generally performed by different persons.

The functional perspective is an attractive one because it links actual behaviors with leadership in groups. It answers the question of what a person needs to do to cause a group to be successful. This perspective is addressed under the topic of how to lead.

Situational Perspective

Support for the situational view had its beginning in the early 1930s and the 1940s. Emory Bogardus[9] suggested that "a person may be generally consistent [in leadership traits] in some situations and inconsistent in others." Similarly, Albert J. Murphy[10] argued that the traits a person demonstrates may change from situation to situation. A person who is assertive in a familiar situation may be reticent in an unfamiliar situation. Those who thought that the situational perspective made sense were given convincing evidence by the Office of Strategic Services (OSS) Assessment Staff Report, published in 1948.[11]

The OSS trained people to carry out secret missions in enemy territory during World War II. Staff members trained candidates to be able to respond to general situations, and they assessed their general aptitude for leadership. The assessment staff solicited ratings of the people they trained from area commanders and fellow returnees, and with that information they generated a leadership score based on actual performance. The correlation between leadership traits and actual leadership was discouragingly low (+.11). Because the trainees were exposed to very specific leadership situations in the overseas areas, researchers concluded that specific situational factors influence the emergence of leaders and their behavior in groups.

Since the initial efforts of the Office of Strategic Services, many other researchers have attempted to discover how various situational variables might affect leadership and leadership emergence. For example, Ralph M. Stogdill[12] and his colleagues investigated the effect of transferring Navy officers to new assignments. They found that an officer's style of interpersonal behavior did not change, but that patterns of work performance did change according to the new requirements of the situation. Contrast the difference in performance that a gruff, impersonal style might make here. An officer is in charge of a unit of recruits. His pattern of handling the task is close supervision. He is transferred to an administrative unit. His interpersonal style does not change, but now the task-handling pattern is more permissive. What difference do you think the situation will make in this person's success as a leader?

C. David Mortensen[13] also believes that leadership emergence is situational. He found that members showed more leadership attempts when they were reinforced and supported by the group. Suppose that you were the leader of a group. You can imagine that you would spend more time guiding the group if members reacted positively to your attempts.

Marvin E. Shaw[14] concluded that leadership emergence is dependent on the person's place in the communication network. Those who occupy a central position in the communication network frequently emerge as leaders. At a table a central place is one in which all members can be seen by this person. This is often the end of a rectangular table. The person seated there will more often emerge as leader.

Finally, Cal W. Downs and Terry Pickett[15] showed that an interrelated set of variables dramatically affects leadership emergence. Leadership style, group compatibility, and the nature of the discussion situation were key variables they studied. As you might imagine, both from our discussion and from your personal experience, leadership emergence is a complex process. There are no easy answers to how it operates, but the research is very promising because it appears to offer hope that we will someday understand how to manage the emergence of leadership. Even given the limits of this research, it is possible to suggest some practical applications:

1. If you wish to emerge as leader, say so, if given the opportunity.

2. Talk often and to all the group members.

3. Locate yourself physically toward the center of the group, or assume a position that will provide you with ready access to all the group members. For example, take a position at the head of the table if you wish to emerge as leader.

4. Know what you're talking about.

Contingency Perspective

Imagine that you are reporting for a job as supervisor in a department of ten people. You are in a relatively weak power position, since they do not know you well and you've had little experience with them. In addition, your job is to supervise a sales force and you know that selling represents a fairly unstructured task. Finally, you recall that you met several of the sales representatives and basically got along. Therefore you believe that word has gotten around that you are a pleasant person and you suspect that people assess your relationship with them as good. Thus your position is like this:

Leader–member relationships: Good

Task structure: Unstructured

Position power: Weak

Once you know these things, what approach would you take to leadership? This is the type of question that contingency leadership research is trying to answer.

Fred E. Fiedler[16] looked indirectly at this question. He identified situation-control dimensions that involved a leader's position power, the task structure, and leader-member relations. Then he ordered these into a continuum of favorableness of the situation to the leader. Table 7.2 displays the ordering based on favorableness. For example, the highest favorableness of the situation for a leader would be when the leader-member relations were good, the task was structured (a step-by-step procedure could be followed), and the leader was powerful (strong).

Next Fiedler measured the effectiveness of two leader motivational orientations—task oriented and relationship oriented—on the basis of the criterion of group productivity. He assumed that an orientation toward task suggests that the person sees the job of leader as especially involving task management. Likewise, an orientation toward relationships suggests that the person sees the job as emphasizing relationships—that is, finding acceptance for self and members. Such a leader might be somewhat more concerned with relationships than with task. Fiedler found that leaders who are highly

TABLE 7.2 The Situational-Control Dimension

Favorable Situation Control						Unfavorable Situation Control	
Octant							
I	II	III	IV	V	VI	VII	VIII
Relations							
Good	Good	Good	Good	Poor	Poor	Poor	Poor
Structure							
Structured		Unstructured		Structured		Unstructured	
Power							
Strong	Weak	Strong	Weak	Strong	Weak	Strong	Weak

Source: Adapted by permission of *Harvard Business Review.* Exhibit from F. E. Fiedler, "Engineer the Job to Fit the Manager," *Harvard Business Review,* September–October 1965, 118. Copyright © by the President and Fellows of Harvard College. All rights reserved.

task oriented function best in highly favorable and highly unfavorable situations. In the favorable situation, the leader can be controlling without arousing negative reactions because things are going well. On the other hand, in the unfavorable situation, when things are going badly, directive leadership is required to keep the group from coming apart. Fiedler seems to be suggesting that the leader place the emphasis on task, allowing maximum effort in that direction.

Relationship-oriented leaders did not function as well in favorable conditions, presumably because of the structured nature of the task. On the other hand, the relationship-oriented leaders were more productive under both moderately favorable and moderately unfavorable conditions. In the moderately favorable situation, the task is unstructured and the leader generates the willingness and creativity of the group members to accomplish their goal by attention to the relationship. In the moderately unfavorable condition, the task is structured but the leader is not well liked. Here the relationship-oriented leader demonstrates care for the emotions of the group members and is successful in generating productivity. The task-oriented leader would presumably not meet these social needs and thus would not be as successful.

Data presented by Fiedler and reproduced in Figure 7.1 show that these conclusions are supported by research findings. Some of these findings may not make sense to you. Why would a task-oriented leader do well in an unfavorable setting? Why would a relationship-oriented leader do poorly under favorable leadership conditions? Several years after the original formulation, Fiedler explained this through his *motivational-hierarchy hypothesis.*[17] This hypothesis makes the assumption that people are motivated to attain more than one goal at a particular time. For example, on graduation, a student may wish to marry, take on a full-time job, begin work on an advanced degree, and so forth. However, he or she cannot pursue all these goals at the same time and with the same amount of determination. Therefore the student decides which goals to pursue first, second, third, and so on. The student could arrange these in a motivational hierarchy.

Fiedler suggests that leaders should arrange goals into categories—perhaps extremely important, very important, important, and not very important. Since there is not time to work on all these goals, the leader works on the ones at the upper range of the hierarchy first and with the most vigor. Further, the leader's hierarchy ought to differ

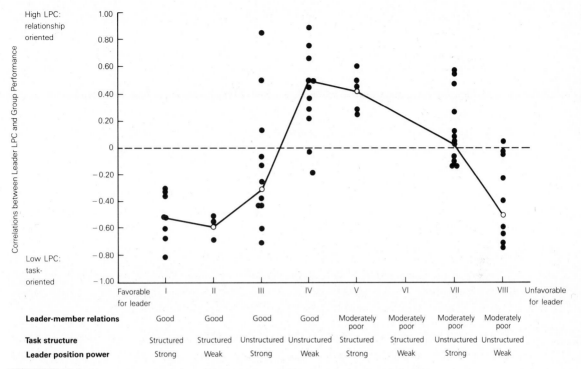

FIGURE 7.1
Fiedler's Data Plotted for Leader Orientation and Group Effectiveness

Source: Reprinted with permission from F. E. Fiedler, *A Theory of Leadership Effectiveness* (New York: McGraw-Hill, 1967).

depending on the person's motivational orientation. Thus a task-oriented leader would be likely to place task goals high on the list, while the relationship-oriented leader would give relationship goals a high placement.

Consider this idea of hierarchy in terms of unfavorable situations. The task-oriented leader would work hardest on moving the group toward completion of its task. The relationship-oriented leader would concentrate on trying to reestablish good interpersonal relationships before concentrating on task goals. On the favorable side of Fiedler's continuum, the task-oriented person can guide the group through its task without much effort. This allows the leader to focus more on being interpersonally supportive. For the relationship-oriented leader, the reverse is the case. The person can focus more attention on task goals. But presumably the person is at a disadvantage as far as quality of task production is concerned, by being less skillful at handling structured tasks.[18]

Cal W. Downs and Terry Pickett[19] examined leadership from a contingency perspective. They investigated the effectiveness of leaders in terms of the degree of social need exhibited by group members. When members had high social needs, task-oriented procedural leaders were most effective. Groups whose members were low on social needs performed best with leaders who were both task oriented *and* person-oriented. Finally, groups whose members had a mixture of high and low social needs performed slightly better when no designated leader was assigned.

What can be concluded from this research is that groups that are heavily involved in the social dimension will benefit from highly task-oriented leadership, but groups whose cohesiveness is low need leadership in both the task and social dimensions. A group that enjoys a balance of high and low social needs will do best if leadership stands out of the way.

It is clear that group members think in terms of contingencies when they describe preferences for leadership style and function. Julia T. Wood[20] asked members of task, social, and mixed task and social groups to respond to a questionnaire. Members of the task- and task-social-oriented groups wanted task-oriented leadership. On the other hand, members of the social-oriented groups wanted a leader high in interpersonal attractiveness and low on task. A moderate level of team spirit was wanted in both situations.

If you have been thinking carefully about these three contingency approaches, you may be discouraged by the idea that a leader has a particular style and thus will be effective only if the particular group situational constraints happen to come together appropriately. There may be some truth to this idea, but it certainly is far from being an absolute. Very convincing evidence shows that *effective leaders are adaptable.* Wood[21] has demonstrated that leaders adapt their behaviors as the situation within the group changes. The leaders in her research changed their behavior from meeting to meeting according to how they perceived the needs and goals of the group. It seems sensible for you to develop the kind of sensitivity and flexibility as a leader to be able to make these kinds of adaptations.

CHARACTERISTICS OF THE EFFECTIVE LEADER

Suppose you are convinced that you would like to be a leader of groups and now you are ready to begin a program in earnest toward the goal of improving your leadership. Where would you start? Are there certain things you can do to build skill in this area? Obviously there are. This section of the chapter will take some of the ideas that have already been presented and use them to generate five general characteristics of good leadership. Specifically, personal communication skills will be presented, and the research evidence to support them will be pointed to. These are skills that you can develop. Here are some specific suggestions as to how you can implement these ideas.

Effective leaders are well informed.   This statement seems noncontroversial, but many potential leaders seem to ignore it. Consider a man who was appointed to head an important policy committee in his department. He spent the first twenty minutes of each committee meeting discovering "what we ought to do today." Thus, when he was finally ready for the group to do something, neither he nor the other members had the information necessary to approach the task adequately. Sometimes he got lucky because one or two members were well informed, but frequently they struggled through the hour. Do not let this happen to you. You must do your homework if you are to be successful. This means investigating the topic, considering alternatives, and perhaps even laying out a complete analysis so that you can have the ideas firmly in your mind. Studies consistently show a high correlation between task ability and effective leadership.[22]

An effective leader provides direction and structure to the group.   This statement has face validity. In most groups you will need to organize and direct the task. But directing is more than giving orders. Good leaders are generally good planners. You must be able to organize a task before you can organize a group. A leader often uses an agenda to accomplish this end. It seems to be good advice to suggest that a leader circulate that agenda—that plan—so that group members can use it while they prepare for discussion. Refer to Chapter 3 for several agendas you might consider.

Effective leaders are skillful communicators.   This means that leaders are, first of all, active participators. Research suggests that leaders have a tendency to talk more than the average member of a group.[23] Not only do they talk more than the average member of a group, they also communicate better. Leaders tend to be more fluent and more confident, and to speak more frequently, than the average group member.

Being a skillful communicator also means being sensitive and adaptive to the changing needs of members. Leading successfully necessitates being aware of where group members are at any particular moment. This is accomplished by careful observation and evaluation of both verbal and nonverbal cues. Wood[24] is among those whose research supports this need. You may recall that she discovered that effective leaders were sensitive to the changes in a group and adapted to them. For example, you might discover through careful attention to feedback that your group is experiencing tension. Perhaps it is frustrated with a particular member. You might take time to talk through this issue with the group. Chapter 10 provides help for making decisions about working through differences with members.

An effective leader is able to adapt leadership style to meet the needs of the group. Fiedler points out the need for different kinds of leadership based on three contingencies: leader-member relationships, task structure, and power position. Recall that a highly task-oriented leadership style seems best under conditions of high and low favorableness for the leader. The social-oriented leadership style works best in situations of moderate favorableness for the leader. A leader can take on the appropriate style as the circumstance changes. (This is the conclusion Wood reached in her research.) A good leader will be sensitive to the group's current situation and adapt to meet changing needs.

Effective leadership results from adopting a "democratic" style.   There are quotation marks around "democratic" for an important reason. Pure democratic style is unlikely to exist in real contexts. There are more likely to be degrees of democracy. The idea that a democratic leader tends to be more effective is supported by extensive research.[25]

Autocratic leaders have a tendency to impose their will upon the group, thus creating a decision-making situation of pseudo-discussion. You have probably attended meetings in a work context where the boss called the group together "to make a decision," but meant instead "to announce a decision and discuss it." Most of us would not call this real discussion.

Much of what is known about decision making suggests that autocratic leadership violates the aims of small group discussion. Groups make decisions to take advantage of available experiences with the situation. Groups make decisions to secure their commitment to the final decision. Groups are called together so that the members can feel included—included in the group and included in the organization. Groups are called together so that the members of the organization will know that they are being taken into account. These are group- and organization-centered goals. Autocratic-style leaders often pursue leader-centered goals.

Some people confuse autocratic leadership with the desire for structure. So one final point remains to be made. Autocratic leadership and structuring behavior are not the same thing. Although leaders generally feel a need to control, there is a very important difference. Autocrats generally try to *impose* their control on a group. Democrats generally approach the matter of control by careful planning of a structure—either by presenting a plan and asking the group to ratify that plan or by asking the group to evolve a task structure on its own.

IMPROVING YOUR LEADERSHIP SKILL

The suggestions presented here are most easily implemented if the leader understands the major responsibilities involved and has a specific plan to implement them. You must know what is involved and how to carry out the duty. Thus there are five major areas of responsibility that a successful leader will attempt to manage:

1. Preparing for the meeting.

2. Structuring and guiding the group activity.

3. Stimulating creative and critical thinking.

4. Managing conflict.

5. Promoting cohesiveness.

Several of these responsibilities will be addressed in detail in separate chapters. Chapter 8 is devoted to a discussion of cohesiveness and how you can work to create it. Chapter 10 focuses on the topic of conflict, suggesting the nature of conflict and several strategies for managing it. Here the remaining issues are addressed: a leader's preparation for a meeting, structuring and guiding the group activity, and stimulating creative and critical thinking.

Preparing for Leading a Meeting

It would be unusual to find a successful leader who did not prepare for a meeting. Most leaders do prepare, of course, but some are more successful than others because their preparation is more thorough. Consider the new manager Carl, who called his supervisors together to prepare a request for his next year's budget. Some prepared a fifteen-minute talk that laid out what they needed. Others did the same but provided justifications and had supporting documents. Those supervisors went away with what they needed for their departments. This outcome might have been different if the unsuccessful managers had had a planning check like the one below. Careful preparation involves formulating a statement of purpose, gathering research and information, soliciting input about purpose and agenda, contacting members, and setting the meeting place. Here is a checklist and comments:

___ 1. *Make a clear statement of purpose or purposes.*

Too often people think they know what their goals are but really do not have a very clear picture. Writing a statement of purpose tends to fix goals more firmly in your mind. You can circulate the statement and ask for feedback from the group members. This will give members the opportunity to ask for clarification if anything is not clear. It may also—and almost certainly will—lead to a more focused and productive meeting. A group might sometimes want to spend a whole meeting clarifying goals. For example, task forces or ad hoc groups often undertake complex, perplexing problems. A meeting or two to lay out goals is clearly in order. A group should always be involved in goal setting if views may differ. Solicit opinions about the agenda. State a tentative goal and ask for feedback. Ask, "Are there any ideas in this statement that seem unclear?" "Is this the direction we should move in to handle this issue?" Sometimes circulating members' comments with the agenda stimulates discussion and provides a context for goal planning.[26]

___ 2. *Take time to do research on the subject or subjects.*

One of the distinguishing characteristics of effective leaders is that they know more about the issues than the other group members. Do you? If you do not—and sometimes even if you do—you need to get informed. Formulate questions that, when answered, will allow you to be informed. Ask experts; read; do some observation in the field. Get informed, whatever it takes.

For several years one of us has been observing the college academic program planning committee. This committee is constituted anew each year. Sometimes uninformed members get selected by this group to lead. They fail miserably. What happens is that a more informed member usually emerges as the group's leader. You see, being well informed is impressive and a source of influence. You can be both an effective and an influential leader by being informed.

___ 3. *Construct an agenda for the meeting.*

Publishing an agenda is an essential part of being a good leader of groups.

Consider the problem created for a group by a leader who does not announce an agenda. The result is ill-prepared members who have to suffer a good deal of discomfort and who cannot contribute in any meaningful way.

The agenda may be a brief list of the topics to be covered. However, if it is expected that a group will be involved in decision making about a complex problem, or will be considering a situation about which members are not informed, wise leadership will include questions under each area of a standard problem-solving agenda. But be sure to adapt the agenda to your group's needs. These questions will help members focus their efforts to prepare, and the meeting will run more smoothly. Chapter 3 provides help in selecting and adapting an agenda. The agenda should be circulated three or four days in advance so that members will have time to prepare. Bring additional copies to the meeting so that forgetful and busy members who misplaced or forgot their copies can be "covered" without embarrassment.

___ 4. *Select members on the basis of their expertise and secure their commitment to attend.*

A group of five to seven people has been shown to be a good size for productive meetings, although a somewhat larger group whose members have experience working together can be very productive too. Selecting members can be a difficult task. Expertise and ability to get along are very important criteria. Asking two people with similar experience and expertise may duplicate effort unwisely, especially in business contexts. On the other hand, such duplication may be wise. Our point is that the matter of duplication ought to be considered. As a general principle, it is important to find willing participants. Tell them directly what they will be doing and listen to what they say. If a person seems reluctant to serve, try somebody else. Look to Chapter 2 for assistance in selecting members.

___ 5. *Review the comments of the participants, revise the agenda, and select a meeting place.*

Review the comments of the participants about your plan and take them into account. This step can save much group time later.

Once you have the agenda set, you are ready to select a meeting place. Be sure the room is appropriate in size. If your group is small, be sure to pick a room that will accommodate them. Too much space and empty chairs detract from a sense of "groupness." Discover whether the group needs work space. If members will need to spread out papers, you need to know that there is space to do so. Location can also be important. It might be wise to hold the meeting in a certain building if most of the group members work there. Occasionally you may have a group member in a wheelchair. Can that person gain easy access? If it is a long meeting—perhaps one and one-half to two hours in length—is there an area for a coffee break? This can help the group relax and thus be more productive. Is the room well lighted and comfortable? Are restrooms close by?

Structuring and Guiding the Group Activity

Observers rate groups whose leaders are skillful at task structuring as better than groups that do not have such leadership. Structure is necessary for planning and coordinating group effort. So the leader should circulate the agenda, write a clear statement of goals, secure group agreement on the agenda, and take responsibility for initiating and maintaining the discussion. Initiating and maintaining the discussion involves such activities as keeping the group goal oriented, introducing new agenda items, encouraging people to talk, regulating participation, summarizing group progress, and verbalizing consensus.[27]

Beatrice Schultz predicted, for eight of nine groups, who would become leader on the basis of the communicative functions members performed. Leaders were more goal directed, direction giving, summary giving, and self-assured than other members. So it seems that members need to cultivate some functional behaviors if they are to emerge as group leaders.[28] Further, Gregory Dobbins and Stephen Zaccaro found that members of groups with leaders high in initiating structure and consideration were more cohesive and satisfied than members of groups whose leaders were low on these behaviors.[29]

These are behaviors that mark the difference between successful and less successful groups. And they are behaviors that any member can contribute to the group process. Certainly every group leader should be able to perform them, and the best way to learn how is to practice.

Inevitably, students want to know what to say or do in order to accomplish the activities just suggested. Some language and strategies that are useful in each of these structuring and guiding activities follow.

1. Keep the Group Goal-Oriented

PROBLEM
Group is digressing too much into social conversation.

LANGUAGE AND / OR STRATEGY
1. Comment on the social issue being discussed and then say, "Now, let's move back to our discussion of causes."

2. "I don't understand how this idea is relevant to our task. Is it? If not, we need to get back to the topic."

PROBLEM
Member persists in an effort to digress from the agenda.

LANGUAGE AND / OR STRATEGY
1. "I've noticed that we seem to keep getting off the track and haven't been making our usual progress. I'm concerned that we might not meet our goal. I'm wondering what the group thinks about this."

2. "How is it we get sidetracked? What can we do about it?"

    3. "What should I do if we get off the subject again?" Then guide the group back to the subject.

2. Introducing New Agenda Items

PROBLEM
Group is ready and needs to move on to the next agenda item.

LANGUAGE AND / OR STRATEGY
    1. "So, we've agreed. . . . [Summarize.] Let's take up the next item."

    2. "So, we've agreed. . . . [Summarize.] Are we ready to take up the next item?"

    3. "The next item asks us to determine what, if anything, should be done about . . ."

3. Encourage Members to Participate

PROBLEM
Member doesn't participate because of shyness or reserve.

LANGUAGE AND / OR STRATEGY
    1. "Recently I was talking with [name of reticent member], who had an interesting [or useful, or insightful] comment. [Name], would you be willing to share your idea?" You need to be sure to discuss some aspect of the issue with this reticent person before the meeting.

    2. "[Name], you heard Susan. Do you agree or wish to add to her comment?"

PROBLEM
Member doesn't seem to be "with" the group; is distracted or working on some private agenda.

LANGUAGE AND / OR STRATEGY
    1. "I think it would be a good idea to take stock of where we are. [Name], will you agree that we've. . . . [Summarize.]"

    2. "[Name], what do you think about [the topic of discussion]?"

    3. "[Name], you seem to be off somewhere. I was wondering if . . ."

PROBLEM
Member appears not to be informed, is fearful others will discover lack of preparation.

LANGUAGE AND / OR STRATEGY
    1. "[Name], will you help me [or recorder] record these ideas? We want to be sure we keep a group memory. [Name], will you review . . ."

Note: Usually you will not be able to know why people are avoiding involvement, so you must proceed with some caution. However, your goal is to involve these people right from the beginning. Often they will not contribute anything if you do not involve them in the first few minutes. So be alert to this problem and do something about it right away. Be careful to encourage without embarrassing. For example, if you ask someone what he or she knows about a particular issue—and the person doesn't know anything about it—you may not be able to get him or her to participate at all. If you anticipate the problem and are able to control seating arrangements, seat that person across from you. Try at first to use eye contact to encourage participation.

4. Regulate Participation

PROBLEM
Member monopolizes the interaction.

LANGUAGE AND/OR STRATEGY
1. Avoid excessive eye contact with talkative person. Establish eye contact with others to encourage them to talk.

2. Ask group members to agree to make only one point when they get the floor.

3. Break in and say, "That is an interesting idea. Let's consider . . . first, John. Then we will come back to your other idea."

4. Approach the talker in private. Tell the person you are concerned about some of the quiet members. Ask the person to help draw them out.

5. Bring it up directly in the group. If the problem seems to persist, you may have to deal with it straightforwardly. Try to be supportive, but make sure that it is seen as a problem for which the group must come up with an answer.

5. Summarize Group Progress

PROBLEM
People get caught up in the interaction and lose track of their progress.

LANGUAGE AND/OR STRATEGY
1. Summarize. "Let's see what we've done so far. . . ."

PROBLEM
Group needs encouragement.

LANGUAGE AND/OR STRATEGY
1. Summarize.

2. Point out the agreement the group has had thus far. Congratulate the group on its progress.

6. *Reducing Tension Levels*

PROBLEM
Tension in the group is high.

LANGUAGE AND/OR STRATEGY
1. "We've been working pretty hard. Let's take a break."

2. Use humor, if you are skillful at humor, to divert the group and lighten the mood.

Some leaders attempt to use humor in their effort to guide the group. If they make this choice, they need to give attention to the type of humor employed. A study by Christi McGuffee Smith and Larry Powell found that the target of the humor made a difference in its effect.[30] When the leader chose himself or herself as the target, the humor was perceived as more effective at relieving tension and encouraging participation, and the leader was seen as being more willing to share opinions. Leaders who targeted their superiors were seen as less helpful to the group and less willing to share opinions. Leaders who targeted subordinates received lower ratings on social attractiveness and lower ratings as tension relievers and summarizers of members' input.

Stimulating Creative and Critical Thinking

There is no magic you can perform to cause people to think creatively or critically. You can encourage people in these directions, but there are no guarantees. Consider what you can do to encourage group thinking.

1. *Stimulate Creativity*

PROBLEM
How to stimulate creativity.

LANGUAGE AND/OR STRATEGY
1. Urge people to go beyond the normal constraints of their thinking. Much of our thinking seems to be boxed in by our private perceptions of an event.

2. Encourage people to listen to others' ideas and to try to expand on good ones they hear.

3. Divide the issue and consider each part separately. This often promotes a more focused and in-depth investigation.

4. Talk members through the process of formally engaging in brainstorming. Using the formal procedure gives people permission to step out of their normal roles.

5. Try to encourage members to provide several alternatives. Actually ask them to say more. Point out the benefits of considering a variety of viewpoints.

2. *Promote Critical Thinking*

PROBLEM

How to promote critical thinking.

LANGUAGE AND/OR STRATEGY

1. Agree with members that each person has the responsibility for helping to evaluate the information.

2. Spend some time asking the group to generate a list of "how" questions. Such a list might include:
    a. How do you know this is true?
    b. How does this information apply to the problem?
    c. How does the source of the information know?
    d. How were the statistics collected?
    e. How well do our criteria apply to these solutions?
    f. How well will this solution work when we try it?

   Once these questions are ready, you might place them on a flip chart where they can be seen.

Obviously you should not memorize the language used here. These suggestions are made to trigger your imagination so that you will be able to develop your own language and strategies for these problems.

SUMMARY

Several issues related to leadership have been addressed. A distinction between the terms *leadership* and *leader* was drawn. Leadership is an influence process that is directed toward group goal achievement. On the other hand, a leader refers to a person who either is appointed to lead or emerges as the leader.

Several leadership perspectives were presented: the trait perspective, the style perspective, the functional perspective, the situational perspective, and the contingency perspective. Each of these has made contributions to the understanding of leadership, but the contingency approaches seem most promising.

Five conclusions about effective leaders were suggested:

1. Effective leaders have more experience and skill with the task.

2. Effective leaders provide direction and structure.

3. Effective leaders are skillful communicators.

4. Effective leaders are adaptive.

5. Effective leaders generally adopt a "democratic" style.

Finally, some straightforward suggestions for improving your leadership were given.

A checklist for preparing for a meeting and language and strategy examples for coping with common leadership problems were presented. Topics included keeping the group goal oriented, introducing new agenda items, encouraging participation, regulating participation, summarizing group progress, reducing tension levels, and stimulating creative and critical thinking.

EXERCISES

1. Describe and analyze your group's leadership. Include (a) task leadership, (b) social leadership, (c) leadership styles, (d) leadership adequacy, and (e) suggestions for leadership improvement.

2. Write your own definition of leadership and bring it to class. In small groups, compare your definition with those of other members of your group. How are they similar? How are they different? Try to come to a definition that all members of your group find satisfactory. Present the group definitions of leadership to the class for discussion.

3. Identify the best leader of a small group that you have personally experienced. Identify the worst leader. Make a list of the characteristics that account for their being categorized as best and worst leaders. Now compare your list with those of your classmates. Is there any similarity? If so, what characteristics are similar? Write a two-page paper that describes this experience and accounts for the results.

4. In a small group, role-play these leadership problems. Rotate the role of leader among group members. Make sure each situation is role-played at least twice. After each role-playing experience, discuss the effectiveness of the leader's actions. Here are the situations:
   a. A leader is trying to involve a nonparticipating member.
   b. A member is continually moving the group away from the task.
   c. A leader wants to discourage an overly talkative member.
   d. A leader wants to resolve an interpersonal conflict and get on with the task.
   e. A leader wants to help members who are engaged in conflict over ideas understand one another.
   f. A leader wants to motivate an apathetic group member.

5. As a group project, prepare a thirty-minute training session on leadership effectiveness. Present your program to the class.

6. Carry out an analysis of the leadership in a group of which you are a part. This could be a group from your small group communication class. Is there a task leader? Is there a social leader? If so, name these people and describe their leadership styles. Identify their leadership behaviors. What is your assessment of the adequacy of the leadership in your group? What suggestions would you make for improving the leadership? Perhaps the leadership is shared. If so, conduct the same analysis, but focus on leadership instead of a particular leader. Write a short essay describing the leadership in your group using these questions as a guide.

7. Work with your instructor to invite to class professional people from the community who are in leadership positions and who work with small decision-making groups. Prepare a schedule of questions that will allow them to talk about their leadership experiences. The idea is to gain insight into how these people handle various leadership problems.

8. Refer back to your responses to the leadership questionnaire presented in Table 7.1. You probably have a dominate leadership style with supporting styles. Paul Hersey and Kenneth Blanchard have called these styles, taken together, your style range, as illustrated in Figure 7.2. This is the extent to which you perceive yourself to be able to vary your leadership style. Record on a piece of paper the column in which each of your responses falls, using the codes in Figure 7.3 as a guide. Now, count up the number of responses assigned to each column. Each column corresponds to the similarly numbered quadrant of basic leader behavior styles presented in Figure 7.2. The quadrant with the highest number is presumed to be your dominate style. Your range is limited if your responses fall only in one quadrant. If the responses are spread over several quadrants, then you perceive yourself to have a wider range of leader behavior.

NOTES

1. Marvin E. Shaw, *Group Dynamics: The Psychology of Small Group Behavior* (New York: McGraw-Hill, 1981), 317.

2. See, for example, R. D. Mann, "A Review of the Relationships Between Personality and Performance in Small Groups," *Psychological Bulletin*, 56 (1959), 241–270; Barbara P. Guyer, "The Relationship Among Selected Variables and the Effectiveness of Discussion Leaders," *Dissertation Abstracts International*, 39, No. 2A (1978):697–698.

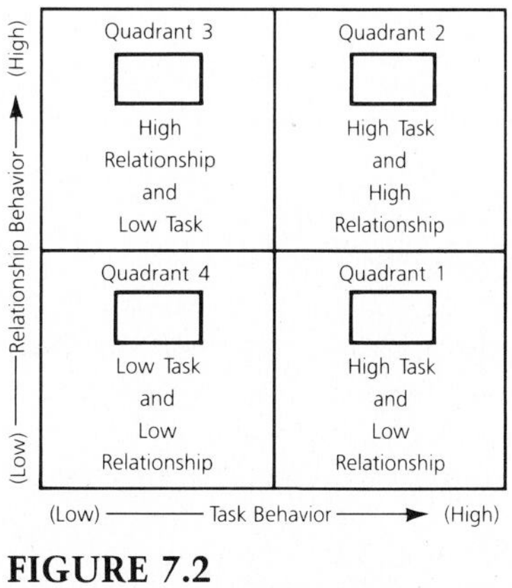

FIGURE 7.2
The Basic Leader Behavior Styles

Source: Paul Hersey and Kenneth H. Blanchard, "So You Want to Know Your Leadership Style?," *Training and Development Journal* 28 (February 1974):23–24.

	(Style Range) Alternative Actions			
Situations	(1)	(2)	(3)	(4)
1	A	C	B	D
2	D	A	C	B
3	C	A	D	B
4	B	D	A	C
5	C	B	D	A
6	B	D	A	C
7	A	C	B	D
8	C	B	D	A
9	C	B	D	A
10	B	D	A	C
11	A	C	B	D
12	C	A	D	B
Subcolumns	(1)	(2)	(3)	(4)

FIGURE 7.3
Determining Leadership Style and Style Range

Source: Paul Hersey and Kenneth H. Blanchard, "So You Want to Know Your Leadership Style?," *Training and Development Journal* 28 (February 1974):23–24.

3. Guyer, 697.

4. Ralph K. White and Ronald Lippitt, "Leader Behavior and Member Reaction in Three 'Social Climates,' " in Dorwin Cartwright and Alvin Zander, eds., *Group Dynamics: Research and Theory*, 2d. ed. (Evanston, Ill.: Row, Peterson, 1960), 527–553.

5. James F. Sargent and Gerald R. Miller, "Some Differences in Certain Behaviors of Autocratic and Democratic Leaders," *Journal of Communication* 21 (1971): 233–252.

6. Lawrence B. Rosenfeld and Timothy B. Pax, "Personality Determinants of Autocratic and Democratic Leadership," *Speech Monographs* 42 (1975): 203–208.

7. William E. Jurma, "Effects of Leader Structuring Style and Task-Orientation Characteristics of Group Members," *Communication Monographs* 46 (1979): 282–295.

8. Robert Bales was the first researcher to demonstrate that the task and social-emotional leadership functions were generally performed by different persons. See "Task Roles and Social Roles in Problem-Solving Groups, in E. E. Maccoby, T. M. Newcomb, and E. L. Hartley, eds., *Readings in Social Psychology*, 3d ed. (New York: Holt, Rinehart and Winston, 1958), 437–447.

9. Emory S. Bogardus, "Leadership and Social Situations," *Sociology and Social Research* 16 (1931–32):165.

10. Albert J. Murphy, "A Study of the Leadership Process," *American Sociological Review* 6 (1941):674–687.

11. OSS Assessment Staff. *The Assessment of Men* (New York: Rinehart, 1948).

12. Ralph M. Stogdill, Carroll L. Shartle, E. L. Scott, Alvin E. Coons, and W. E. Jaynes, *A Predictive Study of Administrative Work Patterns* (Columbus: Ohio State University, Bureau of Research, 1956).

13. C. David Mortensen, "Should a Group Have an Assigned Leader?" *Speech Teacher* 15 (1966):34–41.

14. Marvin E. Shaw and G. H. Rothschild, "Some Effects of Prolonged Experiences in Communication Nets," *Journal of Applied Psychology* 40 (1956):281–286.

15. Cal W. Downs and Terry Pickett, "An Analysis of the Effect of Nine Leadership Group Compatibility Contingencies Upon Productivity and Member Satisfaction," *Communication Monographs* 44 (1977):220–230.

16. Fred E. Fiedler, *A Theory of Leadership Effectiveness.* (New York: McGraw-Hill, 1967).

17. Fred E. Fiedler and M. M. Chemers, *Leadership and Effective Management* (Glenview, Ill.: Scott, Foresman, 1974); Fred E. Fiedler, "The Contingency Model and the Dynamics of the Leadership Process," in Leonard Berkowitz, ed., *Advances in Experimental Psychology*, vol. 12 (New York: Academic Press, 1978).

18. Donelson R. Forsyth, *An Introduction to Group Dynamics* (Monterey, Calif.: Brooks/Cole, 1983), 227.

19. Downs and Pickett, 220–230.

20. Julia T. Wood, "Alternate Portraits of Leaders: A Contingency Approach to Perceptions of Leadership," *Western Journal of Speech Communication* 43 (1979):260–270.

21. Julia T. Wood, "Leading in Purposive Discussions: A Study of Adaptive Behavior," *Communication Monographs* 44 (1977):152–165.

22. G. J. Palmer, Jr., "Task Ability and Effective Leadership," Technical Report No. 4, Contract

No. 1575(05), No. 6, Contract No. 1575(05), Louisiana State University, 1962, cited in Marvin E. Shaw, *Group Dynamics* (New York: McGraw-Hill, 1981), 190.

23. R. M. Stogdill, *Handbook of Leadership* (New York: The Free Press, 1974); R. T. Stein and T. Heller, "An Empirical Analysis of the Correlations Between Leadership Status and Participation Rates Reported in the Literature," *Journal of Personality and Social Psychology* 37 (1979):1993–2002.

24. Wood (1977), 152–165.

25. See Shaw, *Group Dynamics*, 326–331.

26. The issue of goal setting is a very important one for a leader. For an excellent review of the research in this area, see E. A. Locke, K. N. Shaw, L. M. Saari, and G. P. Latham, "Goal Setting and Task Performance: 1969–1980," *Psychological Bulletin* 90 (1981):125–152.

27. One researcher found that groups that spent more time engaged in these activities were judged as more effective. See Randy Y. Hirokawa, "A Comparative Analysis of Communication Patterns Within Effective and Ineffective Decision-Making Groups," *Communication Monographs* 47 (1980):312–321.

28. Beatrice Schultz, "Communicative Correlates of Perceived Leaders in the Small Group," *Small Group Behavior* 17 (1986):51–65.

29. Gregory H. Dobbins and Stephen J. Zaccaro, "The Effects of Group Cohesion and Leadership Behavior on Subordinate Satisfaction," *Group and Organizational Studies* 11 (1986):203–219.

30. Christi McGuffee Smith and Larry Powell, "The Use of Disparaging Humor by Group Leaders," *Southern Speech Communication Journal* 53 (1988):279–292.

RECOMMENDED READINGS

Martin M. Chemers, "The Social, Organizational, and Cultural Context of Effective Leadership," in Robert S. Cathcart and Larry A. Samovar, eds. *Small Group Communication: A Reader*, 5th ed. (Dubuque, Iowa: Wm. C. Brown, 1988), 463–482.

Fred E. Fiedler, "A Contingency Model of Leadership Effectiveness, in Leonard Berkowitz, ed., *Advances in Experimental Social Psychology* (New York: McGraw-Hill, 1967).

H. Lloyd Goodall, Jr., *Small Group Communication* (Dubuque, Iowa: Wm. C. Brown, 1985), Chapter 5, "Leading the Small Group."

Victor H. Vroom and Arthur G. Jago, *The New Leadership: Managing Participation in Organizations* (Englewood Cliffs, N.J.: Prentice-Hall, 1988).

Ralph K. White and Ronald Lippit, "Leader Behavior and Member Reaction in Three 'Social Climates,' " in Dorin Cartwright and Alvin Zander, eds., *Group Dynamics: Research and Theory*, 2d ed. (Evanston, Ill.: Row, Peterson, 1960), 527–553.

Julia T. Wood, "Leading in Purposive Discussion: A Study of Adaptive Behavior," *Communication Monographs* 44 (1977):152–165.

CHAPTER 8

Promoting Group Cohesiveness

OBJECTIVES

After reading this chapter you should be able to:

Describe and explain the relationship between cohesiveness and productivity.

Specify the determinants of cohesiveness.

Identify and explain the sources of member satisfaction in groups, and relate those sources of satisfaction to the particular behaviors that an individual may contribute in a group meeting.

Specify how each of the following bears upon group cohesiveness: leadership style, group size, effective participation, personal commitment to do one's best, commitment to the good of the group, commitment to cooperation, and commitment to careful listening as well as to group goals.

Explain the fundamental idea of Janis's notion of groupthink, and recall and describe the antecedent conditions from which groupthink emerges.

Specify and explain the symptoms of groupthink: overestimation of the group, closed-mindedness, and pressures toward uniformity.

List seven consequences of groupthink, and specify what group members can do to prevent the groupthink syndrome.

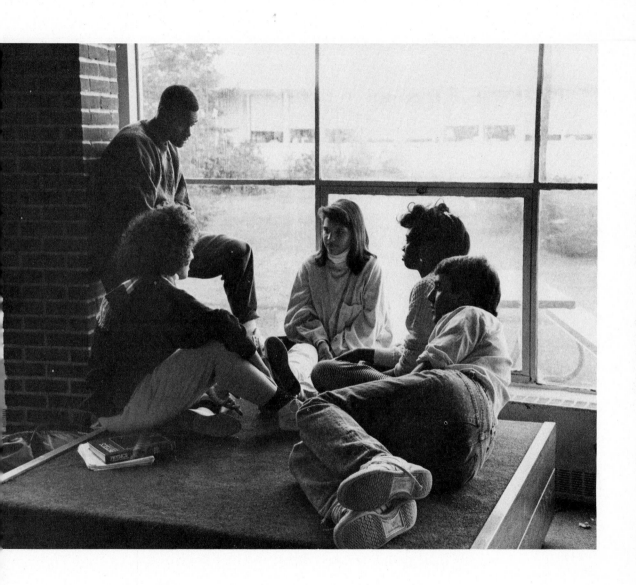

"The best people in our organization are not necessarily the ones we want to call together to solve a problem. Being good is not enough. We need people who can also work together—team players, people who can get along with one another. Get along is not really the right word. I mean people who feel good about one another and want to put together the best answer to the problem they are facing." John Jacobson, a production manager for a mid-sized manufacturing firm, was speaking of what we call cohesiveness. He recognized it as being more important than being "the best people." Certainly he would say that expertise with the situation is important, but experts who cannot pull together are not his notion of an ideal group.

Your own experiences and intuition surely verify this notion. A cohesive group, whether in government or business or in any other context, can consistently perform better than a collection of highly talented individuals. But what attitudes and/or phenomena are at work in cohesive groups? What is missing from groups that are not cohesive?

Recall working in groups that you enjoyed. Undoubtedly those groups were cohesive. The individuals liked one another. They felt committed to some extent to the group's goals. They were willing to work together—to share their successes and their failures. They talked about themselves in collective terms—saying "we" instead of "I" and "our group" instead of "my group." Those characteristics describe cohesiveness.[1] Can you remember how those characteristics evolved? The purpose of this chapter is to describe the determinants of cohesiveness and to suggest how individual members of groups can behave in order to build that sense of cohesiveness.

You may wonder why we want to do this. The answer is simple. An important duty of the leader and members is to build a cohesive group from the raw talents of the members. When they do this successfully, the group has a dramatically improved chance of success. You ought to have the benefits of group success in the groups to which you belong—and you are far more likely to receive those benefits if you know how to build a team. Communication behaviors to affect how groups function—choices well within your ability—will be suggested.[2]

We begin this chapter by describing the relationship between cohesiveness and productivity. Next, we address the topics of determinates of cohesiveness and sources of member satisfaction. From these, we move to consider what leaders and members can do to promote cohesiveness. Finally, the issues of too much cohesiveness and groupthink are explored.

THE RELATIONSHIP BETWEEN COHESIVENESS AND PRODUCTIVITY

Cohesiveness is the degree to which the members of a group are attracted to one another. Productivity, of course, refers to the quality and quantity of a group's output. In every group, both cohesiveness and productivity exist in some degree or amount. Groups may be moderately cohesive or they may be highly cohesive. They may be minimally productive or they may be highly productive. The point is that every group can, to some extent, be described along the lines of its cohesiveness and its productivity.

It is reasonable to suppose that there is a relationship between cohesiveness and productivity. In his review of the literature, Marvin Shaw[3] concluded that, "in spite of some equivocal evidence, it seems evident that the empirical data support the hypothesis that high-cohesive groups are more effective than low-cohesive groups in achieving their goals. The cohesive group does whatever it tries to do better than the noncohesive group." He believed that these two dimensions had a straight-line relationship—the more cohesive the group the greater the productivity. But Shaw provided a word of caution—groups do not always set the same goals for themselves that organizations or outside agencies set for them. Thus, for example, a group might achieve its own goals but be relatively unproductive in terms of the goals that management set for it.

Fisher[4] argues that this dictum—the more cohesive a group, the more productive it is likely to be—is true only up to a point. "The relationship breaks down toward the upper end of the two continuums. Extremely cohesive groups are more likely to have moderate to low productivity." The curvilinear relationship Fisher suggests is illustrated in Figure 8.1. In this figure, the vertical dimension is labeled Productivity. The arrow suggests ever-increasing levels of productivity. Theoretically, the productivity levels that can be reached are without limit. The horizontal dimension is labeled Cohesiveness. Again, the arrow shows increasing levels of cohesiveness.

Fisher suggests that the relationship between cohesiveness and productivity is curvilinear. The curved line in the figure suggests that in a group experiencing low levels of cohesiveness, productivity may be expected to be fairly low. Increasing levels of cohesiveness will yield increasing levels of productivity in task groups—up to a point.

At some point it is possible for a task group to be too cohesive for its own good. If cohesiveness is more intense, productivity suffers, so that the greater the cohesiveness beyond that point, the less the productivity. To illustrate this idea, take a group of friends, all of whom belong to the same church. They have agreed to plan a festival for the church. Their task is clear. They agree to meet at one of the members' houses. One of the members brings refreshments and they snack as they work.

Soon their mood lightens. They begin to enjoy one another's company so much

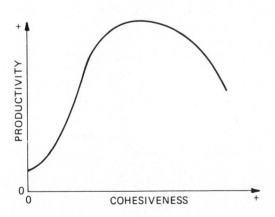

FIGURE 8.1
Relationship between
Cohesiveness and Productivity

that they focus on their relationships rather than on their task. Soon the task group becomes a social group. They are having a party! They set aside their project until another time. Productivity falls dramatically.

Productivity can fall off for another reason when a group becomes too cohesive. Members can value cohesiveness and their relationships with one another so much that they are unwilling to challenge one another's ideas. They fear causing ill will by offending. So they let ideas they have reservations about pass unchallenged. The end product of the group's deliberation may be an inferior decision.

What are the implications of such a curvilinear relationship between cohesiveness and productivity? Members of a task group, and especially those members who wish to influence the success of the group, will do well to monitor the cohesiveness of the group. They should also do everything they can to increase group cohesiveness up to the point at which the group is maximally productive. After that, members who want to help the group succeed will work hard at maintaining the optimum levels of cohesiveness and at keeping the group on the task. Notice from Figure 8.1 that the optimum levels are somewhere in the middle of the horizontal dimension.

Regardless of whether the relationship between the two dimensions is a straight-line relationship or a curvilinear one, the important point is that the dimensions affect each other. That is, productivity has an impact on cohesiveness, and cohesiveness has an impact on productivity. And it is clear that both of these phenomena—productivity and cohesiveness—are the output of the group's work. What, then, can be done by individual group members to affect these important functions of the groups to which they belong? Part of the answer may be found in the evolution of cohesiveness, and that is why this chapter is important to you.

Determinants of Cohesiveness

The evolution of cohesiveness in a group is an enormously complex process. People are attracted to groups for such diverse reasons as the other individuals in the group, the activities that the groups engage in, their own personal need for affiliation, and the like. For example, John very much wanted to join the Junior Chamber of Commerce in the town he had moved to. It is easy to understand that there are good reasons for John to join that particular service and social group. But what is of concern here is why, after joining, he developed such a group loyalty. The explanation lies in the group's cohesiveness, and an analysis of this group's attraction is instructive.

First, John knew that he shared *similar attitudes* with the members of the group.[5] He had shared a dormitory room with someone who was already a member. He spent a good deal of time in social events with members of the group. He was able to identify that he and most Jaycees shared similar value systems—enjoying music and the theater, being rather strongly opposed to violence, placing people and relationships high on their priority lists, and believing that "it's worth working for if it's worth having."

Second, John knew that the group was *successful in its efforts*.[6] The Jaycees were known to be leaders in other contexts. One was vice-president of a local bank. One was sports editor of the daily paper. One had just been elected president of the local ministerial alliance. The Jaycees seemed successful to John in other important and apparent ways. They staged a very popular fund raiser each year called "Blackouts," in which the members sang, played, and danced in a loosely connected series of variety acts. All the parts, all the music, all the scripting, and all the scenery design and directing were carried out by the members. And "Blackouts" was one of the social high points of the year in that small town. In addition, the Jaycees were among the most visible organizations in town, and they regularly came in close to the top in statewide competitions with other chapters. The Jaycees were successful and John wanted to be a part of that success.

Closely related to success, the third characteristic of the group that held John's interest was that it had a *clear sense of how to achieve its goals*.[7]

The members of the group made no bones about their goals. They wanted to be the biggest and the best service club in town. In order to accomplish these twin goals, they focused their attention upon high-visibility activities that produced some evidence of popular judgment—perhaps votes, perhaps trophies, perhaps other kinds of awards. Whatever they could do to get local media coverage was considered important. So was influence in local government if that could be managed. So was mandatory team sports practice. "Blackouts" was a measure of group popularity because the members of the community could tally the number of people who purchased tickets to spend an evening watching the Jaycees. The members of that organization had a very clear notion about how to accomplish their goals.

Perhaps less obvious than similarity of attitudes, success, and clarity of goal path, the Jaycees were attractive to John because of the way they *managed conflict* and because of the kinds of conflict they had.[8]

The members of the Junior Chamber of Commerce were pretty well agreed upon principles. Their conflict almost always centered on the means to the ends and not upon the ends themselves. Thus the regular meetings of the organization included a fairly freewheeling norm. The members debated with one another, using as much evidence and argument as they could muster. Their Wednesday noon meetings thus gave them an opportunity to reinforce one another in the important things—the principles and values they shared—and at the same time to learn about a variety of ways to go about accomplishing their goals. For John, that influence was to become significant later. He joined the Toastmasters Club in order to learn how to present his ideas more effectively in Jaycee meetings.

Finally, the Junior Chamber of Commerce remained attractive to John because the members acted like fraternity brothers. They *reinforced one another*. They talked to one another. They gave one another frequent and positive feedback.[9] They supported one another's personal goal achievements, and they pitched in as individuals to help the group achieve its goals. After each success they staged a well-planned party. In retrospect, its purpose was clearly to provide positive feedback to the members in a symbolically significant and socially pleasant way.

These five determinants of cohesiveness—similarity of attitudes, group success, clear sense of how to achieve goals, conflict management style, frequent and positive reinforcement—are directly applicable to small problem-solving and decision-making groups. Individual members who contribute these functions contribute directly to the cohesiveness of the group. There is a relationship between cohesiveness and member satisfaction in groups, and individual members are largely responsible for the membership satisfaction they and their colleagues experience.

SOURCES OF MEMBER SATISFACTION IN GROUPS

Heslin and Dunphy[10] were concerned about this relationship as early as 1964. As a result of their research, they concluded that membership satisfaction in small groups is dependent upon three dimensions: (1) perceived progress toward group goals, (2) perceived freedom to participate, and (3) status consensus. It seems reasonable to suppose that groups in which these three dimensions of member satisfaction exist will be more cohesive and, consequently, more productive. These three dimensions are generated by individuals talking with one another openly and empathically in an environment in which they feel free to be themselves. And there, in a roundabout fashion, is the key to the whole matter of cohesiveness management. Let us take up these three factors in membership satisfaction one at a time, and then tie them together. This process will yield a set of suggestions for behavior that will promote cohesiveness.

Perceived Freedom to Participate

Anyone who has ever spent time in a classroom (and which of us has not?)—twelve years of elementary and secondary school, and perhaps a few terms at the college level—knows that a typical class includes at least three different approaches to the teaching and learning enterprise. Some students may be counted upon to sit near the front of the room. They may have their pencils sharpened and their notebooks already neatly labeled and catalogued before the class begins. A second group of students may usually be found sitting toward the side of the room. They believe in comparisons, so they talk a lot with one another, refining and focusing their information before they commit to their own conclusions. A third group of students is not a group at all. They scatter themselves around the room. One might take a back-row seat. She listens silently, sometimes taking notes and sometimes merely sitting there. She may never say a word in the classroom. All these students may be enjoying the course, feeling successful as learners, and feeling positive about the instructor and one another. The point is that, while they may or may not talk in the classroom, they believe that they *can* do so if they wish.

Perhaps you have experienced a similar situation. A group to which you belong appears to be making appropriate progress. You feel that you have very little to contribute to the particular conversation so you sit there quietly—sometimes making notes and sometimes just listening. You might be very content about your place in the group, and you might very well feel that both the group and you are being successful. In sum, you are satisfied, even if you do not say anything.

But let the climate change a bit. Suppose that you cannot talk in this group. That is, other members take control and monopolize the floor. Suppose the group climate is such that you do not feel that you are free to participate. At that point, you will experience resentment and dissatisfaction. As long as you perceive that you are free to participate when you choose to do so, you can feel satisfied with a group even though you do not exercise the option to talk. But as soon as the option is removed—or appears to be—you become dissatisfied.

Freedom to participate derives from an environment in which individuals experience themselves as "okay" and, if not equal, at least respected for their views and their essential human dignity. The most important part of that environment, its climate of trust and acceptance, comes from the ways group members talk with one another. They reveal information about themselves and their values. They empathize with one another. They are straight with one another, never coloring the truth, never deliberately misrepresenting themselves or their information. These are functional behaviors that can be learned. It is likely that you have already learned them.

Perceived Progress toward Group Goals

It seems obvious that people in groups must feel that their membership is paying off in some fashion if they are to be satisfied. Given that group goals are one of the primary reasons that individuals become members of groups, it is reasonable to suppose that an individual's satisfaction will depend upon the perception that the group is helping him to achieve what he joined the group to achieve.

Of course, it is easier to perceive progress when progress is being made than when it is not, but either way the perception may be more important than the fact! That perception depends to a large extent upon the conversations that go on in a group. Wise leadership will call frequent attention to progress. "Consider all that we have accomplished," you might say, and then go on to summarize the group's achievements.

Status Consensus

Status consensus is the group's agreement that the roles and relative status of the members of the group are correct. Every group evolves its own status hierarchy. Some members strive to achieve high status. Some members prefer not to be heavily involved— perhaps because they have already made commitments to be heavily involved in other groups. Some members do not wish positions of leadership but care very much about attaining the group goals, so they evolve helping roles that assume responsibility but little leadership. The point is that every member wants to feel that his or her place in the group is right and that it is seen as right by the other members of the group.

The problem is that in a power struggle within a group, if two high-dominant individuals are competing for status, sooner or later one of them will win and the other will lose. Should this happen, the winner, who has thus emerged in the position of greater status, has an immediate leadership problem. The task is to help the loser to accept and adjust to second position—a status that flows from lack of success in the power struggle. Since the loser in that contest may now be the second most powerful member of the group, if that individual does not accept the new, number-two position, he or she may be a very significant potential threat to the group.

Again, for a member to be satisfied with the group, status consensus must occur. Any member can help that to evolve. For status consensus is a function of the talk that passes back and forth in the group. Thus it is reasonable to say that every individual in a group has a responsibility for this important communication function.

PROMOTING COHESIVENESS

Leadership Style

It seems clear to us that effective leadership is essential to building cohesiveness. Everyone in a group can contribute leadership to a group, and each member's willingness and determination to do so is an essential part of team building. The ability to select appropriate task and social leadership behaviors from your repertory, and knowing when it is appropriate to do so, is one of the most important aspects of this skill.

The selection of leadership behaviors and their appropriate and skillful use is a complex issue. Task leadership and leadership styles were the topics of Chapter 7. There alternative leadership styles, behaviors, and skills were presented. The matter of social leadership is developed fully in Chapter 9. How to be supportive rather than defensive, how to meet the interpersonal needs of other group members, and how to listen actively and give appropriate feedback to improve both cohesiveness and productivity receive careful treatment.

Group Size

Group size is directly related to the evolution of a team. That all-important sense of "groupness" and cohesiveness is at risk when a group is too small and when it is too large. Indeed, the size of a group has been linked in research[11] to such group attributes as member participation, leadership, member reaction, a group's ability to achieve consensus, and the effectiveness of group performance. But the literature is not clear about what would be the optimum size for every group. Still, these statements are generally true about group size.

1. The larger the group, the more the variety of skills and abilities available to the group and the greater the knowledge available to the group.

2. The larger the group, the more actual help the group can call upon to accomplish its tasks.

3. The larger the group, the greater the opportunity for people to meet others who seem to them attractive, interesting, confirming, and desirable.

4. The larger the group, the more opportunities for individual anonymity.

Thus clear advantages are related to larger size in working groups, and it makes sense to swell the size of groups when those advantages are needed. But increased size in groups also has clear disadvantages, and we think that those disadvantages will usually outweigh the advantages.

1. The larger the group, the more likely that subgroups will form.

2. The larger the group, the more unequal the amount of member participation.

3. The larger the group, the less time for participation by each member.

4. The larger the group, the more participation centers on the talkative few and the greater the likelihood that those few will address each other rather than the other members.

5. The larger the group, the greater the demands on the leader.

6. The larger the group, the more tolerant the group becomes of leadership's takeover of vital group functions.

7. The larger the group, the more trouble it will have achieving consensus.

Since the limitations that derive from a group's being too large seem to us to outweigh the advantages, when you have an opportunity to do so, try to see to it that the groups to which you belong are not larger than about ten or eleven members. Five to seven members will usually be a good, workable size.

Of course, we recognize that you will not typically be able to influence the size of the groups of which you are member. That is usually done by someone in an administrative position. Even so, you can monitor any group to discover if the advantages—and more likely, the disadvantages—are occurring. If they are, then you may be able to help the group by discussing your perceptions with your group.

An organizer of a town meeting, called to begin the process of identifying ways to improve local schools, handled the size problem this way. The group appeared to have natural subgroups—those concerned with quality of teaching, those worried about the run-down facilities, and those sensitive to the problem of overcrowding. Phyllis, the group's leader, addressed the problem: "I can see that we might profit by dividing into three smaller groups. From your communication so far, I can see that we need to worry about the quality of teaching and facilities, and new construction to ease overcrowding. Let's do that and I'll check with each group after you get started to see how you are doing. I'm going to appoint three people to coordinate these discussions."

Phyllis was able to utilize the resources of this large group to address the potential problems that were developing. It was obvious that the group would be less efficient if it tried to handle all these issues as a large body. Group size can be an important factor in effective decision making.

In summary, the point is that group size can be an important factor in the evolution of cohesiveness—the sense of being a team. Since groups that are too large tend to get into predictable kinds of trouble, if you monitor the groups you are in and alert them to the first hints of those kinds of trouble, you may be able to assist the groups in taking advantage of their size. Such monitoring of work is part of effective participation—another thing you can do to facilitate cohesiveness.

Effective Participation

Obviously, effective member participation is essential to the success of a task group. That statement makes fundamentally good sense at first glance. At a deeper level, we know that the ethical commitment of a group participant bears on both cohesiveness and productivity. People assume that when they join a group, they can expect the other members to behave in certain ways. If their expectations are fulfilled they will be far more likely to experience cohesiveness than if their expectations are unsatisfied. John Cragan and David Wright[12] argue that any group member must make five commitments to fellow group members, and we agree.

Commitment to do your best   You are unique. You have individual skills and abilities. You have special knowledge and insight. You know some things no one else knows. If you make a commitment to do your best, then you will try to share what you know and you will try to participate in the tasks of the group. Without your commitment to do your best, the group will be shortchanged. If your group begins to believe that you are shortchanging it, conflict will almost certainly ensue. You have a responsibility to try to do your best.

Commitment to the good of the group   This commitment is not the same as the last one. From time to time you have been involved in groups in which one of the members was looking out for him- or herself rather than for the group. This seems to happen in many different contexts.

To illustrate, consider this marketing team of a thriving business just outside Boulder, Colorado. One member of the group was an older man who had, five years earlier, personally developed the marketing program for the product being discussed. In addition, this man had a terrible anger—brought about by his awareness that he had never lived up to what he thought was the "promise of his youth." He disliked himself and he blamed the world for his failure. And so he decided that this committee assignment was his chance to gain recompense for all the shortcomings of his career. That private agenda—his goals rather than those of the group—always came before the good of the group. When a member suggested a new marketing approach, this man objected. If another wanted to change any particular item in the original scheme this man obstructed the progress.

Serving with that man was a maddening experience, but it taught a very valuable lesson. Each member of a group can undermine the group's cohesiveness and productivity merely by grinding his or her own private ax or by engaging in self-serving behavior. Individuals and groups have a right to expect that every member will make a commitment to the group good—that every member will put the group before private concerns.

Commitment to straight thinking   Sometimes individuals evolve convictions and beliefs that are very important to them. Sometimes those private truths do not completely square with the facts. When this happens to group members, the results can be trying, both for the group and for the individual. A commitment to straight thinking means that an individual is willing to keep an open mind while the group works toward conclusions. Given the enormous subjectivity of perception and thinking, it very often happens that a group will arrive at conclusions different from those of an individual member. An individual must be willing to test private truth against the arguments and evidence presented by other group members. That sounds easier to do than it is, for it requires personal commitment to rationality.

Commitment to cooperation   When a group member makes this commitment, he or she is making a commitment to cooperative behavior rather than to competitive behavior. Fair play means setting self-aggrandizement aside. It means resisting the temptation to play games. It means avoiding one-upmanship. It means being straight— opening oneself to others, showing the other members of the group who you are. And it means resisting the tendency, especially in larger groups, to struggle for status when what is most important is group achievement of a common goal.

To illustrate the tendency to compete in our culture, quickly think of the names of at least five games you play. List these in your head before you read further. Have you thought of a game that is played in such a way that in order for one player to win, the other player has to win? Very rarely does anyone jot down such a game. Frisbee is the only such game that comes to mind at this moment. Does this make a point about our society's commitment to competition? It probably does, and in a compelling way.

What is common if you check with classmates is that everyone will have considered the names of five games that are played in such a way that one player can win only if the other player loses. It is significant to note that even the games we play for fun reinforce the culture's insistence that the world is a competitive place. Such an orientation can be especially harmful to the cohesiveness and productivity of a group.

Consider the results of this win-lose attitude at a recent meeting of the tenants' association of a condominium complex in Pensacola, Florida.

> FRED: I think we ought to spend the money in our repair fund on a new shell for the swimming pool.
>
> SALLY: I disagree. That's foolish. I insist that we fix the tennis courts. More people use them.
>
> FRED: Since there isn't enough money for both projects, we should wait until there is enough.
>
> SALLY: If you can't support us on this issue, Fred, don't expect our support for your candidacy for city council this fall. I don't want someone with your kind of attitude representing me!

The only way to overcome that damaging tendency to compete is by making a commitment to fair play.

Commitment to careful listening   Have you ever participated in a conversation in which someone else responds to your position in such a way that it appears he or she was not listening to you at all? A group of students engaged in a task one afternoon asked to be observed because group members had been complaining that they were unhappy with each other. Here is part of the discussion in that group. How do you respond to this transcript of language taken from that group meeting?

> TIM: I think we ought to look at our evaluative criteria again. Seems to me that what you're saying doesn't meet . . .
>
> BILL (interrupting Tim):   You're always bringing up those criteria. What's wrong with just laying out a plan—the whole plan—then seein' if there's anything wrong with it?
>
> TIM: Nothing. But the criteria are really relevant on this one point. You want to give a lot of our money to the SGA [Student Government Association], and all I'm saying is that we ought to be sure that's the best way to do it. I mean, are they going to use the two thousand bucks the way we want them to?
>
> BILL: They'll use it right. I'll see to that.
>
> HELEN: You guys are always fighting, and I can't see why. Why don't we just give the two thousand bucks to the SGA and get on with it?

This group was spending more time talking—or planning what they would say next—than listening. Helen's comment makes clear that she was not listening. When Bill interrupted Tim he made clear that he, too, was not willing to hear Tim out. He was not listening. When Tim responded to Bill's question with "Nothing," and then went on to point out that something was wrong with Bill's plan, he said to Bill that he, too, was not listening. Small wonder that the other members of the group complained about having to work with these three!

Making a commitment to good listening means making a commitment to more than just hearing what the others are saying. It involves trying to empathize, to understand not only what is said but what is not said—the feelings and wants of the others. To do so is to contribute to both the cohesiveness and productivity of a working group. Not to do so is to squander the energies of the group and to undermine the sense of team that every successful group needs.

Effective participation is so important to the success of a group that the remainder of this book is devoted to the knowledge and skills involved.

So far, the matter of encouraging cohesiveness has been approached by looking at such variables as leadership style, group size, and effective participation by group members. Perhaps the most important single variable involving cohesiveness, however, is making group progress. You will recall that group members must think they are making progress toward group goals in order to be satisfied with their membership in the group. That all-important *perception* of progress is most likely if the group actually does make progress! Now a closer look at group goals is appropriate. Can individuals do anything to help groups make progress toward their goals?

Commitment to Group Goals

Group goals simply cannot exist outside the individual members of a group. Those individuals must subordinate, to some degree, their own private goals in order to help the group reach its goals. Let us consider this idea further. Individuals join groups because they think they will be able to accomplish some of their own private ends by doing so. Moreover, in the case of most ad hoc groups, individuals join or are appointed because they (or someone with whom they work) believe that they share some common problem that can be resolved only if they work together to resolve it. So the point is that individuals, and not groups, provide all the motivation to accomplish group goals. Together they agree that some of their individual goals should become the property and concern of the group, and they agree to set aside other individual goals in order to accomplish those they share with the other members.

Barbara joined the public relations council because she thought she could receive certain benefits from that group. What she did, in this context, can be put a different way. Barbara joined the council because she believed joining was a means by which she could achieve some of her individual goals. Later she saw that in order to get what she wanted from that council, she would have to set aside some of her other aims and ends. Individuals who join groups seem always to have to subordinate some of their goals in order to accomplish others. This creates the potential for conflict between individual goals and group goals, as well as between individual members.

Group members almost always differ, at least somewhat, when they are asked to identify their group's goals. You can imagine that perceptions of the group's goal might differ in a social sorority, for example. Jill might say that the purpose of the sorority is to provide social activities. Sally might say the purpose is to provide support to a group of sisters as they go through their college years. Pam might say the sorority's purpose is to allow its members the opportunity to sponsor and participate in campus activities. Who is correct? It is a matter of perspective. Each of these members has a different definition of the group's goals.

Moreover, different individuals in groups almost never make the same level of commitment to achieving the group goals. Sometimes, too, individuals join the same group—take the same means—in order to achieve strikingly different ends.

To illustrate, imagine how Lois might feel if she realized that her intense commitment to achieving a certain group goal differs markedly from that of another member? Suppose that—earnestly attempting to help the group—she does a lot of planning and thinking, always comes prepared to provide leadership, and is quick to volunteer her energy and expertise or to spend time (which she takes away from her other projects) to work on the group tasks. Now suppose Lois discovers that Martha really is not very committed to the goal she has been driving toward so hard. Let us say that Martha joined the group because Bill was a member and she was (and still is) interested in an affiliation with Bill. At a group meeting Lois asks Martha if she has brought with her the materials she said she would bring. Martha, somewhat chagrined, perhaps, says: "Oh my gosh! I'm sorry, but I just plain forgot to do that." Lois believes that Martha has reneged on her commitment to bring those materials. So she says: "Martha, darn it. You always seem to be more interested in something else, but not in your commitments to our group. We were counting on your information. Now you've delayed the group for another day, at least. Why don't you ever follow through?" Clearly, Lois feels frustration and anger.

"Now just a minute, Lois," says Martha. "I don't like your tone of voice! And besides, you have no right to talk to me that way. After all, you're the one who makes all the moves. In fact, you made this assignment, and I *never* accepted or agreed to it."

"You didn't disagree with it either, Martha. You never said you *wouldn't* do it. And now, after a week and after we have been counting on you, you've let us down."

"Not so. I resent that you think I'd do that. And I resent your tone. You'll have to find someone else to push around. I'm leaving! Bill, are you coming?"

The point of all this might be that group cohesiveness is at risk when subordination of an individual's private goals creates the potential for conflict between individual and group goals or between individual members. And when this kind of conflict is not managed skillfully, it is very easy for individual members of a group to reject the group's goals altogether.

The second thing we want to say is that group goals tend to be long-range goals. This tendency of groups to develop and evolve long-range goals makes sense, of course. But carrying out long-range goals has been a critical problem for group members because they are not usually stated in concrete, attainable units. But it *is* possible and valuable to break up long-range goals into smaller, more readily attainable units. It is also possible and desirable to talk about those goals in terms of behavior, and to reward every achievement along the way to a group's intermediate goals.

Let us examine each of these practical suggestions in turn, then provide some examples. The first was, *break long-range goals into a series of intermediate goals.* Consider Figure 8.2. Suppose that the long-range goal of the group is somewhere out there on the right-hand side of the continuum. It seems obvious, but worth repeating, that breaking up the task into short ranges creates a series of readily achievable intermediate objectives. These goals should be moderately difficult. This means that they should be difficult enough to provide some challenge, but also attainable. Each successful achievement is reinforcing in itself, because the group can observe its own progress and because the members of the group can experience the benefits of their own success.

Second, *state intermediate goals in terms of behaviors.* In setting up its goals, a task group ought to try to specify *what* ought to be involved and (if the group chooses) *how* the tasks should be accomplished. Part of each meeting's agenda could be devoted to focusing upon what has already been accomplished and what ought to be accomplished next.

As an illustration of how this might work, consider how one group of parents solved a problem through this kind of goal setting. A group of parents decided to organize a Boy Scout troop for their sons. Their long-range goal was to organize a troop that would help their boys to mature and learn the variety of valuable skills that such

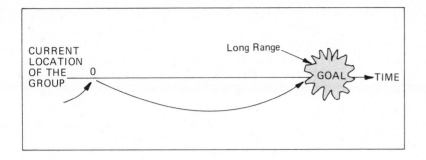

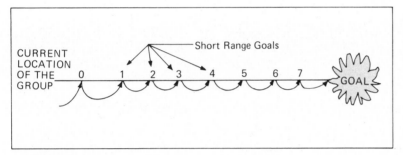

FIGURE 8.2
Illustration of Long-Range and Short-Range Goal Setting

a program teaches. But focusing on this long-range goal did not help them to be productive. They set a series of intermediate goals that led them to the overall goal. Here are some of the intermediate goals that this group actually set down:

1. Conduct a survey to discover who might be interested in sponsoring a troop.

2. Locate a scoutmaster.

3. Publicize the new troop so that all interested boys would be aware of its organization.

4. Meet with local scout officials to charter the troop.

5. Plan and organize an orientation meeting for interested boys and their parents.

The next step was to specify what ought to be involved in carrying out each of these intermediate goals. For example, here are the specifications of short-term objectives for the item "Locate a scoutmaster."

a. Collect names from the scout office by Friday. (Don)

b. Ask the sponsoring agency who from their group might be interested in being a scoutmaster by Friday. (Mary)

c. Call potential scoutmasters and discover their level of interest by Tuesday. (David)

d. Interview the potential scoutmasters by Thursday. (All)

e. Make a selection by Monday. (All)

You can see how this kind of goal setting might work. Regardless of the task, it can lead to increased cohesiveness and productivity.

The point of all this illustration is that any production process includes not only a long-range goal but also a very complex tool for developing intermediate goals. Those intermediate goals ought to be identified in terms of some time sequence, and in terms of the human behaviors required. Note who ought to be assigned.

Thus the questions we learn early in the sixth grade—who, what, when, where, why, and how—provide a clean-cut method for setting intermediate goals and a rationale for identifying the goals that need to be set. A freewheeling system of note taking on stickies, each of which includes at least a noun and a verb, provides a very useful means by which a group can accomplish the task of setting intermediate goals. Brainstorming techniques in this regard are recommended.

GROUPTHINK

Up to this point, this chapter has centered on the beneficial effects that accrue to a group with cohesiveness. The point is that for most task groups you will ever be a part of, the greater the cohesiveness the better. But that idea must be tempered with a very strong note of caution.

Early in the 1970s Irving L. Janis hypothesized that sometimes a decision-making group can get dangerously cohesive. His famous book, which first came out in 1972[13] and in an expanded and revised edition in 1982,[14] offered a title that was both controversial and provocative.[15] The title is still a somber warning about too much cohesiveness: *Victims of Groupthink.* Janis described high-level policy groups in his books—the president and his decision makers in the Kennedy period; the president and his aides in the Nixon-Watergate phase. But groupthink can happen to any group.[16] Indeed, the phenomenon called groupthink is so common to groups that the term, coined by Janis in the early seventies, has become a catchword in the literature on group communication and behavior.

Janis first got the idea for his theory of groupthink shortly after the Bay of Pigs fiasco during the Kennedy administration. Shortly after Kennedy took office in January 1961, he was handed a detailed briefing on a CIA plan hatched during Eisenhower's administration to land a small brigade of Cuban exiles on a beachhead in Cuba, with the idea that they might invade the island and overthrow the government of Fidel Castro. The event, based upon groundless assumptions, was a complete failure from the outset. Yet it was generated by a group of the brightest individuals available to Kennedy and his advisers. How could such a thing have happened?

Janis suggested to his daughter that she write a paper on the topic, and as the young woman began to dig more and more into the question "How could such a thing have happened?" Janis himself became fascinated by the question. In 1965, Arthur M. Schlesinger, Jr., former presidential adviser, published a book on the Kennedy presidency, *A Thousand Days.* His chapters on the Bay of Pigs helped Janis to crystallize his thinking. Says Janis: "At first I was puzzled; how could bright, shrewd men like John F. Kennedy and his advisers be taken in by the CIA's stupid, patchwork plan?" He began to wonder if some kind of psychological contagion had interfered with the deliberate decision making that typically goes into foreign-policy designing.

In essence, the theory of groupthink is that situations can occur in which groups take leave of their senses because they are too cohesive. Instead of testing their group decision making against reality they begin to go collectively crazy. When that happens, the group and its constituents are victims of the malady Janis called groupthink. They make decisions that have no apparent basis in reality. Of course, most of the time, the decision turns out to be a very bad one.

In order to understand the theory, it seems useful for us to review the characteristics of sound decision making. You can scan the table of contents of this book (or of nearly any text prepared for a group discussion course) to find these criteria identified in similar language.

1. The group has thoroughly understood the problems it is trying to solve or resolve.

2. The group has set up criteria against which to evaluate the bits and pieces of the evolving solutions. Members have carefully weighed the costs and risks of any negative consequences of their plan as well as the positive consequences of their decisions.

3. The group has thoroughly studied a broad range of alternative courses of action that might solve or resolve the problem.

4. The group has considered and weighed all the information available, taking into account any expert opinion or evidence that does not support the evolving decisions or the preferred course of action.

5. Having evolved a potential solution in advance, the group has consistently reevaluated it, and both the positive and negative consequences implied.

6. The group determines a final choice and makes detailed provisions for executing the final plan, paying attention to contingency plans that might be required if any of the known risks should occur.

As Janis thought about the problem, other possible fiascos also began to come to his attention. In each case, the burning question Why? repeated itself. His answers to that question became a most influential book. Its tenets are described here, and his suggestions for avoiding the groupthink syndrome are listed and advocated.

Conditions That Promote Groupthink

In evolving his theory of groupthink, Janis described the antecedent conditions that lead to the syndrome. The first antecedent condition is *cohesiveness.* The group that suffers groupthink will experience moderately high to high cohesiveness.

A second condition is *insulation.* The insulation of the group from contradictory sources inhibits members from getting information and expert opinion concerning the subject. Especially, insulation keeps the group from hearing criticisms and skeptical evaluations from others.

A third antecedent condition of groupthink is *lack of a tradition of impartial leadership.* As Janis explains this idea, when group leaders have no traditional constraints to maintain impartial, bias-free relationships with the group on the subject at issue, "the leader of a policy making group will find it all too easy to use his or her power and prestige to influence the members of the group to approve the policy alternative he or she prefers instead of encouraging them to engage in open inquiry and critical evaluation."

Finally, groups that experience the groupthink syndrome *do not have any norms or rules about the methods or procedures* they will use in dealing with the decision-making task. Thus the leadership and the members may proceed as they choose. Almost certainly they will choose a path that is relatively free of criticism or countervailing evidence and argument.

In sum, then, antecedent conditions of the groupthink syndrome have been identified as in Table 8.1. An individual group member can use this information to help the group avoid the groupthink syndrome.

Symptoms of the Groupthink Syndrome

If the antecedent conditions seem likely to generate the groupthink syndrome in any particular group, group members can guard against falling victim to the syndrome merely by examining themselves and their group for the symptoms Janis identified.

Type I: Overestimations of the group—its power and morality In this category of symptoms Janis included a variety of illusions that groups sometimes develop. When the members of a group begin to believe that they are invulnerable (that they cannot be wrong), they will begin to give themselves permissions they might otherwise constrain.

TABLE 8.1   Antecedent Conditions to Groupthink

1. Moderately high or very high cohesiveness
2. Insulation of the policy-making group
3. Lack of tradition to inhibit leadership bias
4. Lack of rules or norms about methods and procedures

The illusion of invulnerability creates an optimism that may not be warranted by reality. Since they begin to believe that they cannot be harmed, group members become more and more willing to take risks. Moreover, a group will sometimes become so cohesive that it begins to believe that its morality is beyond reproach.

Type II: Closed-mindedness   A second dangerous symptom of the groupthink syndrome may grossly be described as closed-mindedness. This kind of problem occurs in groups when the members attempt to rationalize their decisions in order to discount or overcome the skepticism and warnings of people who are critical of them. In addition, sometimes group members rationalize away the adverse implications of information that appears contrary to the group decision. This happens especially under conditions in which group members refuse to reconsider the basic assumptions on which they originally made their decisions, even in the face of countervailing evidence. Groups suffering from the groupthink syndrome do not find such rationalizations obvious.

This same category, closed-mindedness, may be found in situations in which group members identify themselves as "the good guys." They stereotype as "the enemy" those who oppose their views. The enemy is so evil that it does not merit the group's attention or willingness to negotiate. The enemy is too weak or too stupid to counter the decisions of the group—however threatening the group's decisions may be to the enemy, the enemy probably would not understand—and they would try to delay the group from implementing its decisions.

Type III: Pressures toward uniformity   Sometimes it may happen that members find themselves minimizing their own doubts and counterarguments to you. This is one of the most common of the third type of groupthink symptoms. Sometimes members find evidence of the groupthink syndrome when they see the illusion developing that they share a common judgment—even when they do not. In this case, either members do not talk about their reservations (and assume that silence on the part of their colleagues is consent) or they conform to the majority view (or what they think is the majority view), because they trust that the group is invulnerable and morally right anyway.

Janis described the emergence of self-appointed mindguards as one of the pressures toward uniformity that characterizes the groupthink syndrome. These are group members who take it upon themselves to protect the group from any information or opinions that might cause the group to veer away from its course. Mindguards work to protect group complacency about its ethical and moral posture, and about the likelihood of the success of its policy decisions.

Consequences of the Groupthink Syndrome

Imagine what the effects of these symptoms might be on a decision-making task group. If most or all of the symptoms are present, then group members probably will work very ineffectively together. They are not likely to achieve their objectives because their process of decision making will have been highly defective. Janis lists the following symptoms of faulty decision making:

1. Incomplete survey of alternatives

2. Incomplete survey of objectives

3. Failure to examine the risks of preferred choices

4. Failure to reappraise initially rejected alternatives

5. Poor information search

6. Selective bias in processing information at hand

7. Failure to work out contingency plans

Figure 8.3, which appeared first in the Janis and Mann book,[17] *Decision Making*, in 1977, provides a graphic model of the groupthink syndrome. You can use it as a troubleshooting guide when you believe you might be experiencing groupthink.

If the groupthink syndrome happens to cohesive groups, and it happens very often, how can it be avoided? Janis was concerned about this question, of course. His prescriptions seem to us to make excellent sense, so we present them here in abbreviated form.

1. Leaders should assign the role of critical evaluator to each member.

2. Leaders should avoid stating preferences and expectations at the outset.

3. Each member of a policy-making group should routinely discuss the group's deliberations with trusted associates and report back to the group on the associates' reactions.

4. One or more outside experts should be invited to each meeting on a staggered basis. The outside experts should be encouraged to challenge the views of the members.

5. At least one articulate and knowledgeable member should be appointed the role of devil's advocate.

6. Leaders should make sure that a sizable block of time is set aside to survey all warning signals from rivals, and they and the group should construct alternative scenarios of the rivals' intentions.

SUMMARY

In this chapter it was argued that for most groups most of the time, the greater the cohesiveness, the better the group. A curvilinear relationship between cohesiveness and productivity was suggested, and then the job of building a sense of team was developed. The conditions upon which cohesiveness rests were identified, and the idea that there is much you can do to ensure cohesiveness in your own groups was argued. People are attracted to group membership by shared similar attitudes, a clear sense of how to

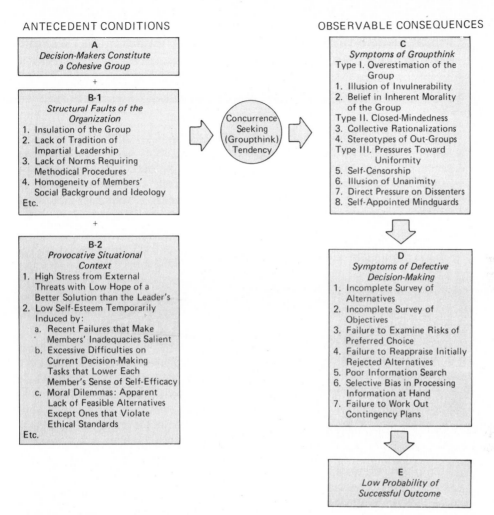

FIGURE 8.3
Model of Groupthink Syndrome

Source: Adapted with permission of The Free Press, a division of Macmillan, Inc., from *Decision Making*, by Irving L. Janis and Leon Mann. Copyright © 1977 by The Free Press.

achieve goals, the kinds of conflict and the ways a group handles conflict, and the frequency and nature of the feedback provided by groups.

Beyond attraction, however, three conditions are necessary for membership satisfaction in groups, without which cohesiveness simply cannot emerge. Group members must perceive freedom to participate; they must believe that they are making progress toward their goals; and they must agree that the status position they hold in the group, relative to the status positions of the other members, is at once right for them and right for their group. What was left, then, was to look at group size, and some of the research findings about group size was detailed. The important point of that discussion was that the information about group size can be extraordinarily useful to individual group members even if they are never directly involved in actually forming a group.

Commitment to doing your best, commitment to the good of the group, commitment to straight thinking, commitment to cooperation rather than to competition, and commitment to careful listening were the next topics developed. All of these commitments led to a discussion of the whole matter of group goals.

Group goals cannot exist outside individual members, who must subordinate some of their individual goals in order to achieve others. This idea sets up the potential for conflict between individual goals and group goals—so much so that it is easy for individuals to lose sight of group goals. Of course, should that happen, group cohesiveness would be at risk.

So the intelligent setting of group goals became an issue. This can best be accomplished by breaking long-term goals into a series of intermediate goals. Those intermediate goals ought to be stated in terms of behavior—specifically who should do what, when, and under what conditions? After assigning carefully defined intermediate goals, the achievement of those goals ought to be monitored by every member of a group. Every time one of those goals is achieved, the achievement should be mentioned and reinforced.

Groupthink happens when very cohesive groups become insulated from criticism, when they lack a tradition of impartial leadership, and when they have no rules about methods and procedures. Under these conditions groups sometimes come to believe that they are invincible and utterly moral. When that happens they may develop closed-mindedness, stereotyping anyone who does not agree with them as "the enemy" and discounting any disagreements on that basis. Typically, such symptoms keep individual members from speaking about their own reservations.

The consequences of groupthink can be summarized in these words: *defective decision making.* The victims of groupthink do not adequately survey their alternatives; they do not survey their objectives or examine the risks of what they are doing. They usually do not reappraise anything they have once rejected. They do not search for information very actively, since they believe that they know all they need to know anyway. They slant their processing of the available information in the direction of what they want rather than what is sensible. Rarely do groups afflicted with the groupthink syndrome ever work out contingency plans. What can you do to overcome the groupthink syndrome? Janis suggested eight prescriptions that will help. What they make clear is that all groups, but especially highly cohesive groups, need to set themselves up in advance to guard the quality of their thought.

EXERCISES

1. Describe and analyze your group's cohesiveness.

2. Consider your experience of cohesiveness in groups. Prepare a list of behaviors that seem to

be indicative of cohesiveness in groups. Now ask yourself another question. What can group members (include any designated leader here, too) do to promote cohesiveness in a group? Make a list of as many suggestions as you can. Bring this list to class.

3. In small groups, using the information you generated above, draw up lists of indicators of cohesiveness and lists of suggestions for enhancing group cohesiveness. Share your work with the rest of the class.

4. Select a group that is known for its high cohesiveness. Interview members to see how they account for the high cohesiveness they experience. Make a list of the factors that they indicate have contributed to their high cohesiveness. Compare these factors with those collected by other members of the class. How are they similar? How are they different?

5. As a class try to answer the question "Why does cohesiveness decrease?" Has anybody been a part of a group in which cohesiveness decreased? If so, ask members to talk about the reasons for the decrease. If not, class members should speculate about factors that cause decreases in cohesiveness. Make a list of causative factors and, for each cause, suggest what might be done to prevent it.

6. What types of conformity are beneficial to groups? Write a three-page essay that discusses the issue of conformity. Indicate when conformity is beneficial and when it is not. Give reasons for your statements about the benefits and liabilities of conformity for small groups.

7. Using periodicals and other accounts of policy or decision making, investigate the Watergate cover-up, the decision to increase U.S. involvement in the Vietnam War, or some other decision of this type. Write a short analysis that identifies any of the conditions of groupthink that may have influenced the decision-making process.

NOTES

1. Marvin E. Shaw, *Group Dynamics: The Psychology of Small Group Behavior*, 3d ed. (New York: McGraw-Hill, 1981); B. Aubrey Fisher, *Small Group Decision Making*, 2d ed. (New York: McGraw-Hill, 1980), 31.

2. We know that the literature has been inconsistent in its findings about the relationship between group communication behavior and problem-solving effectiveness, but we agree with Hirokawa's critique of that literature. See Randy Y. Hirokawa, "Group Communication and Problem Solving: A Critical Review of Inconsistent Findings," *Communication Quarterly* 30 (Spring 1982):134–141.

3. Shaw, 225.

4. Fisher, 33.

5. J. R. Terborg, C. Castore, and J. A. DeNinno, "A Longitudinal Field Investigation of the Impact of Group Composition on Group Performance and Cohesion," *Journal of Personality and Social Psychology* 34 (1976):782–790.

6. F. A. Blanchard, R. H. Weigel, and S. W. Cook, "The Effect of Relative Competence of Group Members Upon Interpersonal Attraction in Cooperating Interracial Groups," *Journal of Personality and Social Psychology* 32 (1975):519–530.

7. A. B. Anderson, "Combined Effects of Interpersonal Attraction and Goal-Path Clarity on the

Cohesiveness of Task Oriented Groups," *Journal of Personality and Social Psychology* 31 (1975):68–75.

8. B. Wheaton, "Interpersonal Conflict and Cohesiveness in Dyadic Relationships," *Sociometry* 37 (1974):328–348.

9. M. Deutsch, "Field Theory in Social Psychology," in *The Handbook of Social Psychology*, G. Lindzey and E. Aronson, 2d ed. (Reading, Mass.: Addison-Wesley, 1968), 412–487; T. D. Schaible and A. Jacobs, "Feedback III: Sequence Effects. Enhancement of Feedback Acceptance and Group Attractiveness by Manipulation," *Small Group Behavior* 6 (1975):151–173.

10. R. Heslin and D. Dunphy, "Three Dimensions of Members' Satisfaction in Small Groups," *Human Relations* 17 (1964):99–112.

11. We are assuming that you will not usually be involved in determining group size, since in most organizational contexts that is a function of management. For greater detail about group size, see Donelson R. Forsyth, *An Introduction to Group Dynamics* (Monterey, Calif.: Brooks/Cole, 1983), 137–138, 152–155, 217–218.

12. John F. Cragan and David W. Wright, *Communication in Small Group Discussions: A Case Study Approach*, 2d ed. (St. Paul, Minn.: West, 1986), 102–104.

13. Irving L. Janis, *Victims of Groupthink* (Boston: Houghton Mifflin, 1972).

14. Irving L. Janis, *Groupthink* (Boston: Houghton Mifflin, 1982).

15. For a critique of Janis's theory, see J. Longley and D. G. Pruitt, "Groupthink: A Critique of Janis's Theory," in L. Wheeler, ed., *Review of Personality and Social Psychology* vol. 1 (Beverly Hills, Calif.: Sage, 1980).

16. Irving L. Janis and L. Mann, *Decision Making* (New York: Free Press, 1977).

17. John A. Courtwright tested student groups in a laboratory. He was able to create situational conditions similar to those of Janis's groupthink and to observe the group decision making. See John A. Courtwright, "A Laboratory Investigation of Groupthink," *Communication Monographs* 43 (1978):229–246.

RECOMMENDED READINGS

Ernest G. Bormann and Nancy C. Bormann, *Effective Small Group Communication*, 4th ed. (Minneapolis: Burgess Publishing, 1988), Chapter 4, "Cohesiveness."

Irving L. Janis, *Groupthink: Psychological Studies of Policy Decisions and Fiascoes*, 2d ed. (Boston: Houghton Mifflin, 1983).

Marvin E. Shaw, "Group Composition and Group Cohesiveness," in Robert S. Cathcart and Larry A. Samovar, eds., *Small Group Communication: A Reader*, 5th ed. (Dubuque, Iowa: Wm. C. Brown, 1988), 42–49.

CHAPTER 9

Managing Relationships in Groups

OBJECTIVES

After reading this chapter you should be able to:

Explain how these three basic assumptions constitute a basic model of human behavior: (1) behavior is caused; (2) behavior is motivated; (3) behavior is goal directed.

Define and explain each of these concepts: perception, cognition, and motivation.

List the four lines of analysis in Schutz's book *FIRO: A Three-Dimensional Theory of Interpersonal Behavior,* and explain inclusion, control, and affection as interpersonal needs.

Specify several ways a group member can use the ideas of William Schutz to make positive contributions to a task group.

Define and explain the terms *empathy* and *trust* and show how each of these concepts bears upon effective group communication.

Name and explain the implications for group discussants of each of the quadrants in the Johari Window.

List and explain each of the six "defensive climates" and each of the six "supportive climates" Jack Gibb described, and show how each list compares and contrasts with the other.

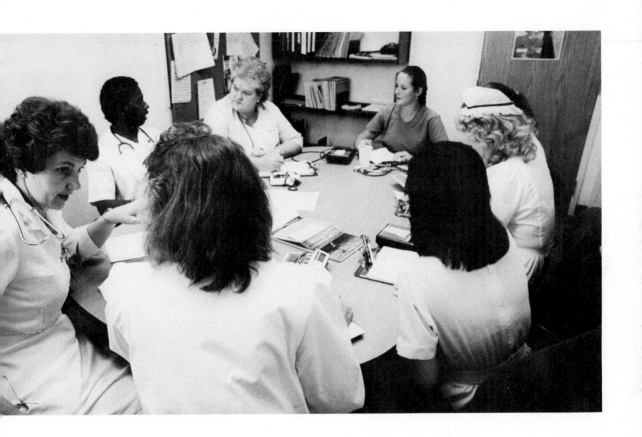

"I do OK with the day-to-day business of communicating," said Ralph Jones, a troubleshooter from the engineering staff group. "What gives me problems is the difficult situations of meeting with a group of engineers from one of our plants to solve a problem. They don't know me and I don't know really know them. And what we have to talk about is a problem that they have been unable to solve. They are feeling defensive. They see me as the enemy." I really have to rely on my relational skills to pull off this part of my job."

"Yeah." Linda Kerr's eyes lighted up. "That's a big problem for me too. And when I try to point out where the difficulty lies, people seem to want to attack me. But in the end, I'm responsible for getting the problem solved and convincing them to implement the solution. When I leave the plant, it's up to them."

Gene Davis, another member of this group of engineers, offered a suggestion. "What I think would be helpful for us is some instruction in how to manage these difficult people situations."

Bernard Jenkins, the group manager, had one final comment, and a good one. "The kind of thing you're talking about is not just a problem that we experience with the plant engineers we work with. It's a problem any time someone is faced with leading a group—it's just intensified because of the nature of our role in this operation."

This short transcript from an actual conversation of a group of engineers focuses on the central theme of the present chapter. In the past several chapters we have described the processes that make groups successful. Logical analysis and argument, verbal and nonverbal messages, and the like, are clearly important to the overall success rate of a group. Clearly, also, groups go through phases and stages, and learning how to identify what stage you are in can be of significant help in learning to facilitate the growth of the group. Finally, of course, the whole matter of cohesiveness—of team building—welds the group together into a unit that can be managed and moved.

Yet what it all comes down to in the end is that all groups are composed of individuals. Sooner or later some very fundamental notions about managing relationships must be addressed. Working one on one is a critical part of a group member's success.

In this chapter we will follow three lines of analysis into the matter of communicating with group members that seem to be most critical. First we will look into how group members, working one on one, can meet each other's needs. It is often said that people spend more time with their colleagues at work than they do with their families at home. Given the typical twenty-four-hour day—in which eight hours are spent at work, about an hour getting to and from work, time out for planning and preparing meals, taking care of the children, and accomplishing all the little chores and tasks that constitute "time off" activity—it is conceivable that working adults do not spend as much time interacting with their families as they do interacting with their colleagues. It follows that the quality of life on the job is essential to an individual's personal and interpersonal health and growth. All of which is important not only to the individual but to his or her colleagues and the good of the group—and ultimately, to the good of the organization as well.

So we will examine how group members can meet one another's needs. Then, taking a closer focus, we will examine defensiveness and supportiveness as people work with one another. Almost always, when individuals behave defensively, it occurs because someone has attempted to manipulate or attack or "lord it over" them. At the very least, defensive behavior can be said to occur when a person thinks or believes or feels that there is reason to be defensive.

And that is a major problem in perception and in drawing inferences. About the only cure, we think, is learning to talk in a different way. Thus information is presented that will help you to know how to remain supportive of the other people in your communication.

MEETING INTERPERSONAL NEEDS

We want to look at the question "How can individual group members, working one on one, meet each other's interpersonal needs?" This seems necessary, since a major reason for joining groups is to satisfy personal and interpersonal needs. The second question we will want to examine is, "What can individual members do to create a positive group climate?" Increasing understanding of how to provide this kind of atmosphere is a central skill for anyone who wants to improve interpersonal communication.

The second question bears directly on the first. A group that manages to generate a supportive climate is able to meet the interpersonal needs of its individual members. A group that is not able to generate a supportive climate cannot meet the interpersonal needs of its members.

If you begin with three basic assumptions, it is possible to develop a model to explain the matter of interpersonal needs satisfaction. These assumptions were first articulated by Harold J. Leavitt[1] and, although they may bear qualification, they still combine to suggest some hard-to-fault logic.

First, *behavior is caused*. Second, *behavior is motivated*. These two assumptions combine to provide the third: *Behavior is goal directed*. These three assumptions taken together suggest that some cause or stimulus motivates a person toward some goal. For a community action group that is meeting to discuss what to do about recent burglaries, this means:

Stimulus:	Burglaries
Motivation:	Concern that residents might be victimized
Goal:	Strengthen neighborhood security
Behavior:	Group meetings

If the assumptions are true, then no behavior is ever completely aimless. It is generated in response to some stimulus that, in turn, is filtered through some system that transforms the stimulus into motivation. This filtering system is critical. It consists, as we have already described in some detail, of language and of perception, cognition, and motivation.

The behavior may be conscious and overt, such as the act of choosing among carefully articulated and researched alternatives, or unconscious, such as habitual coping behavior.[2] Moreover, the behavioral assumptions generalize—that is, the three assumptions bear upon all human behavior of the kind we wish to examine. Of course, some people respond to individual stimuli differently from others. For example, members of the neighborhood association may respond differently to crime in their neighborhood. Some members may respond with alarm; others may not.

Differential behavior patterns must derive from differences somewhere in our understandings of stimuli, or differences in our needs and perceptions of value systems, for instance. Indeed, individual differences are inevitable, and the result of an enormously complex system of variables, including age, sex, perceptual differences, and the like. We want to focus upon some of those variables, which seem to us to be most influential in that filtering system. Figure 9.1 provides a rough sketch of some of them. They may be lumped roughly into three separate, broad categories: perception, cognition, and motivation.

The basic model of behavior illustrated in Figure 9.1 suggests that a stimulus

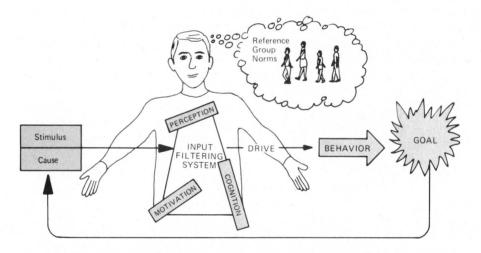

Some Inputs into the Filtering System of an Individual in the World of Work

1. Current health and emotional stability
2. All prior experiences, including what is stored and what is distorted or lost, and the connections that are made among what is left
3. The context (e.g., the location, purpose of a group meeting)
4. Factors in the work place (e.g., available resources, such as people, plant and facilities, materials and energy, money, information, control mechanisms in force, etc.)
5. Interpersonal relationships
6. Organizational variables (e.g., leadership, reward system, structure and the place of individual and/or group within that structure)
7. Intrapersonal variables (e.g., wants, tensions, images of the world, language capability and fluency, etc.)

FIGURE 9.1
A Basic Model of Behavior

triggers, or causes, behavior toward some goal. If you accept the three assumptions, then all of the behavior we are interested in in this book is accounted for in that model of behavior. People take in stimuli, then filter them through a system of perception, cognition, and motivation variables. Then, depending upon their analysis of the stimuli, they experience a drive to behave in some way. Behavior is goal directed.

To illustrate this idea most simply, suppose a group is assigned the task of selecting a vendor for some piece of equipment. Let us say that the equipment is the company fleet of cars. There are three major bidders, as you might imagine: the local Ford dealer, the local Chevrolet/Pontiac dealer, and the local Chrysler/Plymouth dealer. You are a member of the group. You look at the proposals made by each of the three bidders (those are the stimuli), and you begin to process those proposals through your own filtering system. You may have owned one or more cars by the makers represented in the bids. Perhaps you thought your Ford was wonderful, but the Chevy you owned was a lemon. You may never have owned a Plymouth. Your filtering system will include how you perceive the proposals, of course, but also your cognitions and your motivations. Suppose the Ford dealer has offered equipment very close to the specifications, different only in nonessential ways (such as color or weight of certain upholstery materials), and that the proposal is well below the competing figures. At the same time, you know that your boss intensely dislikes Ford products—for no special reason that you can discover— and you want very much to impress him. Surely your position in that group decision- making process will be affected by each of these variables—your cognitions and your motivations—and your perceptions of the proposals and/or the automobiles themselves will also be affected.

But Figure 9.1 does not suggest the implications of these variables. If you want to understand the implications of that sketch in greater detail, you must look at what goes on in the processing system within yourself. That is a difficult task but a valuable one, for it bears directly on people's ability to manage relationships with one another.

Perception

Perception is the only means by which a stimulus can affect an individual. If a stimulus is not perceived, it can have no effect. In interpersonal communication, if the stimulus is someone else's talk or nonverbal messages, then clearly one's own perceptual acuity is critical to the success of that interaction. Thus how we perceive one another is a critical part of interpersonal communication. The important point for this discussion is that people cannot ever perceive the same stimulus in the same way, because their respective filtering systems are unique. Recall that we said in Chapter 4 that selective perception produces a potential problem for communicators. Of course, they can verify some of their similar perceptions through talk. They can agree on a set of facts. They can negotiate and then accept some set of terms or agreements—as, for example, in selecting the evaluative criteria against which a group will choose new cars for the company automobile fleet. But even so, their understandings will be heavily loaded and highly varied from individual to individual. You can imagine how this phenomenon of perception imposes itself upon your ability to communicate with other group members.

In addition to selective perception, two other variables are included in the filtering process—cognition and motivation.

Cognition

Cognition—perceiving, thinking, and understanding—is a process of overwhelming importance. But the concern of this chapter is not individual thinking as much as interpersonal communication. So in the present context, consider cognition as part of the communication process. As we talk to one another, each of us receives and filters the incoming information. This process is a matter of putting new information into the context of what people know about themselves and about the world in which they live.

Cognition evolves out of the interaction of thinking, imagining, reasoning, problem solving, decision making, and the like. The important thing in this discussion is not how it works but what it implies. When we talk to one another in groups, we are actually creating a reality by negotiation—some shared knowledge about the self or the world. Such processes are rational processes, regardless of how they are perceived by others. They exist as a result of people interacting and negotiating a shared view of the world. But they grow out of the truth that each individual carries around within himself or herself.

To put it another way, people always have a good reason for their points of view—at least, they think so. Similarly, every group has a good reason for its understanding of the world—from the negotiated perspective of its members. Individuals behave rationally because they behave in ways that are consistent with their individual perspectives. Groups behave rationally when they behave in ways that are consistent with their perspectives. Every organization behaves rationally—from the point of view of those who are making the decisions. Thus irrationality is a judgment that one person makes about what another person considers to be a rational choice of behaviors.

If you think someone's behavior is irrational, you might say that you just do not know what the other's point of view is. If you "know the truth" and the other person does not believe you, you may feel he or she just does not know any better. More likely, if you "know the truth" and the other person does not believe you, then you do not see it in the same way he or she does. Your cognitive behavior has yielded different truths because your comprehension, your interpretations, and your rationality systems are unique.

Motivation

Not only are our cognitive and perceptual processes likely to generate a unique world view; our motivations will also be unique. If our life motives are different, then our choices of behavior will be different.

The question of what touches off human behavior is a very complex one, and frankly, neither we nor anyone else knows for sure how it works. Even so, it seems clear that differences in what motivates people are the most critical part of understanding what makes individuals behave differently. Here it seems enough to say that there are threads that run through *all* the theoretical conceptualization about motivation. They can be summarized by a fairly simple sentence, but beware. The sentence is simple but the concept is very complex, indeed. The sentence: "People do what they do because they think they will get a payoff that is worth the price they'll have to pay."

Motivating group members requires that you find out what they want from their involvement in a group. What a member may want may be identified in terms of task and relationship goals. Much of what we've said thus far in this book has dealt with task goals. The issue of relational goals—the payoff—is, of course, the topic of this chapter.

The Ideas of William Schutz

In 1958 William C. Schutz published an influential book called *FIRO: A Three-Dimensional Theory of Interpersonal Behavior.*[3] The letters in that title stand for fundamental interpersonal relations orientation. Schutz argued that people need social relationships with other people. His argument included four lines of analysis.

1. Every individual has three important interpersonal needs: inclusion, control, and affection.

2. An individual's interpersonal behavior will be similar to the behavior he or she experienced in his or her earliest relationships—probably with parents.

3. Interpersonal compatibility, defined in terms of inclusion, control, and affection, is essential to the efficient operation of a group, increasing both the desire to communicate and the cohesiveness of group members.

4. As a group develops, it passes through stages that may be identified as inclusion, control, and affection; as it disintegrates, the group retraces its passage from affection through control and inclusion behaviors.

Each of the three needs in Schutz's conceptualization can be understood to exist along a continuum. Some people need a greater degree of each, and some people need a lesser degree of each. Thus the three needs could appear as in Figure 9.2.

Schutz's theory has particular application to communication with group members. He believed that all people have at least three interpersonal needs to some degree or another, and that these needs are interconnected and "fit" along continua described in Figure 9.2. The need for inclusion has to do with an individual's needs for affiliation, which may be measured to some degree by whether or not, and to what extent, the individual attempts to initiate interactions with others.

Clearly, an individual who frequently initiates interaction, and whose interpersonal needs for inclusion are thus satisfied, perhaps optimally so, is taking care of his or her own emotional and relational health. But suppose the person rarely if ever initiates interaction. That individual might very well be undersocial—somewhere in the anxious range, according to Schutz's ideas. What might this mean to you as you attempt to communicate with this person?

	Greater love needed	AFFECTION		Less love needed	
COMPLETE COMMITMENT		Overpersonal Personal Underpersonal			NO AFFECTION
	Originating and initiating much love			Never initiating affection	
STRONG CONTROL	Greater effect upon and power over others needed	CONTROL		Less effect on and power over others needed	NO CONTROL
		Autocrat Democrat Abdicrat			
	Controlling all of own and/or another's behaviors			Controlling none of own and/or another's behaviors	
HIGH INTERACTION	Greater affiliation needed	INCLUSION		Less affiliation needed	NO INTERACTION
		Oversocial Social Undersocial			
	Always initiating interaction			Never initiating interaction	

FIGURE 9.2
The Interpersonal Needs Continua According to Schutz

Similarly, an individual might be completely comfortable—having a sense of being in control of her own life, and satisfied as well that she is able to influence and to exercise power of sorts over the behavior of others. For example, a group member might very well participate in arguments for or against a proposal, offer proposals of her own, and provide evidence and leadership as a group does its work. Such an individual would be within the desired range on Schutz's schema, and enjoying relational and emotional health. But a person could also be an overbearing individual somewhere in the anxious range. An autocratic individual is one who attempts to control too much—both her own behaviors, as in a case where she goes against the consensus of the group "just to show them" that she is in charge of her own decisions, and the behaviors of others, as in a case where she attempts to bully people into argument. Such individuals need help, and constitute a very real challenge when you are trying to communicate with them.

Of course, people cut across a range in their need for affection, too. A person whose needs for affection are well met is called personable. He or she gives and gets affection. He or she interacts freely with others, and both in words and in nonverbal messages asks for and offers warmth and support. Such an individual is an easy-to-get-along-with group member, with whom you will find communicating a joy. But suppose a person is somewhere in the anxious range—either overpersonal, originating and initiating affectionate exchange too much, or underpersonal, rarely initiating affection and rarely seeking it. Either way, the individual may constitute a challenge for group members. As you have seen, the cohesiveness of a group depends, in some measure at least, upon the freely offered shows and signs of "groupness" that flow from affectionate behavior. To round out the thought, the individual in the last illustration could be in the extreme range of Schutz's schema. Someone for whom love and affection displays become the primary motive, to the exclusion of all others, may be a problem group member. Similarly, an individual who never displays affection, turns it away when others offer it, and believes and feels himself or herself unloved and unlovable may also create a problem for a group. Either way, it is easy to see that such a person is in the dysfunctional extreme in this dimension of interpersonal needs.

But what does all this mean for attempting to communicate with other group members? In each of Schutz's categories, what is at issue from your perspective is not motivation but behaviors. A member can choose how he or she will interact with others, and that is the key to successful interpersonal communication.

Reconsider that people do what they do because they believe that they will get a payoff greater than the price they have to pay. If a person's most valued payoff is interpersonal—and that is the basis upon which we usually interact with others—then the payoff most people are looking for will fall into Schutz's three categories. Thus a group member is always in a position to offer other group members the payoffs they need and want. A member can provide evidence to another person that he is included, can choose to affiliate with him. A group member can also acknowledge the efforts of others to affiliate with him, and can confirm them in doing that. As a member of a group, you can assure others that their membership is valued by the group and that their participation is wanted and important. (Of course, this is absolutely the case, since a person who does not participate in a group does not contribute her expertise to the group's goals.)

Similarly, if individuals need, as Schutz suggests, to be in control of their own lives and also to exercise some measure of control over others, you can provide them with payoffs that are valuable both to them and to the group. For example, when another individual makes a contribution—say, an argument that appears to contradict the emerging group consensus—you can acknowledge and value that contribution. Given the tendency of some groups toward conformity to one another's views, the individual's contribution really *is* valuable. Even if the group ultimately decides in a way that is contrary to the person's arguments, still, by treating him or her seriously you can contribute to the individual's sense of control. You may be able to think of other ways to help individuals to satisfy their need to control. At their best and healthiest, such interactions—which treat substantive ideas seriously and thoroughly, while at the same time valuing the individuals who make those arguments—are the essence of democratic decision making. The more of that you can encourage the better.

So, as one individual communicating with another, you can provide the other person with payoffs in the dimensions of inclusion and control. It must be obvious, too, that you can do that in the dimension that Schutz called affection. Yet in our society we do not often go about asking for and giving shows of affection. You might find the following conversation a bit discomforting if it happened in one of your group meetings!

MARY: Jess, I need a little affection this morning. Will you accommodate me?

JESS: Gosh, Mary. Sure thing. Ahem. Uh. I give you affection. I have affection for you. I really like you a lot.

MARY: Thanks, Jess. I needed that.

JESS: You're welcome, Mary. Now, the next item on our agenda is . . .

Learning to talk about our affections is a valuable but difficult-to-acquire skill. As a very practical matter, giving and getting affection can make the difference between wellness and sickness. We are talking about physical health as well as mental, psychological health. Shows of affection are absolutely essential to every living person. And shows of affection can be critical to every human relationship—including relationships at work, in service organizations, and in so-called nonintimate settings.

But we live in a culture that punishes clear talk about feelings, especially feelings of affection. It would seem awkward, therefore, for Mary and Jess to talk to each other in a meeting as we suggested above, although they might say those things privately.

Similarly, you would be unlikely to hear the following dialogue at the office, although there is no reason—except cultural rules against such talk—for Sam and Dale not to say these things to each other:

SAM: You know, Dale, we've worked together for a long time. I just want you to know that I am very fond of you. I think about you quite a bit and worry and care about your well-being. I want you to be happy, as I have real affection for you.

DALE: I know that, Sam. I like you, too. A big part of why I like my job is that I enjoy working with you; getting and giving strokes from each other. Knowing you, having you for a friend, really picks me up.

Although nothing is really wrong with such an exchange, and although it probably does both parties great good to share their feelings with each other, and although those feelings are very clearly present in many same-sex working relationships just as they are present in opposite-sex relationships, such an exchange is very rare indeed. The unwritten rules of the culture make it very difficult to talk about feelings.

Group members can give one another signs of affection. A member might approach another upon his arrival at the group's meeting with, "It sure is good to see you tonight, John." Or perhaps a member might address the whole group at the end of a meeting. "I'm really glad that everybody could be here tonight. It's fun to work with the group." Finally, a group might express its affection more freely through attention to the social dimension. Perhaps someone will say, "Let's go for a pizza now that we have finished." That member is saying, in effect, "Let's continue to enjoy each other in a social setting."

SELF-DISCLOSURE, EMPATHY, AND TRUST

Self-Disclosure

In his important book *Transparent Self*, Sidney M. Jourard[4] posed a concern that *self-disclosure*—revealing information about yourself—is discouraged, especially in our culture. We teach individuals to close themselves. Jourard believed that it would be far better for individuals to become transparent. He said that people ought to tell others who they are—how they feel, what they want and expect, what their intentions are, what images they have in their heads, and the extent to which they feel open to topics and persons at any given moment. But, he said, we learn to distrust one another early on, and it is difficult to overcome that distrust.

In task groups a person can be too open or not open enough. The appropriate degree of self-disclosure depends upon the nature of the group and the norms it has evolved. Still, as you will see, learning to manage self-disclosure is very important to the group.

How can you know what a group member wants if she will not tell you? Her telling you what she wants is part of disclosing herself. If what she wants is important to the climate of the group, and she is feeling frustrated because you are not giving it to her—and if she will not communicate that want in some unequivocal fashion—then what is to become of the group? The group cannot know what she wants unless she discloses herself to the group.

A scholar named Joseph Luft[5] was very concerned about the importance of self-disclosure to the success of working groups when he wrote his influential description of what he called the Johari window. Figure 9.3 illustrates his ideas. You will see that the window has four areas, each of which may be larger or smaller than the others, and each of which may change size. For example, the first quadrant would include information that is known to the individual and also known to the individual's group.

At first, perhaps only a person's name and other demographic information would be included. A group member can *see* how tall a person is, so he does not have to ask. He can *see* what color a person is. He can *hear* the person's tone of voice and accent. The other group member does not have to verbalize this information. Thus the information is known to the individual and known to the group. It would be part of the information in quadrant 1 of Figure 9.3.

That is not very much to go on, is it? More information is needed to know the group member—the information that is included in the third quadrant. Here you would

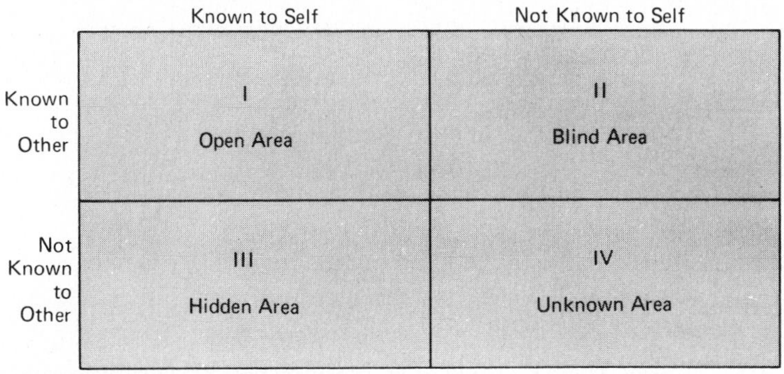

	Known to Self	Not Known to Self
Known to Other	I Open Area	II Blind Area
Not Known to Other	III Hidden Area	IV Unknown Area

FIGURE 9.3
The Johari Window

Source: Joseph Luft, *Group Processes: An Introduction to Group Dynamics* (Mountain View Mayfield, CA, 1984).

find information that is known to the person but not known to the group. For example, included here might be that the person is very knowledgeable—perhaps something of an expert—in an area of concern to the group. Unless the person is willing to bring that information over to the first area—that is, unless he is willing to disclose himself— then the group simply cannot take full advantage of his knowledge and he loses opportunities to contribute to the group's success and to its cohesiveness.

We can imagine that there would be information that the person would need, too. Perhaps he needs information about how the group is experiencing him. That kind of information, information that is known to the group but not to the individual, would be in the second quadrant. To illustrate, Don had just been appointed to a committee to study how to reduce energy costs at Teledyne Continental Motors. He had been at Teledyne for six months and considered this an important assignment. A colleague, Joe, the committee chair, approached him when it was time for the first meeting.

> Joe: I'll walk with you to the meeting, Don. Are you ready to go?
>
> Don: Sure. Let me finish this little chore and I'll be right with you.
>
> Joe: I decided to meet informally for our first meeting, Don.

Joe steered toward the cafeteria across the street, rather than to the conference room in their own building.

> Joe: I want to introduce you to some of the people that are going to be working on the committee with you. They haven't met you, but they've heard you're a bit of an opportunist and they're feeling threatened. I think it would be a good idea for you to spend a little time chatting with them to see if you can't do something about that image.

That statement came as quite a surprise to Don, who received it with mixed feelings. How could they have formed an opinion without ever meeting him? Don wondered. And what could be done about it, if anything? For that matter, what *should* be done about it, if anything?

> Joe: Just be yourself, Don. They'll like you when they get to know you.

Information from quadrant 2 in the Johari window is difficult to discover, but it can be very valuable. You might say Joe was disclosing himself in an effort to shrink this area and to increase the size of the known area, quadrant 1. Don listened, heard the message, and was grateful. Joe began the meeting by asking members to introduce themselves and describe in some detail their experience and expertise. He was causing them to enlarge the relevant area of open self by moving information from the hidden self. This helped the group members get to know one another in the area important to the group's success.[6]

The point about disclosure, using the Johari window as illustrative material, is this: In any group, appropriate disclosure norms are important. A wise group member will attempt to monitor the known and the unknown and to adjust the Johari window according to his or her own needs and the needs of the group. But that cannot happen without empathy and trust.

Empathy

Empathy refers to understanding another person well enough to know what the person is feeling and saying. Individual group members need to learn to make an effort to empathize, and they can learn to do that only by talking with one another. If they do so, then the other individuals in the group can come to know and understand them. If they do not do so, then the other individuals cannot. For how can individuals experience any motivation to communicate with you if you give no signs of understanding—not only what the others think about tasks, but also what those understandings mean to them?

Suppose, for instance, that Joe had been unable to empathize with Don. Without empathy, Joe might not have "known" how important the others' perceptions of Don were to Don. Joe might not have been able to put himself in Don's shoes. He might never have determined to introduce Don to the members of the important group he was to join. Joe might never have been able to anticipate or understand what the expressions of distrust he'd heard from the others about Don could mean to Don personally in the coming months and years.

Beyond all this, empathy serves as the counterbalance of power in interpersonal relationships.[7] The counterbalance allows people to trust one another and to work together. Without empathy, group members would be unable to give weight to other colleagues' interests as well as to their own.

And consider this. If you believe that another person feels what you feel and has your attitudes about things, are you not more willing to disclose yourself to him or her?

Empathy, then, like self-disclosure and trust, is very important to the success of a group. It is nearly impossible to imagine a group having any cohesiveness if the members cannot listen empathically. When groups are cohesive, their members display themselves to one another—not only intellectually, but without very much censoring of their emotional selves. Even if an individual is presenting a string of facts and proofs, the group needs to be able to hear the tone of voice, the phrasing, and the pausing, all of which say, "This is important to me. I feel strongly about it. I want your approval and support." Beyond these fairly obvious statements, it seems reasonable to suppose that empathy is a key to effective group activity.

To illustrate, if you imagine a group at the local YMCA working in a brainstorming session, you can readily see empathy at work. One member offers a suggestion—a half-baked idea at best, but a suggestion nonetheless. A second member hitchhikes on the idea of the first. A third member tunes in to the emerging idea and offers a new facet. The first member, feeling support and now in better control of his own idea, adds a phrase or two. Someone from the group jumps in with another statement, and so on. The group members create a puzzle of idea fragments out of their own experiences— lending, blending, and sharing in the creation of the brainstorm. The members have become a single working unit whose creative task is a shared phenomenon because they are able to empathize—and for no other reason. The point Deutsch[8] made in his 1960 essay applies here: They could not work together without trust.

Trust

The reason Deutsch gave to support his argument is interesting and relevant. *Trust* refers to the confidence we have in other people that we believe we can predict their behavior and rely on our predictions. Trust is central to cooperation because once people begin to cooperate (and the more they do so), sometimes their *individual* gains can be maximized by *not* cooperating rather than by cooperating! Deutsch illustrates this argument by describing a group of men who agree to build houses for one another. Once the first house is completed, the individual whose house it is has no physical reason to continue to cooperate. His payoff (completion of his house) is already a reality. If his only reason for cooperation was to get his house built, he has no reason to continue to cooperate. Deutsch speculates that if he quit the group at this point, then no other houses would be completed. Moreover, if the group had foreseen that he would quit, it is unlikely that any of the houses would have been built.

The agreement to build houses by mutual cooperation, then, is an act of faith and trust. Each participant puts himself into a position in which he can both suffer damages and gain benefits. Typically, in trust situations, the risk is that the potential for damage from betrayal is greater than the potential benefits to be gained if betrayal does not occur.

After reviewing the extensive literature on trust and cooperative effort, Alexander[9] concluded that careful communication can make a big difference to people's willingness to trust one another. But Alexander knew that in order to gain the maximum benefits of the ability of communication to contribute to the evolution of cooperative efforts, individuals need training in communication skill. "Individuals should be complete and credible in their communication," he said. "Likewise, they should emphasize messages intended to coordinate action and to communicate positive affect or trust. Messages which communicate negative affect or distrust or threaten should be avoided."

It takes but a small step to realize that if we cannot or do not trust one another, we quickly put up our defenses. Perhaps we stop listening to one another and begin thinking about what we will say next. Perhaps we become rigid in our own positions on issues that matter to us and about which we are feeling defensive. Defensiveness refers to a feeling of being threatened, dominated, or afraid. If we are feeling defensive about others, then we may become rigid in our positions on issues we were talking with those others. We try to find some way to get even—sometimes even lashing out. And sometimes, if the situation is important enough, we end up regretting that we let things get out of hand. Let's explore this notion of defensiveness in greater detail.

CREATING AN EFFECTIVE COMMUNICATION CLIMATE

If you feel threatened, your first response (like ours) will probably be to defend yourself. If someone is attacking our self-concept or if someone is denying our personal worth, we defend ourselves.[10] If we suspect but are not quite sure that either of these things is happening in a group setting, or worse, that they are both happening at the same time, the situation becomes intolerable. We defend ourselves. At least, we defend ourselves unless we make a conscious decision not to do so. And that is the key concept. We can choose whether or not to defend ourselves. We can also choose whether or not to discount others. Creating a climate in which communication can occur involves making intelligent choices about how we will talk with others, and about how we will interpret what others say to us.

When we determine consciously or unconsciously to defend ourselves, we can use a number of available strategies. We can avoid the other person. When in a group situation, this might mean simply avoiding eye contact. We can also confront the other person: "Dave, I'm wondering why you come late to our meetings. We don't like to start without you. Our meetings are almost always fifteen minutes late." We can attack the other person, believing the popular wisdom that a good offense is the best defense. Perhaps Dave follows this strategy: "Sue, you're always on my case. You aren't such a hot-shot group member yourself! You always get us off track and waste time." Sometimes, of course, it is sensible to avoid the other person. Dave might quit coming to the group's meetings. If the other person's judgment is unimportant or insignificant, it will not be worth worrying about. Perhaps Dave responds as if Sue hadn't said anything at all: "Well, let's get started." Or perhaps he says: "Well, that's one opinion. I can't see that it's a problem." Any unpleasantness that can be avoided under these situations ought to be avoided. So *defensive behavior* consists of acts designed to ward off what is perceived to be an attack by another.

Sometimes, however, we tend to avoid when we might more wisely choose another strategy. For example, we tend to avoid others when we do not like what they are saying, or when we do not want to hear their judgment. But if that judgment is important, it might be wiser to listen, even if the other person does not put his judgments very tactfully and even if we do not like hearing the other's assessment of us.[11]

Sometimes we attack others in order to win in a situation that we define as competitive. In fact, this is a very common method of handling our own defenses, but we do not recognize it in every communication event. One of our students vividly illustrated this strategy in the context of a paper she wrote to analyze an interpersonal communication problem. She had been dating a group member. As she reported it, on one of their study dates they had been arguing about "some aspect" of her participating in their group meeting. She was offended by one of his remarks.

When James came on so strong about me being lazy I knew that I had to do something. He was wrong, and beyond that, it hurt. Well, I couldn't think of anything else to do, so I went for his jugular—but in this case I really knew how to hurt him. He was attacking me, so I attacked him. I went for his self-image in male-female relationships. I told him that both his jokes and his conversation are boring, not only in group, but also on dates. I pointed out that he's not nearly as charming as he tries to be. Then the knife! I told him that he didn't even measure up to average men. Actually, I didn't have anybody to compare him against, but I said it anyway. Of course, he was very hurt. I may have "won" something, but I also lost; it was our last date.

The passage is interesting for its own sake, of course. But it is also a helpful illustration of behaviors that Jack Gibb recommended against in his now-classic and much-anthologized essay on defensive and supportive communication behaviors.[12]

Defensive Climates

We have a natural tendency to react to the "argument context," rather than to the actual disagreement. Stephen Alderton and Lawrence Frey suggest that we react more to the "argument" than to the actual arguments.[13] We become defensive when we perceive that we are having a difference and stop listening to the actual points the other person is making.

Gibb studied what happened when people in groups began to get defensive, and he discovered six behaviors that seemed to appear regularly under those circumstances. The first of these is *evaluation*. James suggested to his friend that she was lazy. He engaged in evaluation. When she told James that he was not nearly as charming as he tried to be, she was evaluating him. When she told him that both his jokes and conversation were boring, in group meetings and on dates, she was evaluating him. When she suggested that he did not even measure up to average, she was evaluating him. In no case was she talking about James's ideas about objects or events in the world. She was talking about James's ideas about himself.

A second category of behaviors, which Gibb called *control*, included all those behaviors that occur when one individual attempts to manage what the other person believes about himself, or what the other person believes about the world. You will surely recall that Schutz's theory of motivation included the idea that people have an inherent need to control others as well as their own destinies. If he is right, then we have an inherent need to control what others believe. And it must be obvious from your own experience that if someone is trying to control you, and you become aware of it, you will surely try to resist. That resistance is defensive behavior.

Was the student who wrote the paper on interpersonal communication trying to control James's behavior or self-image by her actions? We suspect that she was. Indeed, she says: "When James came on so strong about my being lazy I knew that I had to do something." Then she says: "I went for his self-image in male-female relationships." This is a very clear and straightforward example of what Gibb was talking about in the control category.

Gibb found out that indifference tends to generate defensiveness on the part of other people. He called this third category *neutrality*, by which he meant treating people without consideration for their personal identity or uniqueness. You may have experienced neutrality in situations where someone else treated you as though you simply did not matter.

In a group situation, neutrality most frequently occurs when someone makes a contribution that the others just ignore. For example, an accountant in a training session complained about his group experience: "Heck with the group I'm in. I want *out* of there! Every time I say something, they just pay no attention to me. I can't possibly continue in that group."

The demand to be removed from the group is a clear example of one kind of defensive behavior we are identifying—withdrawal. The accountant could no longer tolerate being ignored—he could no longer tolerate the group's neutrality.

A fourth category of behaviors that seem to create defensiveness occurs when someone takes on superior airs. *Superiority* implies behaviors that suggest a person is better than others—wiser, perhaps, or stronger, or more creative. If you pretend that you can overrule another, you are acting superior. If, to illustrate, a member of a group repeatedly plays the game of "Yes, but . . ." he or she is acting out superiority. "Yes, but my way will work more efficiently." "Yes, but you have overlooked this information." "Yes, but don't you see that your argument breaks down at that point?" "Yes, but how do we know that this evidence is reliable?" "Yes, but . . ." and other shows of superiority create defensiveness in group settings.

Certainty—the fifth category of behaviors that create defensiveness—implies or frankly states that a behavior is clearly and unequivocally right. "I am certain that I am right, and therefore you are certainly wrong." Such behavior leaves no room for negotiation. It eliminates the possibility that anyone else's notions have value. Thus, in the face of certainty, the other group members usually look for ways to defend themselves or their ideas.

Imagine how James felt when the student he was dating made it clear that he was below average. If he had any doubts about himself, her apparent confidence in her statement—made without hesitation, made with no sense of doubt—must have been very threatening. How could he ignore such an attack? His withdrawal from the relationship was virtually guaranteed by her behavior.

Gibb identified a sixth category of behaviors that tend to produce defensiveness in group members. He called the category *strategy*, in which he included any attempt by one person to manipulate another in order to implement a plan. If someone in your group tries to manipulate your behavior, and if you discover him or her in the process, you will almost certainly become defensive. The idea that others would try to trick you instead of just asking for what they want ought to be enough to build distrust. Such a behavior will clearly contribute to a climate in which effective group interpersonal communication will just not occur.

Consider this group, in which one member was using a strategy on another over a two-month period. Listening to audio tape recordings of their group meetings and examining journals that the members wrote regarding each meeting made it clear that one member, Jess, was determined to strategize his way through the group assignment. Indeed, his candor as he wrote in his journal makes clear not only that he set out to manipulate, but that he was doing it as an intellectual exercise. Here are three excerpts from his journal that demonstrate the point:

> January 18. If it's true that these people are having difficulty in selecting a topic—and that's what [the professor] said today—then maybe I can trick them into discussing the bookstore pricing problem. Anyway, that's what I am going to try for the next several meetings.

> January 19. It works! And, it's easy! I set out, in this afternoon's meeting, to manipulate Kip's thinking—he seemed least interested and involved in the group, and I thought he'd be easiest. So I arranged to "bump into" him outside the building. Told him I was frustrated that our group wasn't getting anywhere, and that I thought he could really make a contribution by suggesting a solid topic that everyone could run with. He asked what, and I told him the bookstore price policy. I said I couldn't bring it up because it would look like I was trying to run things, and that, anyway, he hadn't said much yet, and that put him in an excellent position to have clout. He brought it up almost immediately, and with surprising force, given that he never talks much in the group. And the group bought it. Moral of the lesson: It works.

> February 9. Kip is so easy! Today I talked him into going along with Janice's idea about forming a student government bookstore, even though his first inclinations were that the SGA couldn't possibly support it. I am continually amazed at how easy some people are to manipulate.

But ignoring any moral judgment for the moment, Jess's strategic successes were not entirely without cost. Consider this entry from the journal that Janice wrote that day:

> February 9. Jess is such a phony—and so slick. Today he got Kip to back me. Poor Kip— no mind of his own. But, Jess, UGH! He's a snake, and you can't trust him for anything. I don't think he believes in anything.

These six categories, then, comprise the kinds of behaviors Gibb found in groups that experienced defensiveness. Looking closer at the interacting groups, Gibb came to believe that there must be an equal number of categories that would reduce defensiveness— behaviors that contrasted in some way with the six categories that generated it. Table 9.1 presents the two contrasting lists. They are presented to help you compare and contrast—and remember—the behavioral categories.

Supportive Climates

The behaviors that tend to diminish defensiveness in groups include reacting to the individual as okay, although this does not necessarily imply agreement with the other's ideas. You can describe only what you can observe—and you can only observe what goes on in the world that is available to you. Thus you cannot observe such judgment calls as "beautiful" or "intelligent" or "correct." What you can observe is behavior or

TABLE 9.1   Categories of Behavior That Generate or Reduce Defensiveness

Behavior That Generates Defensiveness	*Behavior That Reduces Defensiveness*
Evaluation: Judgments or assessments of another that imply the other's "not okayness"	*Description:* Statements or questions that confirm the other as okay, and that treat the other's ideas and his image and self-concept with respect
Control: Behaviors that attempt to manipulate others—to impose upon them a point of view or attitude or some behavioral restraint	*Problem orientation:* Behaviors that make clear to the other that you wish to collaborate in defining a mutual problem and seek its solution; cooperation, not competition in approach to others
Neutrality: Behaviors that show little or no concern for others, and that treat the other as a *thing,* capable only of functions, rather than as a person capable of choices and emotions	*Empathy:* Behaviors that show an attempt to identify with the other's thinking and feeling, and that show respect for the other's value-belief system and affirm his human dignity
Superiority: Behaviors that expressly state or imply a "one-up" position and that discount the other; behaviors that state or imply "I'm okay but you're not okay"	*Equality:* Behaviors that expressly state or assume "I'm okay and you're okay, too"; behaviors that minimize differences in status, ability, power, and the like
Certainty: Behaviors that show rigid commitment to a point of view, and that suggest or imply that the other's ideas are wrong if they don't conform to that point of view; behaviors that create a win-lose definition of the situation	*Provisionalism:* Shows of one's own willingness to be tentative, to suggest that additional information might result in change of mind; behaviors that show willingness to cooperate in problem solving and that create a win-win definition of the situation
Strategy: To preplan a goal, then manipulate the other into believing he or she is making the decision; to imply caring that does not exist	*Spontaneity:* Straightforward, candid expressions of one's own attitudes, beliefs, and feelings

Source: Adapted from Jack R. Gibb, "Defensive Communication," *Journal of Communication* (September 1961):142–145.

existence, and then you must compare what you observe with some set of evaluative criteria. What constitutes beauty? What constitutes intelligence? What constitutes correctness? You might be able to make those judgments, of course—we all can, and we continually do so—but presenting them as judgments tends to create defensiveness. A better strategy is to attempt, rather, to describe the behavior or the reality being observed, and then, if it seems appropriate, to describe as well the evaluative criteria against which the observations might be judged.

To illustrate, this exchange occurred in a group meeting. Notice how Bill's response to Rick's evaluative statement not only softens the blow but is probably also far more accurate.

> RICK: Honestly, Joan. Sometimes I think you're spaced out. That question didn't make any sense at all—you weren't even listening to what I said.
>
> BILL: Wait a minute, Rick. That doesn't seem fair to me. You may think her question wasn't any good, but I bet she thinks it was! It seems to me that any question about something she doesn't understand is a good one. I can't understand why you think Joan wasn't listening—her question seemed to me to be relevant to what you were saying.

Notice, also, that Bill's comment is *descriptive.* It is characterized by references to his own observations and his own inferences. When he makes any judgmental statement, he labels it as such (" . . . doesn't seem fair to me," ". . . I bet she thinks it was!" ". . . her question seemed to me to be relevant"). He respects Rick but challenges Rick's ideas. There is no attack in Bill's remarks; that is, Bill does not attack Rick although he does confront him. Bill defines what he thinks "fair" means (". . . any question about something she doesn't understand is a good one"), thus to label the question as not making sense, and to brand the speaker as "spaced out," is unfair.

A *problem orientation* seemed to Gibb to be the opposite of control. When some people engage in conflict, take on a win-lose definition of a situation, and set out to win, they are trying to control others. But when they make clear that they want to cooperate rather than to compete, and when they show that they want to share in identification, definition, and solution of a mutual problem, they are taking on a problem orientation.

Once you have experienced the difference, you will see immediately how the problem orientation is likely to reduce defensiveness. Suppose you were in this finance committee meeting with Carl, a fellow who truly believes that the world is a hostile and competitive place. Suppose further that the topic you are working on in that group is the budget for the coming year. You say: "Well, it is clear that there just isn't going to be enough money to do everything that we want to do. How will we solve this problem?"

If Carl tries to control, and he has probably already made up his mind about how the money should be spent, and he has set out to have his way, he might say: "There doesn't seem to be any problem to me; we've got to meet our number-one goal as best we can. That means we've got to spend whatever it takes to meet it. We've already said that our first goal is to get a personal computer. So let's get on with it and get the computer."

If Carl wanted to take a problem orientation, he would make clear that he had a mutuality of interest and wanted to work with you. He might say: "Well, we have listed some priorities, but that was when we didn't know how much our budget would be. This low figure might change things. Should we reconsider our priorities before we make any final decisions?"

Carl's first statement—his attempt to control—would cause the other members of the group to become defensive, especially if they had some other priority for spending the limited funds. Carl's second statement offers collaboration; it invites redefinition of a problem the whole group shares; it suggests that Carl is thinking more of the group than he is thinking of his own private preference. The other group members are far less likely to become defensive in response to Carl's second statement.

Notice also how Carl's second statement shows empathy. It implies an attempt to identify with the other group members' thinking and feelings, and to respect what they value. Moreover, it clearly implies equality and provisionalism. *Equality* is the presentation of ideas in such a way that others see the presenter as acting like them in status. *Provisionalism* is behavior that suggests tentativeness in presenting ideas.

Carl's first statement, on the other hand, discounts the others. There is little evidence in that first alternative that Carl cares about the others. Moreover, the first alternative clearly implies that Carl thinks he, and not the others, is right. He is committed to the point of view, and he implies that any disagreement from the other group members would mean that they are wrong. His second statement makes clear that Carl does not believe he has any more prerogatives, and any more claim to the limited budget, than anyone else in the group. That is, the second statement shows equality.[14] Moreover, the statement shows that Carl is willing to be tentative and eager to create a win-win situation in the face of a difficult problem—a short budget.

Consider the differences between strategy and spontaneity. Imagine a little more of the conversation from this group meeting. Recall, that strategy suggests an attempt to manipulate. *Spontaneity*, on the other hand, is a straightforward candid expression of attitudes, beliefs, or feelings.

SUSAN: Well, it is clear that there just isn't going to be enough money to do everything that we want to do. How will we solve this problem?

CARL: It was pretty easy to list priorities when we didn't know how much our budget would be, but this low figure might change things. Should we reconsider our priorities before we make any final decisions?

WENDY: (thinking to herself, "Hmm . . . I know Carl wants to buy a computer, and I'd like that too, but I don't want to be the one to suggest spending all our money on one thing"): But, Carl, didn't you have something in mind the other day? Seems to me you said we ought to be careful not to water things down and I thought that was a pretty wise suggestion. With a limited budget we can't be all things to all people.

Here is a clear case of pursuing a strategy. Wendy has set out to manipulate Carl. She suggests by implication that she cares about Carl. She encourages him without taking a position of her own. A far more spontaneous comment would have made clear that Wendy was speaking for herself:

WENDY: (speaking as she is thinking in a game-free expression of her position): Well, I'm not sure that we ought to try to be all things to all people. I mean, I don't think it's a good idea to water down anything. I'd like to buy a computer, but I wouldn't like to buy a cheap computer just so we can also do other things.

Wendy's second statement, far more open and honest than the first, might bring out some controversy, but it would not create defensiveness. Her first comment might not call attention to itself, and she might be able to pull it off. But if Carl or anyone else ever got the notion that Wendy was strategizing the group, their defenses would go up immediately. That, of course, is the risk that Gibb was talking about.

Once you have analyzed the appropriateness of a dominating ego state for a particular situation, you will know whether to do something about it. If it is your own behavior, then simple determination to change, and some practice, will make the difference. If it is another person's behavior, then you have to make choices among tolerating, withdrawing, confronting, or attacking the behavior. Attack is not a very good strategy under any circumstances. Sometimes, of course, withdrawal or merely ignoring the behavior makes the greatest sense. But in those difficult cases where confrontation seems to be in order, you will be most successful if you have already been working to develop a climate in which effective communication can take place.

In situations in which defensiveness is the most likely outcome of the communication event, the climate will not lend itself to confrontation. Jack Gibb's classic research on group behaviors that produces defensiveness suggested six dichotomous categories of behaviors. Learn those behaviors that tend to minimize defensiveness, and learn to avoid those that tend to maximize it. Over several pages, behavior in each of the categories was characterized and illustrated in order that you might fully understand them and make the appropriate choices. It is a good idea to work on the climate of all the groups you work with, and to do this by using supportive language.

COMMUNICATION NETWORKS

The evolution of communication networks is a function of the evolving social structure of the group—its members' power relationships, for example, and task concerns—leadership being one of these. This last section examines communication behavior across time and space, the sequence of events that reflect what's going on in the relationships among group members as they work on making decisions.

Of the many hundreds of studies of group communication, perhaps the most common approach has been to study the sending and receiving of messages across space. These studies have been called *network studies*, and they have in common a focus upon the patterns of connection, or linkages, among the individual members of the groups studied as numbers transmit and receive messages. Interestingly, most of these studies are unconcerned with the content of those messages, and they aren't concerned about the means by which the messages are transmitted. The focus is on the pattern of connections—the networks.

Communication networks can evolve over time or they can be prearranged. For example, in most complex organizations, the chain of command specifically establishes a hierarchy for its members, including preordained channels of communication. And the saying is commonly heard: "Go through channels." Of course, even within this more formal context, informal channels often arise to meet the information and social needs of group members.

At the other extreme, groups often form without any prior notion about the communication patterns that will work best for them. In these groups the networks arise out of trial and error, reflecting the evolving social structure of the group—its members' power relationships, for example, and the leadership positions.

Most commonly, authors present highly stylized, five-person networks. Of course, group membership may exceed this number greatly or may be as few as three people. The five-person networks, however, are descriptive of the most common concern of those scholars who study group structure—centrality and its opposite, distance. Figure 9.4 presents the most common networks in five-person groups.

Centrality is a term used to describe the measure of distance from one group

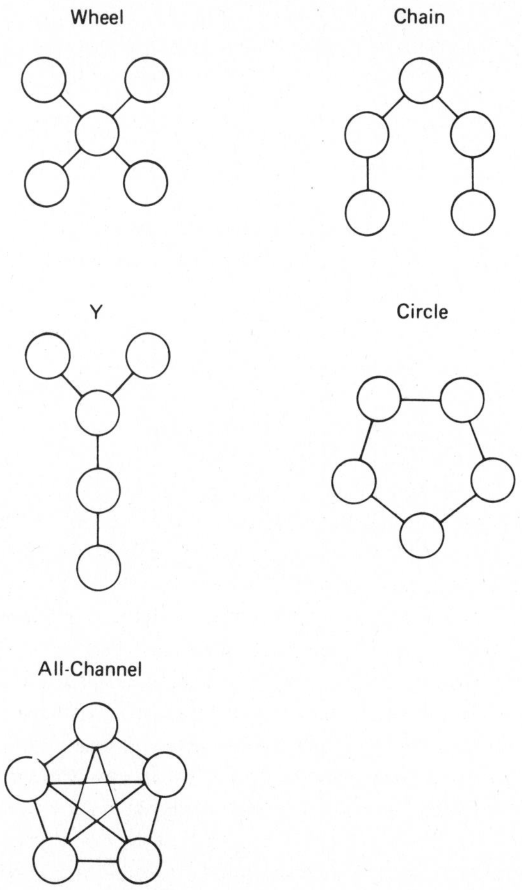

FIGURE 9.4
Communication Networks

member's position in the communication network to another. The measure most commonly used is the total number of connections, or linkages, required for one person in the network to send a message to another. To illustrate, imagine a two-person network (X-----Y). In this case there is only one link between X and Y. Thus only one linkage is required for X to send a message to Y. Every member of a network has some relative degree of centrality in the network. The most central individual is the person who can communicate with every other member in the network through the fewest linkages.

In a three-person group (X-----Y-----Z), for example, Y can communicate with X through a single linkage, and with Z through a single linkage. So Y requires only two linkages to communicate with the other members. On the other hand, X must go through Y in order to communicate with Z. You would count the linkages as follows:

$$X \text{ to } Y = 1$$
$$\underline{X \text{ to } Y \text{ to } Z = 2}$$
$$\text{Total} = 3$$

Since both X and Z require three linkages to communicate with the other two members, and since Y requires only two linkages to communicate with the other two members, Y has the greatest relative centrality.

With two- and three-person groups, of course, the matter of centrality is fairly obvious. It is not so obvious in the real world, however. Which is the central position in Figure 9.5?

Let's look again at the five networks in Figure 9.5, this time to identify the number of linkages each position requires to communicate with every other. Remember that the lowest number of linkages means the greatest relative centrality.

Notice that the all-channel network is a peculiar case. It implies that each member has equal access and equal relative centrality. We believe that the all-channel network constitutes a beginning state—a potential. But people evolve networks over time, so the all-channel network must be viewed as a beginning state—before a network has evolved.

Network studies have been interested, primarily, in the effects of centrality upon networks. For example, the literature generally suggests that a centralized network (the wheel; the chain) is more efficient and works faster than a decentralized network (the circle). In addition, centralized networks are better at solving very simple problems. But decentralized networks are better—more accurate—at solving complex problems. In terms of the social life of the groups studied, decentralized networks generate greater satisfaction among group members than do more centralized networks. If you take these findings at face value, you might wish to control the networks available to a group in order to ensure the best chance of group success. But the findings have not been clear because of a number of problems with the research. Thus, while you might want to keep the findings in mind, we don't think it is a good idea to restrict group interaction to achieve similar results. You might want to encourage full participation by all the members within a decision-making group, since many problems taken on by such groups

Wheel

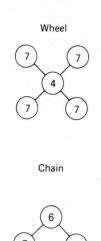

Circle

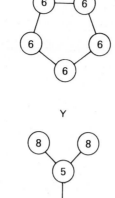

FIGURE 9.5
Central Positions
in Networks

Chain

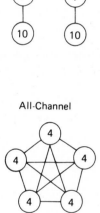

Y

All-Channel

are complex. Remember that decentralized networks tend to be better at solving complex problems *and* generate greater group satisfaction.

SUMMARY

Members of groups meet one another's needs through their communication behavior. Three assumptions about communication behavior were presented as a basis for understanding communication behavior in small groups. First, behavior is caused. Second, it is motivated. Third, it is goal directed. Group members behave in certain ways because they perceive needs and are motivated to meet those needs in order to meet certain goals. These needs are a function of each individual's personal perception. Perception must be understood as selective. It is selective as information is filtered through cognition and motivation.

Members meet one another's needs through communication behavior. William

Schutz believed that all people have at least three interpersonal needs that are met by members of a group: inclusion, control, and affection. When group members recognize these needs and meet them through communication, they provide satisfaction for group members and enhance the group experience.

Beyond meeting the group members' needs through communication, members' communication behaviors affect the group climate. A member can behave supportively by adopting behaviors that demonstrate descriptiveness, problem orientation, spontaneity, empathy, equality, and provisionalism. On the other hand, a member can generate defensiveness by adopting an alternative set of behaviors. These include evaluation, control, strategy, neutrality, superiority, and certainty. As group members talk to one another about relational problems, this communication can be more productive if the members follow the suggestions offered by Jack Gibb for creating a supportive climate.

Communication networks develop in groups as a result of the evolution of social and task structure. The key idea in network studies has been centrality, the measure of communication linkages between parties in the network. This is because people in more central roles tend to be individuals who can exercise power and leadership more easily. Moreover, groups with clear centrality tend to be more efficient and effective at handling simple problems than decentralized networks. But decentralized networks are better at handling complex problems, and their members tend to be more satisfied with membership.

EXERCISES

1. Describe and analyze your group's communication climate. Include both defensive and supportive behaviors.

2. Consider the idea of meeting members' needs. In a small group, generate a list of ways members might meet one another's needs for inclusion, control, and affection. Once all groups are satisfied with their lists, write the suggestions on the chalkboard. Compare each of the suggestions. Which of these seem to be the most effective? Try to come up with a list of five of the best suggestions for each category.

3. Observe a group outside class. Keep track of any instances that seem to be attempts to meet members' needs for inclusion, control, and affection. Write a short essay that presents your analysis of the ways this group attempted to meet these needs.

4. During an in-class discussion, serve as an observer and rate the group on the supportiveness-defensiveness dimensions. Create a rating form for each participant that looks like the one below. Place a check mark on each continuum to describe where you believed the group was on the dimension.

Evaluative   __:__:__:__:__:__:__   Descriptive

Controlling __:__:__:__:__:__:__   Problem oriented

Strategic   __:__:__:__:__:__:__   Spontaneous

Neutral   __:__:__:__:__:__:__   Empathic

Superior   __:__:__:__:__:__: Equal

Certain   __:__:__:__:__:__ Provisional

Evidence for my evaluations:

Write a two-page report giving your evaluation of the impact of supportive and defensive behaviors on this group.

5. This experience is also suitable for use with Chapter 10. Role-play the following incidents in a small group to which you are assigned. Be sure to apply the communication skills presented in this chapter. After each role-playing situation, evaluate the communication about the particular situation.

A member is continually late for group meetings.

A member displays superiority when talking to other members.

A member's need for inclusion is not being met by the group.

A member's need for affection is not being met by the group.

A person believes that the group moves off the topic too much; the person wants more control.

A person resents the childlike behavior that another member adopts when talking to her.

A person resents the fact that one member wants to play, rather than work.

NOTES

1. Harold J. Leavitt, *Managerial Psychology*, 4th ed. (Chicago: University of Chicago Press, 1978), 8–10.

2. Leavitt included *all* behavior in his paradigm, including such involuntary human behavior as respiration and, we suppose, heartbeats. We think that there is no sense in arguing this point. We are concerned with interpersonal behavior, and we think that interpersonal behavior may be described by these three basic assumptions.

3. William C. Schutz, *FIRO: A Three-Dimensional Theory of Interpersonal Behavior* (New York: Holt, Rinehart and Winston, 1958).

4. Sidney M. Jourard, *The Transparent Self*, 2d ed. (New York: Van Nostrand, 1971).

5. Joseph Luft, *Group Processes: An Introduction to Group Dynamics*, 2d ed. (New York: Holt, Rinehart and Winston, 1978).

6. Knowing others and being able to predict what they will say are important aspects of group communication. Knowing the other person increases accuracy of prediction. See James M. Honeycutt, Mark L. Knapp, and William G. Powers, "On Knowing Others and Predicting What They Say," *Western Journal of Speech Communication* 47 (1983):157–174.

7. See William S. Howell, *The Empathic Communicator* (Belmont, Calif.: Wadsworth, 1982), for an excellent analysis of the role of empathy in communication.

8. Morton Deutsch, "The Effect of Motivational Orientation Upon Trust and Suspicion," *Human*

Relations 13 (1960):123–140. See also his earlier essay "Trust and Suspicion," *Journal of Conflict Resolution* 2 (1958):65–79.

9. Elmore R. Alexander III, "Communication and Conflict Resolution," in Richard C. Huseman, Cal M. Logue, and David L. Freshley, eds., *Readings in Interpersonal and Organizational Communication*, 3d ed. (Boston: Holbrook Press, 1977), 297.

10. C. R. Rogers and F. J. Roethlisberger, "Barriers and Gateways to Communication," *Harvard Business Review* (July–August 1952):28–34.

11. William H. Baker, "Defensiveness in Communication: Its Causes, Effects, and Cures," *Journal of Business Communication* 17 (1980):5–17.

12. Jack R. Gibb, "Defensive Communication," *Journal of Communication*, 11:3 (September 1961):141–148. This research has been supported in more recent studies. See W. F. Eadie, "Defensive Communication Revisited: A Critical Examination of Gibb's Theory," *Southern Speech Communication Journal* 47 (Winter 1982):163–177.

13. Steven M. Alderton and Lawrence R. Frey, "Argumentation in Small Group Decision Making," in Randy Y. Hirokawa and Marshall Scott Poole, eds., *Communication and Group Decision Making* (Beverly Hills, Calif.: Sage, 1986), 157–173.

14. Research shows that defining relationships as equal contributes to an atmosphere of inquiry and freedom to participate. See Donald G. Ellis, "Relational Control in Two Group Systems," *Communication Monographs* 46 (1979):161.

RECOMMENDED READINGS

Jack R. Gibb, "Defensive Communication," *Journal of Communication* 11 (1961):140–148.

Gerald R. Miller and Mark Steinberg, "Empathic Skills and the Development of Interpersonal Communication Effectiveness," in Robert S. Cathcart and Larry A. Samovar, eds., *Small Group Communication: A Reader* (Dubuque, Iowa: Wm. C. Brown, 1988), 421–428.

William C. Schutz, *FIRO: A Three-Dimensional Theory of Interpersonal Behavior* (New York: Holt, Rinehart and Winston, 1958).

CHAPTER 10

Managing Conflict in the Group

OBJECTIVES

After reading this chapter you should be able to:

Explain the nature of a situation that produces conflict.

Distinguish among intrapersonal, interpersonal, and intergroup conflict.

Identify substantive and affective conflict in decision-making groups.

Contrast conflict resolution with conflict management.

Describe the circumstances when conflict is dysfunctional.

Explain the functional uses of conflict in groups.

Identify the sources of conflict in group discussion.

Specify the conflict-management strategies that are not helpful.

Explain techniques that are viable for managing both ideational and interpersonal conflict in groups.

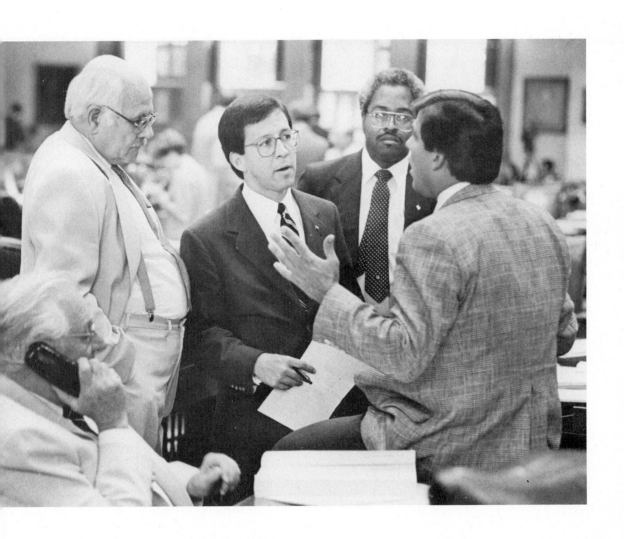

EVOLUTION OF CONFLICT IN A SMALL GROUP: A MEMBER'S REPORT

First Meeting

"The group of people from the Maryknoll Neighborhood Association got together today for the first time. I immediately noticed that members were lounging around in a rather loose circle. I suggested that we move in closer and we did. Carol got us started by suggesting that we introduce ourselves and tell where we work. This broke the ice. It turned out that Sue, Carol, and Nancy are all close neighbors and socialize frequently. Sue works as a speech pathologist at the local hospital. Carol works in her home, while Nancy works at a local bank as a manager. Jim is from Mississippi, working as the manager of a fast-food store and living alone. Doug is a coordinator of recreation for the city park department.

"I suggested that we could always get along without a leader. People seemed satisfied with this suggestion."

Assume that you are part of this neighborhood group and that you were taking those notes. Sue, Carol, Nancy, Jim, and Doug are also members. The group's members were volunteers, but you know the others from talking. Some know one another better than others. Your group has been asked by the president of the association to select several projects to propose to the whole association. These ideas for neighborhood improvement are to be presented to the next general meeting. We would like you to suppose that you took the following notes, too.

Second Meeting

"Doug missed this meeting. Jim said we ought to elect him 'leader.' Some folks laughed, but I thought that Doug's missing might be a sign of a problem. Carol suggested we get started picking projects. Jim wanted us to talk about the bad lighting at the corner of Hillcrest and Maryknoll. He apparently had a recent visitor who could not see the street signs. After a long silence, I said we ought to investigate what could be done to get better neighborhood park facilities. Sue wanted to know what I meant by 'better facilities.'

"I said I've never heard of parks without sandboxes for the kids, and baseball diamonds. She agreed with me; Carol and Nancy nodded in agreement. Jim asked if we should agree to this project without consulting Doug. We all agreed that Jim will talk to Doug before the next meeting and see what he thinks. We are to meet on Friday at seven o'clock."

Third Meeting

"Doug, Jim, and Nancy hadn't arrived by 7:45. I knew this was a bad sign! Carol was really ticked off at her neighbor, Nancy, for not showing. Nancy finally arrived a few minutes later with an apology. She had to work an extra half hour when someone didn't show up. We really didn't feel like doing anything since two of the members weren't there. Sue said that she thought Jim was cutting our meeting because the group didn't treat his idea for a project seriously. Carol said that maybe Jim didn't even talk to Doug—just to get even.

"She said that some guys couldn't accept female leadership. After elaborating for several minutes on this idea, she concluded with: 'They are just going to have to accept it this time.' I felt very uneasy with all this. I didn't object, but didn't agree. We ended the meeting with a vow to do a good job even if Doug and Jim didn't join in."

Fourth Meeting

"All of the members were present. I got there a few minutes late and found Sue, Carol, and Nancy sitting close together on one side of the living room. They had obviously reserved an empty seat for me right next to them. It was as if Sue, Carol, and Nancy had talked and agreed to fight Doug and Jim. I sat down. I could sense the tension. There was quite a lot of small talk, with Jim making several jokes and no one laughing. It seemed as if a coalition had formed against Doug and Jim. We were making no progress. Finally, I . . ."

How would you complete this sentence? What would you do in this situation? What would you have others in the group do if you were the leader? Remember that this is the fourth meeting and the group hasn't been able to pull together yet. It doesn't seem that the group is going to complete its work in time. What would you do? We think that depends on your attitude about conflict.

Self-analysis is an important step for you to take if you want to improve your ability to manage conflict. Self-analysis helps you to discover your attitude toward conflict and how you might manage it. For example, if you believe that conflict is evil, you might try to avoid it. If you have a positive attitude, you might make the best of it. We urge you to consider the various aspects of your attitude and compare them with what we have to say as we present our ideas.

We'll begin with a discussion of the nature of conflict. This will include some definitions and introductory material. Next we develop several ideas about the role of conflict in groups, which leads to a distinction between functional and dysfunctional conflict. Then we identify the major sources of conflict in groups. Finally we move to several practical suggestions for managing conflict in small groups.

THE NATURE OF CONFLICT

Conflict can be defined as a struggle involving opposing ideas, values, and/or limited resources. Morton Deutsch stated this idea more formally when he said that conflict exists when there is an "action that is incompatible with another [and it] prevents, obstructs, interferes, injures, or in some way makes the latter less likely or less effective."[1] Conflict has also been conceptualized as a struggle over values and claims to scarce status, scarce power, and/or scarce resources.[2] The goals of those involved in the struggle are to damage, neutralize, or actually eliminate one another. The important ideas in these definitions are (1) the incompatibility of opposing ideas or values; (2) the struggle over perceived scarce status, scarce power, and/or scarce resources; and (3) the goal of preventing, obstructing, interfering, injuring, or in some way making it less likely that the opposing goal will be achieved.

Incompatibility of ideas, values, and/or goals must be present to provide the motivation for conflict. The incompatibility may be either real or imagined, but there must be a sense that the differences exist and are important. This leads to an attempt to prevent, obstruct, interfere, injure, or in some way intervene to achieve the desired end.

The intensity of the conflict, and thus the stress involved, is related to several contextual variables. First, the more important and attractive the individual goals, the more intense the conflict is likely to be. If I am the leader of a group and know that the evolving decision is going to be really difficult to implement, and if I think the decision will cause me a great deal of grief, I will fight hard to defeat the proposal.

Second, the relative attractiveness of the options affects the intensity of the conflict. If the group perceives two ideas to be equally attractive, there is likely to be great conflict if the members also see the alternatives as being important. Conflict of this type has been called *approach-approach conflict*. On the other hand, when one alternative seems somewhat more attractive than the other, there is less conflict.

Third, a group may find that the ideas it is considering have both attractive and unattractive features. A solution to a parking problem at a local plant might provide more space for people to park but then cause them to walk much farther to their work stations. Such a situation produces *approach-avoidance conflict*.

Finally, the number of ideas to consider may affect the conflict. The group that sees several possible alternatives as equally attractive *and* sees its decision as an important one may experience very intense conflict. Members want to make the best decision, but they are likely to have trouble sorting through the many possible alternatives.

THE EFFECT OF CONFLICT IN GROUPS

The term *conflict resolution* reflects an attitude of the user about conflict. To resolve something is to settle it. To resolve conflict is to bring it to an end. The attitude is that conflict is something that can and ought to be settled. Conflict resolution is just not possible, sometimes, and may not even be desirable. For example, suppose that we have serious differences with Phil and John, co-chairs of a city council subcommittee, over the content of a report from their subcommittee. Suppose further that each of us is committed to his position. We know that in the end we will need to come to some agreement, but the active conflict is something that can produce benefits. It may cause John to be extra careful as he drafts the report and documents his ideas. It may also lead Phil to be extra critical as he reads what John writes. The best that they might hope for is to manage the conflict. They may never resolve it, and in fact resolving it might not be desirable at all, for the end result of this conflict could be a better report.

The term *conflict management* is used to refer to handling conflict. This term does not imply that conflict necessarily ought to be brought to a swift conclusion. Nor does it promote the idea that conflict is good or bad. To suggest that conflict must be swiftly resolved denies that it might be "good" and implies that it would be "bad." A more sensible approach is that conflict can be functional and/or dysfunctional for a group.

Functional and Dysfunctional Conflict

A number of people have grown up with the idea that conflict is an evil that should be avoided. Many students believe in harmony in their group interaction. They seek interaction with little or no conflict, as if conflict were bad.[3] This attitude can easily be understood. It may have its root in the fact that conflict is often a painful experience. The argument goes something like this: "Pain is bad. Conflict is painful. Therefore conflict must be bad also." This argument is an easy one for people to believe because it is sometimes true. Painful experiences are sometimes bad, but they can also be good. Likewise, conflict can be bad for us, but it can also be good.

Whether conflict is bad or good depends in part on how skillfully it is managed. Skillfully managed conflict has a good chance of being functional for the group. Poorly managed conflict may tear the social fabric of the group and be quite painful. Poorly managed conflict is usually dysfunctional.

The objectives of those involved may affect the usefulness of the conflict. Conflict is most likely to be functional when members value both the group task and each other. This valuing produces a need to work through differences. When members do not value each other, they undertake conflict more easily, with self-centered goals as the end, sometimes adopting an all-or-nothing attitude. When members possess the wrong goal orientation, conflict is likely to be dysfunctional.

Finally, conflict seems to be functional for some kinds of group activities and dysfunctional for others. Leonard C. Hawes and David H. Smith[4] came to this conclusion when they examined the results of several studies. They concluded that conflict is functional when a group is searching for and evaluating information. Conflict facilitates the search-and-analysis processes. On the other hand, conflict is dysfunctional in choice activity (selecting outcomes). Successful groups avoid this kind of dysfunction by concentrating most of their conflict in the middle of their group process, where they are searching for and evaluating information. The emergence phase marks the end of most of the conflict and is a period of substantial agreement.

INTRAPERSONAL, INTERPERSONAL, AND INTERGROUP CONFLICT

People in groups experience intrapersonal, interpersonal, and intergroup conflict. Our concern in this chapter is with interpersonal conflict. *Intergroup conflict* is conflict between opposing groups within the societal system. On a college campus you might discover several groups, such as fraternities and sororities, engaged in intergroup conflict—as, for example, when the fraternities compete for prizes in the homecoming float contest each fall. Sometimes those who believe strongly in particular political views may band together in groups and engage in conflict—as, for example, when Democrats and Republicans each try to elect their own candidate for governor. In a work context struggles of this type are illustrated by labor-management disputes. Intergroup conflict is an intriguing area of study, but beyond the purposes of this book.

Intrapersonal Conflict

You experience *intrapersonal conflict* when you engage in a psychological struggle over opposing ideas or actions. People frequently engage in intrapersonal conflict. We weigh alternatives in order to decide what ideas we ought to present and which ones we can support as others are presented. We discover that we are attracted to more than one alternative (approach-approach). We discover that we are attracted to an idea but that its consequences may be too risky (approach-avoidance). We discover that neither of the available choices is suitable and so we are stuck with having to choose the "least worst" (avoidance-avoidance).

The intensity of the conflict is determined by the importance of the ideas and situation and whether we are experiencing approach-approach conflict, approach-avoidance conflict, or multiple ideas or solutions. Intrapersonal conflict and its intensity create problems for groups because group members often conceal intense intrapersonal conflict. Groups can only be aware of intrapersonal conflict going on inside an individual member if it emerges in the form of interpersonal conflict. For this reason we will deal with conflict on the overt, interpersonal level rather than focusing upon intrapersonal conflict. By dealing with observable behavior, we can suggest some things group members can do to address conflict intelligently and turn it into an asset for a group.

Interpersonal Conflict

Recall the example you read at the beginning of this chapter. Sue, Carol, and Nancy were attempting to confront Jim and Doug nonverbally. They seemed to be trying to draw you into the conflict by providing a seat near them. The group was experiencing interpersonal conflict.

Interpersonal conflict takes place when group members openly express their differences over ideas, values, and scarce resources and/or goals. This expression usually leads to an attempt to prevent, obstruct, interfere, injure, or in some way intervene to achieve their ends. So interpersonal conflict involves some kind of directly observable sequence of communication behaviors. These behaviors do not have to be verbal. In fact, we suspect that in its initial stages most conflict is expressed nonverbally.

SUBSTANTIVE AND AFFECTIVE CONFLICT

Several years ago, Harold Guetzkow and John Gyr[5] conducted a classic field study of conflict in decision-making groups. They collected data by observing over one hundred groups from business and government. Two dimensions of conflict were identified—substantive and affective. These dimensions coincide with the task and social dimensions of communication. This distinction is important because these different types of conflict produce different effects in groups.

Typically, *substantive conflict* involves opposition related to ideas or issues. The focus is on the content—the ideas. Suppose the director of the mental health center calls together his staff to discuss follow-up support groups for their chemical dependence program. George thinks they should meet in support groups at least twice a week for approximately one hour. Joy thinks they should meet for a longer period, approximately two hours, once a week. These staff members are engaged in substantive conflict.

Affective conflict, on the other hand, is rooted in emotional and interpersonal relations. Consider again the staff meeting of the mental health center. Suppose, instead, that after lengthy debate about the composition of these self-help groups, Bill says, "Joy, you want to meet only once a week because it would be convenient for you to do so. You know that these folks need more contact than that. I really resent your attitude about this." You can imagine how Joy responded to a remark that seemed to challenge her professionalism. "I can't imagine that you would say anything like that, Bill. Who do you think you are to be able to read my mind and tell me what I think? You're dead wrong about all of this!"

Bill and Joy are engaged in affective conflict. This type of conflict is often characterized by clashes over self-oriented or personal needs. Perhaps both Bill and Joy seem to have a need to dominate. Thus the focus on the interpersonal and social rather than substantive and topical.

Guetzkow and Gyr found that the type of conflict affected how the group best achieved consensus. They summarized their findings as follows:

> A group in substantive conflict tends to achieve consensus by emphasizing those factors that positively promote consensus. A group in affective conflict tends to achieve consensus by reducing those forces that hinder the achievement of consensus. This reduction is largely achieved by withdrawing from a situation in which these forces are present.[6]

The group that is experiencing primarily substantive conflict solves its conflict largely through availability and use of facts and through efficient problem solving. Such groups are aided by warm, friendly, and nonrestrictive interpersonal relationships.[7] George and Joy might have solved their substantive conflict by presenting their reasons for wanting different formats for meetings. Groups experiencing affective conflict, on the other hand, seem to handle conflict best by avoidance. They often withdraw in order to avoid meeting the issue head on. Withdrawal in this case reduces the force hindering consensus.[8] In the case of Bill and Joy, after the brief interchange Bill withdrew from the conflict. In fact, he remained silent for the rest of the meeting.

Edward E. Sampson and Arlene C. Brandon[9] confirmed these findings in a study they conducted. They called group members who engaged in substantive conflict "opinion deviates"; the members who engaged in affective conflict were termed "role deviates." They found that an opinion deviate was met with increased interaction, presumably in order to exert pressure toward conformity with the majority opinion. This interaction is largely affirming, since it focuses upon the person's ideas through rational discussion. Others may ask for reasons, suggest alternatives, explain their own positions, and the like. But behavior toward the role deviate was not affirming at all! Role deviates were almost completely ignored by the other group members. This ignoring behavior serves as a punishment of the role deviate.

FUNCTIONS OF CONFLICT

Conflict is functional when it serves useful purposes in the group. Some of these useful purposes might be:

Conflict Increases Involvement

Consider the last conflict you experienced. It is likely that you cared about the issues. (If not, you would have been unwilling to engage in a struggle.) Most of us are willing to risk the pain of conflict over an important issue. This caring provides the stimulus for our initial involvement. But beyond this, hearing the issues and presenting and arguing for our position increase this involvement.

A group of local church members met to discuss their strengths and weaknesses. These were leaders of the various groups in the church. Thus, as you might imagine, they had a high level of commitment. They came to this meeting with a certain level of involvement. But, as they clashed over their differing views, they became even more interested and involved with their task. The clashing—that is, conflict—drew them into a commitment that was deeper than their initial level.

Once we become involved we are likely to risk more, say more, and to draw others into the discussion of an issue. Lively debate is often satisfying, especially if conflict is managed satisfactorily.

Conflict Provides an Outlet for Hostility

Groups can develop deep-seated hostilities that can be damaging to both the social climate and task achievement. If a group can permit conflict, it can be a healthier group. Members realize they are accepted as whole people who express both positive and negative feelings. That same group of church leaders profited from airing their views. They discovered their differences, were willing to disagree with one another, and thereby came to a new level of understanding. They came to the meeting feeling a bit apprehensive. There was tension in several of the group members. Engaging in conflict in this supportive atmosphere allowed them to release their tension. If the atmosphere had been nonsupportive, they could have released some tension but might have added new tension related to interpersonal relationships. They would have traded tension related to content for tension related to affect.

Conflict Promotes Cohesiveness

Many factors promote cohesiveness, and several of these are related to successful conflict management. A group establishes a history of being successful under difficult conditions by working through conflict. Beyond this, successful conflict management often means increased productivity, which also promotes cohesiveness. Finally, when groups manage their conflict successfully, members develop a feeling of commitment to one another.

Conflict Increases Group Productivity

The primary reason that we engage in group decision making is that we seek a quality decision. We expect that a group can make a better decision than an individual in a particular case. If speed rather than quality were primary, we would ask one individual to make the decision.

The time spent in conflict often yields a better product and therefore greater productivity than conflict-free decision making. L. Richard Hoffman and his associates[10] investigated how groups that were engaged in conflict used their time. Conflict about ideas causes a group to search for more alternatives. The searching is responsible for improved quality of decisions. Further, Thomas Beisecker[11] discovered that as the conflict from clashes over issues increased, the group's members increased their effort to arrive at solutions. Thus it seems clear that conflict over issues promotes critical thinking and thereby increases group productivity.

Conflict Increases the Chance of Genuine Commitment

The commonsense view of conflict is that a clash might cause members to retreat and thus be less committed to their decisions. This commonsense view appears to not be the case.[12] If group members feel free to express their opposition and their arguments, and if consensus is achieved, that announcement of support motivates group members to support the decision. B. Aubrey Fisher concludes, "If members are committed enough to sustain social conflict over issues, they should remain committed once consensus is achieved. Superficial or false consensus is more likely to result from suppressed conflict than from expressed conflict."[13]

A group that avoids conflict has much to lose. Interpersonal conflict in a group increases involvement, provides an outlet for hostility, promotes cohesiveness, increases productivity, and increases the chances for genuine commitment. But perhaps all of these benefits presume successful conflict management. Conversely, conflict that tears the social fabric of the group is generally dysfunctional.

SOURCES OF CONFLICT

Knowing the source of conflict may help you to isolate its causes. Once you know the source of a conflict, you can sort through alternative strategies and decide what to do. We think the major sources of conflict are ideas, status, power, and goals.

Ideational Conflict

Decision making requires the presentation and testing of ideas. In this process, differences become evident and arguments may ensue, creating a conflict that is useful. Thus productive groups will encourage ideational conflict as a channel for emerging consensus.

Ideational conflict may sometimes focus on the values that underlie preference for a particular idea. Observe the intensity and length of conflict. Value-related conflict is generally more intense and prolonged than purely ideational conflict.

For example, a case study used by teachers of small group communication is entitled *Nat Bronson*. This involves a fourteen-year-old boy who has been caught taking a car for a joy ride. The discussion question is "What should the court decide to do with Nat Bronson?" You can see that this is certainly a question of value—and very intense discussion, often turning into debate, often results. The decision revolves around religious and moral questions that center on the participants' values.

Value conflict centers around goals and means. If your group is having trouble making a decision, ask if members agree on basic goals. Sometimes members submit one proposal after another and are rejected each time. This is usually a sign of a goal problem.

Verbally aggressive people attack both the ideas and the self-concept of others. Although we do not wish to speculate about the causes,[14] we want to point out that such behavior in groups violates the ethic of being a good group member. The effect of aggression on the group is usually to dampen the spirit of free discussion and, thereby, reduce the quality of the group's decision.

Sometimes the problem is a basic disagreement about how the group is proceeding; for example, when overall goals are clear but no agreement has been reached about procedure. However, be aware that sometimes a group member will choose to create procedural conflict to mark either interpersonal conflict or disagreement regarding the solution.[15] Nevertheless, value questions must be met before a group can productively weigh important issues.

Status and Power Conflict

Status is the position of a member in a group hierarchy—a ranking of each member on the basis of the person's perceived importance. *Status consensus* is agreement on where various members fit in this hierarchy. It is one of the important conditions for promoting cohesiveness. Dissatisfaction with one's status will generally lead to tension and conflict.

All groups, as they meet to complete a task, work out a status hierarchy and sometimes two. The status the group members work out among themselves is called *achieved status.* Members weigh one another's contributions, personalities, and so forth and come to some sense of their importance to the group. This, of course, is usually not a topic of discussion, but people do size up other members. One of the high status roles, for example, is that of leader. A person may make attempts to influence. If the group accepts this influence, it is saying, "We give you status in this group." In addition, some groups have an *ascribed status* hierarchy. This status is based upon designations given to members by the parent organization. In a business context, for example, the ascribed status would come from the organization's management—they have promoted people to their various levels. The achieved status would come from the relative importance members give to one another. Conflict can occur as the group members work through the process of establishing a status hierarchy.

Power is intimately related to status. *Power* is the perceived influence one person has over another. Conflict can arise when members think a person is using power inappropriately. For example, a member might try to use coercive power to gain acceptance for some plan. Group members might resist and cause conflict. At a different level, group members will not usually follow a person who is not prepared. Conflict ensues when someone with appointed rank tries to lead without preparation. You may be able to think of many other examples of power abuse. Disregard for appropriate use of power is an important source of conflict in groups.

Goal Conflict

Of course, you may not always be able to identify a single source of conflict. Indeed, when conflict occurs in a group it is usually drawn from more than one source. At other times, conflict may derive from someone who is pursuing private goals—goals that are not shared with the group. (You may wish to review the Chapter 8 discussion on individual and group goals.)

Stanley E. Jones, Dean C. Barnlund, and Franklyn S. Haiman[16] assert that one source of conflict is the *hidden agenda.* This refers to goals or objectives that a member or members have, and choose not to reveal, that differ from those of the group. For example, a member may try to dominate the group in order to increase his or her status. Goal conflict from a hidden agenda is likely to take one of two forms. "It may be a *status conflict* masquerading as an ideational dispute." Or, "although the issue is purely a *socioemotional* one at heart, it surfaces as ideational conflict."[17]

In the status dispute, a person may want to be more influential and so challenges ideas in order to seem influential. Perhaps the person wants to be taken more seriously but cannot say that directly, so he or she tries to gain status by challenging the ideas of the higher-status members. A socioemotional problem happens when a person, disliked by some group members, challenges their ideas in order to impede the group and to get even.

But how do you know when a member is pursuing a hidden agenda? Look to nonverbal behavior, and watch for the excessively negative. Suppose a person makes several judgmental statements in a row. Perhaps the person can't seem to see anything positive about a particular person and/or her ideas. Expect disagreements to be couched in antagonistic terms, but notice overly cutting and negative remarks. You might observe one member not respecting another. Perhaps the person makes remarks that directly call into question the other's intellect, competence, and so forth. Perhaps the person jokes about the other's personality. Disagreements can happen without negativism and personal attacks. When they do happen that way, though, they may signal a hidden agenda. Also, watch the patterns of interaction. Two high contributors vying for status will sometimes attack each other. A challenger will direct attacks at the high-status person.

A hidden socioemotional agenda is more difficult to spot. The person may avoid eye contact while engaged in ideational conflict. Such behavior, coupled with argument, may signal a hidden socioemotional agenda.

You can tell from our discussion that there are many sources of conflict, and that it may be difficult to discover an exact cause. It makes sense to try to understand as much about conflict as possible. But what method might best help you to manage conflict? The next section of this chapter addresses conflict-management strategies.

MANAGING CONFLICT EFFECTIVELY

The manager of a marketing department handled conflict by raising his voice to shouting level. Then he reminded the others of their respective status in the department. He made it clear that whatever they had to say was not really important to him. This man generally won the issue at hand because he had the necessary power. He lost whatever respect his opponents might have had for him. His way of managing conflict was not an effective strategy. It was not effective because he damaged relationships. The resentment created also affected the department's members, who had to carry out decisions that resulted from such sessions. They were reluctant to put in their full effort.

We begin this section by pointing out some kinds of conflict management to avoid. Then we will turn to appropriate strategies that you can learn without difficulty. But first, a word of caution: You must weigh a situation carefully to make judgments about what will work for you in a particular group context. For example, in a work group under some circumstances, a strategy of using power and confrontation to make things happen may be the best. Change the situation or the context and this forcing strategy can become the worst of all possible alternatives.

Dysfunctional Conflict-Management Strategies

Do not say, "Communicate more."   Some people naïvely believe, "If we would just communicate more, then we would understand one another and agree." More communication may occasionally be the answer, but not often. I may understand perfectly and still be in hot disagreement! When people suggest this they usually mean that we should communicate differently. Good advice. To communicate differently is to turn to one of the other potential strategies.

Do not say, "Cooperate more."   We are certainly for cooperation, but it is not easy, and it may not be enough. People in conflict are usually unable to cooperate on an issue. Telling them to cooperate is not particularly helpful. Can you imagine how effective this strategy might be when two angry group members have been abusing one another over one's hidden agenda? Harold finally says: "Okay, bub. If that's the way you want it, you'll have to do it over my dead body!" Kenneth says: "Step outside, you turkey." You say: "Aw, come on, guys, cooperate more!"

Do not blame the other person or the group.   Even if you believe the other person is the cause of your differences, blaming behavior leads to defensiveness. Defensiveness leads to a rigid position, which leads to poor communication, which often leads to destructive behavior such as lashing out. The people you blame will not be at a loss for a response. They are likely to blame you back! Then where do you go for help in managing the conflict?

Do not attack the other person or persons.   Name-calling is a very common mode of attack, a mode of self-defense—a common reaction as conflict escalates.[18] We do not mean name-calling in the usual sense; we mean making judgmental statements about another person. To illustrate, you might say: "You're so lazy. You never come to the meeting prepared." By our understanding, this would be attacking the person by calling him or her lazy. This behavior would produce defensiveness, not a very helpful strategy for dealing with conflict.

Do not be too general.   Some people figure you're better off stating your complaint in general terms. They reason that the more specific the complaint, the easier for an opponent to argue against it. The idea that general statements do not give the opposition ammunition with which to fight back is right in one sense. This kind of behavior confuses an opponent. But it also makes constructive action practically impossible to begin. Defining the conflict in specific terms—stating the specific behaviors that are annoying—gives members a place to start in discussing the problems.

Do not avoid conflict.   Groups often create a norm that emphasizes the need for agreement. For example, the boss we talked about above (the one who tried to manage conflict by shouting) also tried to head off all conflict in public meetings. Some of the strategies he employed would make amusing stories if they were not true. This boss seemed to believe in these strategies—at least, he often used them! He would:

1. Tell them they are in danger of losing something and therefore must present a united front.
2. Tell those who disagree they are not "team players."
3. Tell the group members that he knows they will do the "right thing."
4. Hold the controversial agenda item until the end of the meeting when members of the opposition may have left or are tired.

You can see that a strategy of heading off conflict can create resentment and can decrease productivity.

Do not try to keep people talking so long that they give up.   Group members who use this strategy will try to manage conflict by sustaining it. They often make statements that appear to be group centered but that are actually designed to keep people talking. One might say: "I'm glad we are able to take as much time as we need to resolve this problem. It's good to get it all out." This may seem like a legitimate strategy, but if they have ever experienced a "keep 'em talking" strategy before, the group is likely to feel considerable tension next time it meets. People often vote yes just to bring an issue to a close! Considerable hostility and distrust may result from the experience. "Keeping 'em talking" is usually a most ineffective conflict-management strategy.

Strategies for Managing Conflict

A small group can use a number of strategies to manage conflict. You can probably compose such a list yourself by recalling your last several experiences with conflict. How was the conflict approached? Your list might look something like this one:[19]

1. *Forcing:* Using power to force the other person to accept a position; each party tries to figure out how to get the upper hand, causing the other person to lose. For example, "I think we've talked long enough about this. As chair, I'll settle the issue. We will recommend installation of a light at the corner of Maryknoll and Hillcrest."

2. *Withdrawal:* Retreating from the argument. For example, "Let's not talk about that today. I'd rather move on to something else."

3. *Smoothing:* Playing down the conflict (differences) and emphasizing the positive (common interests), or avoiding issues that might cause hard feelings. For example, "I know that we have our differences, but I hope we can put these aside, be professionals, and get on to making a decision."

4. *Compromise:* Looking for a position in which each gives and gets a little, splitting the difference if possible; nobody wins all, each loses something. For example, "It looks like Joe would like to give the Athletic Boosters $1,000. Cindy would like to give the Intramural Programs the $1,000. Let's give each $500."

5. *Confrontation–problem solving:* Directing energies toward defeating the problem and not the other person; open exchange of information is encouraged; parties try to reach a solution that is optimal to all; the situation is defined as one in which everyone wins. For example, "I can see that we have a difference of opinion as to where to spend $1,000 for athletics. What are some of the options for handling this?"

In his book *Interpersonal Conflict Resolution*, Alan Filley[20] has given us some insights about these methods. He classified them according to their likely outcomes: win-lose,

lose-lose, and win-win. A win-lose outcome occurs when one party in the conflict achieves his or her goal when the other loses. Lose-lose outcomes occur if, as a result of a conflict-management episode, both parties lose or fail to achieve all or part of their goals. A win-win strategy results in conflict management that is to be applauded. If two parties in a conflict manage their differences so that both parties achieve their goals, they have employed a win-win strategy. Since most of the time we are better off when both parties can achieve their goals, we are interested in aiming for a win-win strategy.

Win-lose methods   *Forcing* is viewed primarily as a win-lose situation because it calls for one person's view or goals to be accepted and the other's to be rejected. Small groups employ a number of forcing strategies. For example, the very powerful leader of a work group may let it be known that those who do not go along will suffer in some way. A not-so-obvious method of forcing in groups where a vote is appropriate is the majority vote. The neighborhood PTA may tire of discussion and take a vote in order to force a decision. Voting forces one group to accept the other's views or goals or solutions. If the minority complains too much, the "good loser" ethic is often evoked—this states that it is not appropriate to complain after the majority has voted. Although voting can be an acceptable method of conflict management, a win-win method might be attempted initially. *Withdrawal* is often employed as a method of obstructing a decision. Often the withdrawing person only obstructs the effort, and those who remain in the group win the issue. This is a win-lose method because withdrawal of support is rarely effective. Instead, there is now no opposition and by his or her absence, the person is in effect giving tacit support—a kind of permission for the group to do what it wants. On the occasions when this is effective, it is usually so because the group actually needs the person's support in some way. Thus once in a while the "loser" actually becomes the winner.

Lose-lose methods   Alan Filley suggests that *compromise* is generally a lose-lose situation. Sometimes it may be necessary to evoke a compromise, but if this is the initial effort at managing conflict we think it creates a problem. The problem is that each gives something *and* may resent having to do so. Compromise implies some reluctance, unless people have been genuinely unsuccessful at achieving consensus. If they have worked hard at consensus and failed, then they may be less resentful at having to strike a compromise. Compromise is usually a second-best, but often necessary conflict-management method.

   Smoothing is also a lose-lose strategy. Playing down, or perhaps "burying," the differences rarely dissolves the underlying tension in the group. Instead it allows the problematic situation to simmer and fester. This is apt to undermine the group's potential. The conflict may even emerge later at an escalated level. The conflict may only be set aside for the time being; thus both parties are potential losers.

Win-win method   Aubrey Fisher[21] has said, "When in doubt, confront." *Confrontation–problem solving* is a win-win strategy because it allows the group to collaborate in an attempt to find consensus. When the members of the group are not particularly far apart, they may be able to make a decision merely by focusing on goals and discussing information that relates to the problem. *Consensus*—the agreement of all the group's members—may be relatively easy to achieve under these circumstances. However, when parties are polarized in opinions or when there are a variety of possible solutions that seem equally acceptable, a more systematic approach is needed. The key here is to shift attention from solutions to goals. We will have much more to say about this in the next section, which addresses conflict management directly.

MANAGING INTERPERSONAL CONFLICT

Most of us find it much easier to confront ideas than people. This difficulty is easy to understand. Consider the difference between saying, "I disagree with you" and, "I believe that you are obstructing the group by your continual objections." Most of us would find the first statement easier to make than the second.

Interpersonal problems may be group problems because they hinder goal achievement. But they are also personal problems between people. Thus they necessitate a decision about whether they are best handled in the group or individually. It may well be that one person can find an effective channel through some other group member to the second party in an interpersonal conflict. Individuals can be unnecessarily embarrassed when you approach them about their behavior in an open meeting. A member who possesses good interpersonal skills, is respected by the disruptive person, and is willing to approach him or her may be successful in managing the conflict with a private conversation. If a private conversation doesn't work, the group can move on the problem as an agenda item. Rensis Likert provides a clear statement of how this can be done and its likely results. He indicates:

> At such times, it may be necessary for the group to stop its intellectual activity and in one way or another to look at and deal with the disruptive emotional stress. After this has been done, the group can then go forward with greater unity. . . .[22]

Open confrontation, then, involves making the interpersonal problem an agenda item. When the group has managed the conflict, positive results generally accrue.

Preliminary Considerations

There are some general guidelines that you might find useful if you decide that you are going to confront another member. These suggestions review much that we said in Chapters 8 and 9.

1. *Talk with other members of the group to confirm your perceptions and conclusions.* Your attempt to confront may not be successful if others in your group disagree with you.

2. *Make a list of the specific behaviors you have observed as being disruptive.* Presenting general statements about the disruptive behavior is likely to produce arguments from the person involved. Description of days, times, and actual behaviors may minimize both defensiveness and argument.

3. *Have some tentative suggestions in mind to present if needed.* The person may say, "You've said what you don't like about me in this group. Now tell me what you want." Beyond this possibility, it is important that you have some tentative, positive suggestions.

4. *Be prepared to listen carefully to the other person's view.* Listening is very important in confrontation. Most people have what they think are good reasons for their behavior. They want you to hear those reasons. When you have listened carefully and the other person knows that you have, the person feels understood and may be more open to change.

5. *Be prepared to use supportive communication behaviors.* Review the discussion of supportive and defensive communication in Chapter 9. Supportiveness in interpersonal conflict is essential to its skillful management.

6. *Attempt to integrate the views of others when possible.* It appears that a certain type of argument facilitates consensus. Daniel J. Canary and his associates found that the only argument structure that proved to be statistically different between consensus and dissensus groups was the convergent argument.[23] This is the argument that integrates the views of others while the issue is being contested.

Aubrey Fisher[24] has suggested another method of confronting a person with his or her own behavior that we think has considerable merit. This is especially useful when the person may not be fully aware of the impact of the behavior. Another member may choose to act out the disruptive behavior so that the other person can see the impact of the behavior. Fisher reported an experience in which a woman was particularly annoyed with a male group member's behavior. The woman chose to role-play that man's behavior—being overly critical without contributing any better suggestions—for an entire group meeting. We can imagine her saying, "I really don't believe that will work for the following six reasons." And then later, "I don't really know what we ought to do, but I don't like any of these ideas much." Then, at the next meeting, she confronted the person with what she had done. Here is her report of what she did: "I confronted the member I disliked with just that. I told him I had stolen his role at the last meeting to give him the feeling of despair and put him into another role that forced more responsibility on him. I like to be deviant. It's much less work to just sit back and oppose everyone's ideas than to create your own. But I will assume my regular position from now on because I put over my point."

The reaction to this confrontation by the deviant individual was remarkable. He wrote, "I feel closer to [the member who did the role-playing] in that because of our conflict and interaction we have developed a more meaningful group relationship."

A final suggestion for managing interpersonal conflict involves the group discussing how it is doing. Some ongoing groups are able to spend some time during each meeting—

usually at the beginning or end—to discuss how they are getting along. The leader of a weekly meeting of religious leaders might say: "Let's take a few minutes to review our progress and see how you think our last meeting went for you." If the leader can promote this kind of activity, then the group can gain a sense of progress as well as handle interpersonal issues. But concerns will not come out unless the group is convinced that it is all right to talk about feelings and the problems members might be experiencing. A session in which the group successfully manages conflict provides an advantageous time to initiate this sort of procedure.

But the skills of direct confrontation have not yet been described. Is there a better way to confront someone? Is there a skillful way to be clear about another person's disruptive or boorish behaviors in a group? We think there is.

Effective Confrontation in Groups

Suppose you have decided to confront an individual in your group. Experience and a good deal of research suggests the following advice, which might take years to acquire by trial and error.

Be sure you want to confront.   Very often people get themselves into trouble in groups because they act too hastily. Something occurs that creates a conflict situation and then, without thinking things through, one group member confronts another. We think every confrontation is important enough that you ought to make sure you want to confront. But how do you do that? What should you consider in deciding whether to confront?

First, put some time between the conflict moment and your decision making. This allows you to examine your own motives for the choice to confront. Here are some questions you might ask yourself: What do you want to accomplish? What is motivating you? Is there some perceived injustice that another is imposing upon you or the group? Are you grinding a private ax? Do you have a private hidden agenda? What are you feeling that triggers the inclination to confront? If what is motivating you is the good of the group, you might go ahead. If you are trying to get even, you may want to reconsider.

Second, examine the situation from all relevant points of view. You may not be fully aware of your own point of view. Of course, that is the reason for the first comment above. But you may not be aware of the other's point of view either. Perhaps there are reasons for his or her behavior. You might examine the situation from the other person's perspective. Ask yourself if you have discovered, so far as you are able, what the individual is thinking about. What motives could there be for the behavior you want to confront? For example, does Herb know something you do not know? Is his point of view correct? Even from his point of view, what does he want from the group? What is he feeling? Suppose that his child has been hospitalized? Would that be important to know?

Third, determine whether or not confrontation is appropriate from a common-sense perspective. Ask yourself these questions: Is the payoff worth the price? For example, in the task dimension, are you likely to get what you want by confrontation? In the relationships of the group, will confrontation create greater problems than it solves? Perhaps Herb will become disruptive if confronted. Is there a power relationship that creates an ineffective payoff-price ratio? (For instance, perhaps Herb is the chair of this committee. Is it wise to confront him on this issue?) And in the final analysis, are you likely to achieve enough of your goal by confrontation to justify going ahead? How much of what you want would you be likely to get without the confrontation?

Set your goals. Do not confront someone until you are pretty clear about what you want to accomplish by doing so. What do you want that you are not getting? Do you want Herb to come fully prepared, even if his son is hospitalized? Do you really mind if he needs to be a little late? Sometimes people do things you do not want. So the question is, What do you get that you do not want? Ask these questions about the tasks of the group and about your own task goals, as well. Then ask them about your relationship with the other person. Do you want to feel differently? Do you want Herb to change any of his attitudes? Maybe Herb is short tempered and not tolerant of other members.

If you determine that you want to feel differently, there is something that you can do for yourself, and something that confrontation may not be able to accomplish for you. So after you have identified your goals in the most primitive way, put them into positive statements about the other person's behavior.

The other person can choose to behave differently if you are able to ask in particular terms about the behavior you want changed. For example, you might write, "I want Herb to be more tolerant, tentative, and considerate of others' ideas when he talks." That would be much more helpful to Herb than telling him (and writing down), "I want Herb to stop bullying the group." To you, both statements may mean the same thing. To Herb they will mean quite different things indeed.

When you have identified the goals you want to accomplish by the confrontation, the next step is to determine if the other person can give you what you want. If the other cannot do so, there does not seem to be any reason to confront. Perhaps the fact that Herb's son is hospitalized leaves him no alternatives about being late and being unprepared. If the other person can give you what you want, then it makes sense to go to the third checkpoint.

Select the right channel. Given the goal you have identified, and your determination that a confrontation is appropriate, are you the right person to do it? If not, who? And if so, either way, should the confrontation be oral? Written? Both? Should it be face to face? By telephone? There may be very good reasons to confront a person face to face, but there may be other, equally good reasons not to do that. Similarly, it might be wise for you to confront the individual personally, and it might be wise for someone other than you to do the confronting. For instance, suppose that you have been a very verbal group member. You have taken an opposing position to Herb before. There might be a risk that now, if the confrontation comes from you, it will be perceived by Herb and by the group members as a continuation of earlier disagreements. If that should occur, it might also diminish the power of the confrontation. Thus you would be well advised to get someone else to do the confronting on the present unrelated matter.

Set the time for the confrontation carefully.   Almost always, confrontation follows a conflict situation. If the appropriate time is not selected, you run the risk that neither party will be open to communication with the other. Moreover, emotions may still run high immediately following a conflict situation or one that has the potential for conflict. Thus the latitude of acceptance of both parties is down. This can be a critical issue in selecting the time for a confrontation. But it is by no means the only one.

Do not confront someone when there is not enough time for the confrontation to take place. A thirty-minute conversation cannot occur in a ten-minute time period. If you cannot anticipate how much time will be required, err on the side of too much time in your estimate. For example, you may suppose that you can handle the situation in about half an hour. Do not select a time when you have only thirty minutes available. You cannot know how things will go during the confrontation. So select a time when closure has plenty of time to occur.

Do not confront someone while the flood of feelings is still running high. Rather, put enough time between the conflict moment and the confrontation to allow both parties to get their emotions under control and to get some perspective on things. Perhaps, if you decide to confront Herb, you should do so at the end of the meeting. Assume what is almost certainly the case—that the other individual is working on the conflict situation just as you are. Allow time for that to happen.

Allow enough time for advance planning to occur. If you are going to confront an individual, asking for a goal that will take time to implement, it makes no sense to ask for that goal if there is no time for the implementation.

A sign on the wall of an executive office at International Paper Company reads: "We can manage difficult problems in a couple of days. The impossible ones require a little more time." If you ask another group member for something you want, allow that person enough time to give it!

Choose the location and setting carefully.   Where you elect to confront Herb may make all the difference in success or failure to achieve your goals. Clearly, you want to maximize the chances that you will be successful. Should the location be neutral? Should the location lend support to you, at the risk of being perceived as threatening by Herb? Should the location give the advantage to Herb? For instance, a person's office or home is his territory. He probably feels comfortable there. He probably has arranged the space so that he can control the flow and ebb of power and interaction. He may have a barrier he can choose to use. Should the confrontation occur in a private or a more-or-less public setting? If you take Herb to lunch, will that setting allow for the full range of expression that must occur if you are to be successful? With that thought in mind, would it be best to put the confrontation into a setting that will impose itself upon the confrontation? If Herb is prone to making scenes, will the setting invite that? If so, will that help or hinder your ultimate goal achievement?

Stay in the present tense.   You have now determined to confront; you have a clear set of goals in mind, stated in terms of the other's behaviors. You have determined to meet the individual through a particular select channel, and you have carefully set the time and location for the confrontation. You are ready to talk. Resist talking about the past.

Herb cannot do anything to retrieve past behaviors. If you are confronting, you are beyond the conflict moment. But that does not mean that you must dwell on that moment. Neither you nor the other can restructure the past—and you do not have to. In any case, the past is gone, and you have stored it in your memory. Your relationship with the other individual, including what you remember of any conflict situation, is a present-tense phenomenon. So stay in the present. Perhaps you can tell Herb how much the group needs his help. You might ask him if there is anything you can do to help in the future.

And negotiate for future behavior changes. Herb cannot take back something he said or did yesterday, but he can agree not to say or do it again. He cannot undo what he did yesterday, but he can agree to behave differently tomorrow. And it is clearly the case that, if he cannot take back or undo the past, neither can you. If you try to hold Herb to his transgressions and omissions, you create an impossible situation for both of you. Stay in the present and talk about the future.

Personalize the confrontation.   By the term *personalize* we mean talk about yourself. Personalized talk makes clear that the person doing the talking is owning up to his or her own responsibilities, feelings, weaknesses, and strengths.[25] It is characterized by references to your own feelings and wants and judgments, rather than references to the other person's feelings, wants, and judgments. If you make a judgment, that is a function of your own activity, not the other's. Thus if you say to Herb, "You behaved foolishly," you are putting your judgment on him. It would be far better to refer to your own feelings: "I think your behavior was foolish."

To provide you with a means of internalizing this important notion, we have constructed Table 10.1, which provides both personalized and other-directed versions of the same sentences. In places we have exaggerated in order to make the point. You will see instantly that the underlying principle is that effective communication is honest and self-aware. Learning to talk honestly may take some practice, and it is absolutely essential if you are going to confront someone like Herb.

Be supportive.   We have come full circle. If you are going to confront Herb successfully, you must learn to be supportive. The kinds of behavior that minimize defensiveness and that tend to maximize supportiveness have already been described. Review Table 10.1 very carefully. A large part of learning to be supportive is learning to talk to another person in ways that are descriptive, problem oriented, spontaneous, and empathic. You cannot be supportive if you are also suggesting superiority. Equality and tentativeness thus characterize supportive discourse as well.

We have drawn these ideas together into a checklist to help you manage

TABLE 10.1   Some Personalized and Other-Directed Sentences

Other-Directed Sentences	*Personalized Sentences*
You make me angry.	I get angry when I see that behavior.
You're always acting silly and horsing around.	Your behavior seems silly to me. I don't like it.
That idea doesn't make sense.	I can't make sense out of that idea.
I can see the point you're trying to make, but you're wrong. The issue is, really, whether to . . .	I can see the point you're trying to make, but I don't agree. From my point of view . . .
There isn't enough evidence to make that claim.	I don't think the evidence is sufficient to support that claim.
You're late again. Looks like you don't care very much about this group.	You're late again. I'm guessing that you don't care very much about this group.
It's important that we meet before next Wednesday.	I'm not satisfied, and I think we need another meeting before next Wednesday.
It's just not fair for you to shirk on your share of the group effort.	I'm feeling resentful. Based on what I can tell, you have chosen not to follow through on your commitment to do these things.
You ought to say what you mean.	My guess is that you are not saying what you mean, and I have a rule in my head that I would like to impose upon you.
You simply must learn to prepare for these weekly meetings.	I don't believe you have been preparing for these meetings, and I am feeling frustrated.
I can't do that . . .	I choose not to do that . . .

confrontations better. Table 10.2 presents a confrontation checklist that you can use to organize your thinking.

Managing Ideational Conflict

There is a sequence of choices with respect to managing ideational conflict. The sequence looks like Figure 10.1.

Confrontation–problem solving   Ideational conflict needs to be confronted and kept at the ideational level if possible. This kind of conflict can easily escalate to the interpersonal level if people become ego-involved. Stanley Jones and his colleagues[26] have suggested a method of managing ideational conflict that attempts to avoid this problem. They call this process the "cone of consensus seeking."

Jones argues that issues have their beginning in assertions of group members. For example, if we were sitting in on the deliberations of a personnel committee, such an assertion might be: "We should fire Smith." This might be countered by: "No, we

TABLE 10.2   Confrontation Checklist

I.   Am I sure that I want to confront?

   A.   Have I examined my own motives?

   B.   Have I examined the situation from the other's point of view?

   C.   Is confrontation appropriate in this case?

      1.   Is the payoff worth the price?

      2.   Have I examined the power relationship?

      3.   If the confrontation is successful, what percentage of the goal will I be likely to achieve?

II.   Have I set a clear statement of my goals?

   A.   Have I stated my wants and expectations in terms of the other's behavior?

   B.   Have I stated my wants in terms of both task and relationship?

   C.   Can the other person give what I want?

III.   Have I selected the appropriate channel?

   A.   Face to face?

   B.   In writing?

   C.   By telephone?

   D.   Should someone else do the confronting?

IV.   Have I selected the best time for the confrontation?

   A.   Latitude of acceptance?

   B.   Closure?

   C.   Emotions under control?

   D.   Enough time to implement what I am asking?

V.   Have I selected the best location or setting?

   A.   Private or public?

   B.   My space, the other's space, or a neutral space?

VI.   Have I committed myself to the present tense?

VII.   Have I rehearsed the situation, taking to care to personalize my talk?

VIII.   Have I practiced being supportive?

should give her another chance." Then the discussion of Smith's job performance might go on in this manner for a minute or two. If the differences are merely semantic, the members might be able to resolve their differences at this level. However, when groups do not achieve consensus, members may find their discussion moving from assertions

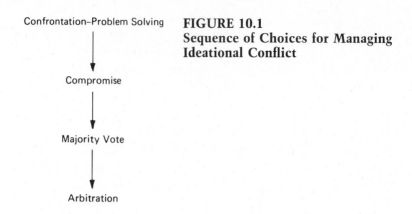

Confrontation–Problem Solving

Compromise

Majority Vote

Arbitration

FIGURE 10.1
Sequence of Choices for Managing Ideational Conflict

about the issue to assertions about one another. One such comment might be: "You know, Pete, you really do not understand this issue. If you did, you couldn't possibly believe as you do." See how the ideational conflict has moved to the interpersonal level. Interpersonal conflict is generally harder to deal with than ideational conflict. Shifting the conflict to the interpersonal level might be avoided by moving the argument to the next level of ideational conflict—reasoning.

Reasoning involves more rationality than assertion. The group leadership should ask those in the conflict to provide the reasons behind their assertions. This strategy forces members to expose the logic behind their ideas, providing a new area for discussion and potential agreement. In the case of firing Ms. Smith, the group might agree to one more year when it discovers that a member believes this is reasonable because Smith has not been adequately informed of the expected standards.

Members may believe that no particularly valid argument has been presented at this level, and before long may move toward a premature vote. Conflict should be moved to the third level rather than voting. Evidence needs to be provided. The group may need to go out and conduct more research. In Smith's case, perhaps she needs to be interviewed, and observed, and her work carefully studied. Armed with this evidence, the group may be more ready to continue its discussion. A stalemate at this point suggests that the group needs to move to a final level—values.

People who hear the same evidence and arrive at different conclusions may be in conflict over values. An individual's willingness to accept a particular idea may hinge upon what he or she thinks is good or proper or desirable. This is the most difficult of the levels of ideational conflict, but values can and should be questioned. Values ought to be subject to critical examination just as ideas are.

The easiest way of testing a value is through direct observation. To illustrate, suppose the president of a tennis club believes that strong, autocratic control is not a desirable method for leading a group whose membership is voluntary. But Don Johnson, who is chairperson of the membership committee for the tennis club, is fond of this style of leadership. The president of the club could attend one of Don's meetings and observe his style. Objective observations allow him to test the value of the method in the specific context involved. He might even formulate questions that would allow him to examine the underlying basis for this value. He might ask: Why is the autocratic leadership method undesirable to me? What is my basis for believing this? Is this basis valid? Why? So you see that the suggestions offered by Stanley Jones, Dean Barnlund, and Franklyn Haiman can be used to guide your group through a logical sequence as you address ideational conflict. Some groups do this quite naturally and without prompting. Other groups need leadership. We believe, of course, that you ought to provide this leadership when it is needed.

There is other evidence that Jones's suggestions really work. Researchers Harold Guetzkow and John Gyr[27] produced the following conclusions from their extensive study of groups in conflict:

1. A degree of conflict is necessary and helpful when related to the task.

2. Facts and expert judgment help resolve substantive conflict.

3. An orderly treatment of topics is helpful.

4. Members should discuss one issue at a time rather than discuss several issues.

5. Members must understand what is being said.

6. Leaders of groups with substantive conflict should do much more direct seeking for information of an objective factual nature, largely by questioning, and should offer more solutions and usually tentatively.

At this point, if the conflict still persists, a group may have exhausted its ability to reach consensus. The question becomes: Is there some middle ground in which those involved are willing to give what it takes to move together? Notice that the assumption here is that further talk will not yield consensus, and that no particular position that has already been stated should emerge as the decision.

Compromise   Compromise can result in pseudo-consensus. Once a group has compromised its original position and agreed upon a decision, members may still have reservations about the decision. When people give up something, they lose and they may not be at all satisfied with the outcome. If you were to question group members privately, they might say: "We couldn't reach an agreement so I gave in for the sake of the group. I don't really like the outcome and I don't agree with the decision."

You might conclude that compromise ought to be avoided in all cases, but this is not true. Compromise may be necessary when confrontation–problem solving does not work. When a group has met and struggled with a problem *and* talked back and forth about the issue and cannot achieve consensus, then compromise is an appropriate alternative.

The problem you face beyond actually finding some acceptable middle ground is achieving as much commitment to the decision as possible. It is a good idea to reestablish commitment to the group's goals. People have been willing to participate in a struggle to attain consensus. They apparently value the group's goals. You might say something like: "We've been struggling hard to come up with a decision and haven't been able to do it. Is that how other people see it?" (Stop here and see if you have agreement.) "It seems like we could abandon the project or try to work out a compromise. What do you think?" (Pause and let group members affirm the group's goal or say that they want to abandon it. If they show commitment, confirm their commitment.) You might say: "I'm glad you think the project is important enough that we continue. One of the problems that I've experienced with compromise is that everyone gives and takes. The taking is usually easy; the giving is hard and it creates disappointments. Are you folks committed enough to seeing us complete our work that you are willing to give and take?" (If the answer is yes, you are ready to discuss a compromise.)

Keep in mind that the language suggested here is only a sample. Our students often ask for some model—a concrete sense of how to verbalize the suggestions we make. If you decide to try it, you should carry out this idea using your own words. By the way, we suggest that you practice many different ways of saying the same things.

Majority vote   Stanley Jones, Dean Barnlund, and Franklyn Haiman[28] provide three very good questions that will help you decide if a majority vote is called for to resolve conflict.

> First, are the motives of the members really so much in conflict that, given more time for exploration, they might not be able to come to an agreement?

You might size up how close member positions are. Are there some points of agreement? Do members seem to be moving closer? Are their statements becoming more general? Often as groups are moving to agreement they drop the presentation of evidence and make less absolute statements. For example, "The best way of handling the increase in violence in our neighborhood is a crime watch patrol. And here is why . . ." may become "One way to handle the violence is a crime watch patrol." You might also ask the group if it wishes to continue talking or if it is ready to vote.

> Second, is time really at a premium?

Is there a deadline for a decision? If not, try to discover if members have time to meet again. Ask if they think it would be valuable to continue discussion by either extending this meeting or calling another. If they think further discussion is a good idea, proceed with it.

> Third, will a majority vote truly produce the greatest good for the greatest number when the members of that majority have not had an opportunity to come to a full appreciation of the minority's feelings?

Often a vote is taken without adequate opportunity for the minority to be heard. Decide if the minority position has been fully explained. You might do so by trying to summarize the minority position, including their arguments, in your own words. Ask if other members believe you have accurately reflected the minority's ideas.

If you can answer yes to all three of these questions, your group can appropriately take a vote. But keep in mind these problems:

If the vote seriously disadvantages the minority, then resentment sets in.

If the minority is needed to carry out the plan, minority members may resist.

If membership in your group is voluntary, minority members may quit.

If you answer no to some of these, your group may need to employ third-party intervention.

Arbitration   Arbitration involves the presentation of the group's arguments to a neutral third party, the group agreeing in advance to accept the decision the person makes. The assumption on which arbitration rests is that the group *cannot* work out its problem and that voting would not work either. It is also assumed that the neutrality of the third party will produce a fair decision, without causing either side the embarrassment of having to give in.[29]

Obviously this method of managing conflict is open to the same criticism as compromise. Members will have given and taken and thus are likely to be less than satisfied with the outcome. But sometimes it is possible to use a member of the group in this role. The group may recognize an uncommitted member whom it trusts to make a fair decision. The role of arbitrator requires a very exceptional member, and it also places the person under extreme pressure. It is better to find an impartial outsider if possible. Perhaps the group might even adopt an advisory role and allow the person who called the group together to make the final decision.

A Parting Plea

Conflict is generally uncomfortable and tension producing. This is why people avoid it if possible. Problems that produce this high level of tension are not likely to go away unless they are addressed. Confronting the differences usually produces beneficial results. Screw up the courage to confront the differences your group members have.

SUMMARY

Your personal definition of conflict can make a difference in the way you approach conflict. If you think of conflict as evil, then you are likely to try to avoid it. If you think of it as good, then you may approach it directly and attempt to manage it skillfully. We think that conflict has potential for being beneficial to groups if you understand it and are able to manage it well.

Conflict can be defined as a struggle involving opposing ideas, values, and/or scarce resources. This definition implies (1) the incompatibility of opposing ideas or values; (2) the struggle over perceived scarce status, scarce power, and/or scarce resources; and (3) the goal of preventing, obstructing, interfering, injuring, or in some way making it less likely that the opposing goal will be achieved.

People experience intrapersonal, interpersonal, and intergroup conflict as they interact and associate with groups. Our concern is with interpersonal conflict, as it is the overt level of conflict we experience in groups. Interpersonal conflict takes place when group members openly express their differences over ideas, values, scarce resources, and/or goals. This usually leads to an attempt by the parties involved to press their position in an attempt to gain acceptance. Conflict may be over substantive issues—ideational conflict—or over affective issues—social conflict. The locus of the conflict will affect the way the group responds to it.

Conflict can be functional or dysfunctional, depending on how skillfully it is managed and its outcome. Conflict is more likely to be functional if group members value each other and the group's goals. Conflict also tends to be functional when the group is searching for and evaluating information. It tends to be dysfunctional when a group is in the process of generating information and selecting outcomes.

Conflict can serve many useful functions for a group. When managed skillfully it (1) increases member involvement, (2) provides an outlet for hostility, (3) promotes cohesiveness, (4) increases group productivity, and (5) increases the chance for genuine commitment to the decision.

There are four sources of conflict: ideas, personality, status, and power. Understanding the source of conflict is the first step in managing it. These four fall into two basic categories: ideational and interpersonal conflict.

Sometimes those who suggest how to manage conflict give bad advice. We think that it is not helpful to suggest communicating more, cooperating more, blaming the other person, attacking the other person, keeping the talk general, or trying to keep others talking long enough that they give up. There are other strategies that are often not productive. These include withdrawal, smoothing, compromise, and forcing. The strategy we think is the most promising is confrontation–problem solving.

Interpersonal conflict is usually best handled by confrontation. We presented several things you ought to do if you decide to engage in confrontation: (1) talk with other members of the group to confirm your perception and conclusions, (2) make a list of the specific behaviors you have observed as disruptive, (3) have some tentative suggestions in mind to present, (4) be prepared to listen carefully, and (5) be prepared to utilize supportive communication behaviors. Beyond these you need to decide whether to confront the person in your group meeting or privately. A private confrontation may be successful if the person doing the confronting is a respected and skillful communicator. We presented a confrontation checklist to help you manage interpersonal confrontation.

As an alternative, you might consider bringing up the behavior in the group. One creative way to do this is to role-play the disruptive behavior of the other person. The person may realize that he or she is creating a problem and be able to correct the situation.

There is a sequence of strategies that you might follow when your group experiences ideational conflict. First, try confrontation–problem solving. You can use the "cone of consensus seeking" as a model for confrontation–problem solving. Move from the assertion level to the reasons behind the assertions to the evidence and finally to the underlying values. Then move to compromise if your group cannot achieve consensus. If this doesn't work, your group may need to take a vote and go with the majority opinion. If a vote seems unwise, you might submit the data to a neutral third party for arbitration.

Compromise can result in pseudo-consensus. It is therefore a second-best method. It is appropriate if members cannot achieve consensus and are willing to give and take. Majority vote forces the minority to accept their view. You might resort to this if the good of the group is likely to be achieved and the minority has had sufficient opportunity to present its view. Arbitration might be the answer when members believe they are sufficiently biased that they may not make a decision that is for the good of the group. Arbitration may also be wise when members know that strong feelings may keep the minority from supporting the decision of the group. Both the minority and majority may be able to agree to support the decision of a neutral third party.

Finally, confrontation can be facilitated by creating a norm and a time in the group to discuss the group's progress and problems. This provides a forum for interpersonal conflict. If you decide that the conflict is ideational, you will want to move the group through the "cone of consensus seeking." This involves the relative attractiveness of the options in relation to each other, and the mixture of positive and negative outcomes related to the options.

EXERCISES

1. Describe your personal style of conflict management. Analyze its effectiveness in your group. Complete your analysis of conflict by describing any sources of group conflict that you have observed.

2. As a small group, design a role-playing situation that involves the potential for conflict. Assign some members the task of bringing up arguments that are likely to be controversial. Assign other members the task of managing conflict in this group. After twenty minutes of discussion, analyze the conflict management employed by each of the members who were actively attempting to manage the conflict. What techniques did they use? How well did they work? What alternative strategies might have been employed?

3. Conduct a class discussion where the idea of conflict being good is discussed. Do class members agree that conflict is usually good? Why? Why not? Under what circumstances do you see conflict as being functional? Dysfunctional?

4. Write a short paper that analyzes your personal style of conflict management. Describe your style. Describe what usually happens when you employ this management strategy. How do you feel? How does the other person feel? Would you describe it as a win-win, lose-lose, or win-lose strategy? Is the relationship between you and the other person usually strengthened as a result of the conflict? Is it weakened? Based on the information presented in this chapter, describe what you believe to be the best conflict management strategy for you personally.

5. A group is discussing the problem of plagiarism. One member says, "I think there is nothing wrong with cheating. Everyone does it. That is the way people survive." Another member says, "I am shocked that you would admit that you believe such things. Don't you understand that there is more to morality than just doing what others are doing? I can't believe you said that!" You know that both participants are likely to believe strongly in their positions. You know that they will need help in working through this conflict. Describe the steps you might take to manage this conflict.

6. Role-play the following incidents in a small group to which you are assigned. Be sure to apply the confrontation checklist presented in this chapter. After each role-playing situation, the communication about the behavior should be critiqued.

A member is continually late for group meetings.

A member displays superiority when talking to other members.

A member's need for inclusion is not being met by the group.

A member's need for affection is not being met by the group.

A person believes that the group moves off the topic too much, the person wants more control.

A person resents the parentlike relationship that another member adopts when talking to her.

A person resents the fact that another member wants to play rather than work.

7. Find a meeting of a group that involves a number of special interests related to a controversial topic. Perhaps this group is a city council, student government, or some policy-making group. Discover an interchange that you would characterize as conflict. Write a short paper that describes the conflict, discusses how the conflict was managed, and critiques the method used for its effectiveness.

NOTES

1. Morton Deutsch, *The Resolution of Conflict* (New Haven: Yale University Press, 1973), 10.

2. Lewis Coser, *The Functions of Social Conflict* (New York: The Free Press, 1956), 8, 41, 49.

3. Victor D. Wall, Jr., Gloria J. Galanes, and Susan B. Love, "Small, Task-Oriented Groups: Conflict, Conflict Management, Satisfaction, and Decision Quality," *Small Group Behavior* 18 (1987):31–55.

4. Leonard C. Hawes and David H. Smith, "A Critique of Assumptions Underlying the Study of Communication and Conflict," *Quarterly Journal of Speech* 59 (1973):423–435.

5. Harold Guetzkow and John Gyr, "An Analysis of Conflict in Decision-Making Groups," *Human Relations* 7 (1954):367–381.

6. Ibid., 373.

7. Ibid., 377.

8. Ibid., 379.

9. Edward E. Sampson and Arlene C. Brandon, "The Effects of Role and Opinion Deviation on Small Group Behavior," *Sociometry* 27 (1964):261–281.

10. L. Richard Hoffman, Ernest Harburg, and Norman R. F. Maier, "Differences and Disagreements as Factors in Creative Group Problem-Solving," *Journal of Abnormal and Social Psychology* 64 (1962):206–214.

11. Thomas Beisecker, "Communication and Conflict in Interpersonal Negotiations" (Paper presented to the annual meeting of the Speech Communication Association, New York, December 1969).

12. Henry W. Riecken, "Some Problems of Consensus Development," *Rural Sociology* 17 (1952):245–252.

13. B. Aubrey Fisher, *Small Group Decision Making*, 2d ed. (New York: McGraw-Hill, 1980), 239.

14. See Dominic A. Infante and Charles J. Wigley III, "Verbal Aggressiveness: An Interpersonal Model and Measure," *Communication Monographs* 53 (1986):61–67, for a discussion of causes of aggressive behavior.

15. Linda L. Putnam, "Conflict in Group Decision Making," in Randy Y. Hirokawa and Marshall Scott Poole, eds., *Communication and Group Decision Making* (Beverly Hills, Calif.: Sage, 1986), 175–196.

16. Stanley E. Jones, Dean C. Barnlund, and Franklyn S. Haiman, *The Dynamics of Discussion: Communication in Small Groups*, 2d ed. (New York: Harper & Row, 1980), 140.

17. Ibid.

18. Virginia G. Waln, "Interpersonal Conflict: An Examination of Verbal Defense of Self," *Central States Speech Journal* 33 (1982):557–566.

19. Ronald J. Burke, "Methods of Resolving Superior-Subordinate Conflict: The Constructive Use of Subordinate Differences and Disagreements," in R. C. Huseman, C. M. Logue, and D. L. Freshley, eds., *Readings in Interpersonal and Organizational Communication*, 3d ed. (Boston: Holbrook Press, 1977), 254–255.

20. Alan C. Filley, *Interpersonal Conflict Resolution* (Glenview, Ill.: Scott, Foresman, 1975).

21. Fisher, 252.

22. Rensis Likert, *New Patterns of Management* (New York: McGraw-Hill, 1961), 176.

23. Daniel J. Canary, Brent G. Brossmann, and David R. Seibold, "Argument Structures in Decision-Making Groups," *Southern Speech Communication Journal* 53 (1987):18–37.

24. Fisher, 253.

25. One group of researchers discovered that this type of language is perceived as more supportive than other types of pronoun construction. See Steven Winer and Randall E. Majors, "A Research Done on Supportive and Defensive Communication: An Empirical Study of Three Verbal Interpersonal Variables," *Communication Quarterly* 29 (1981):166–172.

26. Jones, Barnlund, and Haiman, 146–151.

27. Guetzkow and Gyr, 367–381.

28. Jones, Barnlund, and Haiman, 151.

29. Jeffrey Z. Rubin, "Experimental Research on Third-Party Intervention in Conflict," *Psychological Bulletin* 87 (1980):380.

RECOMMENDED READINGS

Alan C. Filley, *Interpersonal Conflict Resolution* (Glenview, Ill.: Scott, Foresman, 1975).

Roger Fisher and William Ury, *Getting to Yes: Negotiating Agreement Without Giving In* (New York: Penguin Books, 1983).

J. L. Hocker and W. W. Wilmot, *Interpersonal Conflict*, 2d ed. (Dubuque, Iowa: Wm. C. Brown, 1985).

Linda L. Putnam, "Conflict in Group Decision Making," in Randy Y. Hirokawa and Marshall Scott Poole, eds., *Communication and Group Decision Making* (Beverly Hills, Calif.: Sage, 1986), 175–197.

Victor D. Wall, Jr., and Linda L. Nolan, "Small Group Conflict: A Look at Equity, Satisfaction, and Styles of Conflict Management," *Small Group Behavior* 18 (1987):188–211.

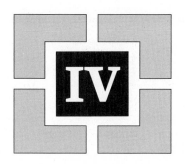

Analyzing Small Group Decision Making

CHAPTER 11

Observing and Evaluating Groups

OBJECTIVES

After reading this chapter you should be able to:

List and explain the ground rules for observing a group discussion.

Utilize an interaction diagram in observing a group.

Tabulate categories of interaction using Bales's interaction process analysis (IPA) category system, and specify the effect the categories had for the task and social dimensions.

Identify the various roles being played in a group, and analyze the effect of these on the group's progress.

Evaluate the leadership of a group using the Barnlund-Haiman leadership rating scale.

Evaluate the decision making of a group discussion.

Utilize discussion participant evaluation and postmeeting reaction forms to make conclusions about a group discussion.

Evaluate the cohesiveness of a group using the Seashore index of group cohesiveness.

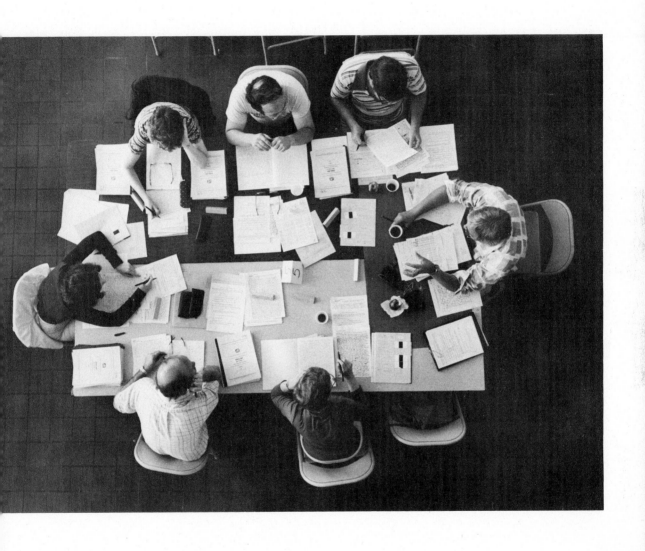

Paul Smith has been a manager in a research group of a food canning company for five years. His way of working with problems assigned to his department is to hand them over to members of a research team. He frequently sits in on parts of their meetings to check on their progress. If you could listen to him talk to himself, you would hear something like this: "I don't understand how it could take them so long to deal with such a simple problem. I sure wish I could help them. Well, I'm not sure how they got where they are and what I might suggest to help. I better keep out of it this time." Paul Smith is a real person who expressed a thought like this one day. What he was trying to say was, "I wish I had some way of being able to tell what is going on in situations like this. And beyond that I wish I had the knowledge to know what to do to help these groups when they are having trouble."

The first ten chapters of this book provide information to you and people like Paul Smith to help you analyze what is going on in groups and know why and understand what your options are for helping. This chapter focuses on the other half of Paul's dilemma. He must be able to observe and collect data to use in attempting to help with a group's problem. The chapter's aim is to give you the skills and tools to systematically collect data about a group. The chapter begins with some basic suggestions about observing groups and collecting data about them. Then a variety of data-collecting instruments are presented. We offer a variety so that you can choose those that will allow you to look at the particular aspect of a group that is of most interest to you.

The content of this chapter was selected with several assumptions in mind. First, we assumed that you are not interested in observing groups for the purpose of constructing theories. We also assumed that your interest is not in doing formal research. Rather we assume that you are interested, as was Paul Smith, in observing groups and collecting data in order to make sense out of what is going on in them. Further, we assumed that you are collecting data for the purpose of improving on a group's performance and making the experience better for the group's members. Consequently, the data-collecting tools we present are developed as simply as possible. Several of them have been used as research tools; for those of you who might have an interest in that use, we present the citations for the reports that describe the instruments and their use in greater detail.

OBSERVING SMALL GROUP INTERACTION

Observing a small group in a classroom setting is usually quite a different experience from observing a group out in the community or at work. The classroom setting allows more freedom for the observer and a variety of observer interventions. In the classroom the observer might interrupt the discussion at predesignated points and discuss with the group what he or she has observed. Sometimes an observer is assigned to a particular member and whispers suggestions based upon his or her observations to the member. This kind of observer intervention is normally inappropriate in community or work groups.

Ground Rules for Observing Groups

The roles of observer, analyst, and critic can be quite frustrating if you do not know something about observation techniques. Here are some suggestions.

First, decide what it is that you want to observe. You might want to observe the interaction, the roles being played, the leadership, the problem-solving process, or overall effectiveness. But you are unlikely to be effective in an effort to examine all of these. Set a goal for your observation and criticism. Focusing allows you to examine much more closely and make more refined judgments.

Second, be careful to distinguish between judgments made on the basis of your data and judgments that go beyond your data. The data serve as evidence for what you have to say. Use them to describe the group's behavior and then suggest your conclusion. When you move beyond the data, cue the group in to that fact. You might say, "Here is what I saw. I am wondering if the group also . . ."

Third, do not try to comment on everything you observe. Focus your criticism on key points. Your major reason for observation and criticism is to help groups improve. If you comment on everything, they will not know how to focus their effort to improve.

Fourth, balance the positive and the negative. Being too negative can adversely affect the climate of your critique. Groups expect that they have faults and are usually ready to hear them. But they also expect that they are doing some things right. Keep a balance, and be careful not to give too much negative criticism. Perhaps you can give them two or three things to work on for their next effort.

Finally, avoid focusing on one particular discussant. Try to give a balanced critique that includes comments for all members. Show trends and group characteristics when possible. This will help you avoid singling out a particular member for criticism.

INSTRUMENTS FOR COLLECTING DATA

Groups will generally profit from periodic observation and evaluation. A typical time for reflection in groups outside the classroom is on completion of a project. This seems like an appropriate time for the leader to ask members to fill out reaction sheets and to discuss how they experienced the group. The group can take note of any difficulties they experienced and reinforce each other for their achievements.

Groups that meet in a classroom setting, where the focus is on learning to be better discussants and studying small group theory, can profit by more frequent observation and criticism. Sometimes the instructor will ask these groups to fill out reaction forms, discuss group progress, and set goals about once a week. At other times, the groups will be subject to a "fishbowl" discussion. Here other class members serve as observer-critics. The various instruments we present are applicable to both in-class and out-of-class discussion groups. Some are suited to self-evaluation, and others are especially useful to an observer.

Interaction Observation Forms

Interaction observation serves a variety of purposes. One purpose is to discover how much individual members talk and to whom they talk. The most efficient form for gathering this kind of data is the *interaction diagram.* Here the observer draws a series of circles on a paper to represent the various group members. Once the members are represented, the observer draws arrows to represent the initial interaction of a member with another. Members' comments that seem to be made to the whole group are shown by arrows pointing toward the outside of the paper. Then each subsequent interaction is coded by a slash mark across the appropriate arrow. An example of this kind of observation sheet is found in Figure 11.1.

Consider this completed interaction diagram. Can you identify the most vocal member of this group? Which group members tend to talk to each other most? Can you identify the member who is not contributing verbally to the group? What kinds of inferences can you make from these interaction patterns?

A second kind of interaction observation instrument is represented by Bales's interaction category scheme, shown in Table 11.1. The purpose of this kind of assessment is to identify what kinds of behaviors are being performed in a group. With an understanding of the behaviors that are needed for a group to perform well, the observer is able to discuss with the group how it might improve. This category system allows the observer to identify comments, and can be set up to record who made them and when they were made.

Notice that certain items relate mostly to the social-emotional area (categories 1, 2, 3, 10, 11, and 12), while others (categories 4–9) fall mainly into the task area.

A tabulation sheet is set up to list the twelve categories down the right-hand side of a paper. The categories are set off by horizontal lines. Vertical lines are drawn from

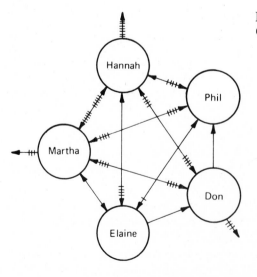

FIGURE 11.1
Completed Interaction Diagram

TABLE 11.1   Bales's Interaction Categories

1. *Seems friendly:* Raises others' status; provides assistance and rewards

2. *Dramatizes:* Jokes; tells stories; gives indirect suggestion

3. *Agrees:* Head nodding; verbal suggestions of commitment about information, opinion, or suggestion

4. *Gives suggestion:* Takes the lead; tries to assume leadership on the task

5. *Gives opinion:* Provides evaluation, analysis, expression of feeling or wish

6. *Gives information:* Provides orientation, repetition, clarification, confirmation

7. *Asks for information:* Requests orientation, repetition, clarification, confirmation

8. *Asks for opinion:* Requests evaluation, analysis, expression of feeling or wish

9. *Asks for suggestion:* Requests direction while maintaining a submissive position; questions designed to call for initiative of others

10. *Disagrees:* Gives passive rejection, mild disagreement; failure to respond

11. *Shows tension:* Laughter; signs of emotional anxiety; holding back

12. *Seems unfriendly:* Reduces others' status; defends or asserts self; conveys negative feelings

the top to the bottom of the page, across the paper. A member's name or code number is then placed in each column.

A more elaborate analysis can be made of the categories if you use a wide paper with one column for each comment. This allows you to keep track of the flow of discussion comment by comment throughout. That is, you can tell what kind of comment follows what kind of comment. And if you assign a number to each group member and a separate number to the group, you can tell to whom a comment is addressed and by whom it was made. For example, a 2–0 would be a comment from member 2 to the group. A 3–2 would be a comment from member 3 to member 2.

Once you have completed charting the interaction, you will be able to answer questions like these: What kind of balance do you have between social-emotional and task behaviors? Do certain members engage in certain behaviors more than others? Do the kind of comments vary from phase to phase as suggested in Chapter 5? And, finally, do some members address other members more frequently?

Role Analysis in Discussion

Kenneth Benne and Paul Sheats are responsible for one of the oldest category systems for classifying roles. We discussed their work in Chapter 6. Recall that they divided roles into three broad classifications: task roles, group-building and maintenance roles, and self-centered roles. An observer can keep track of the kinds of roles played by each member, and then analyze the effect roles had on the interaction.

Task roles are those functions members contribute that directly help the group with its work. They include contributions of information, opinion, elaboration, orientation, evaluation, and the like. An observer can keep track of the kinds of task behaviors members contribute by constructing a form like the one displayed in Figure 11.2.

Group-building and maintenance roles are behaviors that contribute to the social dimension of the group. The person who seems to play these more frequently than any other is usually identified as the social-emotional leader. The performance of these roles is important to a group because they enhance the group climate and help to build cohesiveness. Construct a form like the one in Figure 11.3 to observe and record the social-emotional roles of your group. You can discover what roles are being played and by whom. See what kind of attention is being paid to the climate of your group.

Recall that *self-centered roles* are behaviors performed to satisfy personal goals rather than group goals. Sometimes these goals produce behavior that is disruptive. For example, aggressor, blocker, and dominator are disruptive roles. Other self-centered roles merely deprive the group of the energy and input the person might have contributed if he or she had not engaged in them. Examples of these rules are the playboy/playgirl, special-interest pleader, and self-confessor.

When you are concerned about members who are playing nonfunctional roles, construct a form like that in Figure 11.4 and collect data about member roles. Once the roles and role players are identified, the group can choose to do something about them.

Participants' Names

Functional Task Roles							
1. Initiator							
2. Information seeker							
3. Information giver							
4. Opinion seeker							
5. Opinion giver							
6. Elaborator/clarifier							
7. Coordinator							
8. Diagnostician							
9. Orienter							
10. Energizer							
11. Procedural technician							
12. Recorder							
13. Evaluator-critic							

FIGURE 11.2
Functional Task Roles of Discussants

Source: Based on Kenneth D. Benne and Paul Sheats, "Functional Roles of Group Members," *Journal of Social Issues* 4 (1948):41–49.

Participants' Names

Social-Emotional Roles

Social-Emotional Roles							
1. Supporter/Encourager							
2. Harmonizer							
3. Tension releaser							
4. Compromiser							
5. Gatekeeper							
6. Feeling expressor							
7. Standard setter							
8. Follower							

FIGURE 11.3
Functional Social-Emotional Roles

Source: Based on Kenneth D. Benne and Paul Sheats, "Functional Roles of Group Members," *Journal of Social Issues* 4 (1948):41–49.

Leadership Rating Form

Leadership can be supplied by a number of different members. It does not matter so much whether one person provides most of the leadership or not. What is of concern, however, is whether the leadership is sufficient for the group to perform its task. The Barnlund-Haiman leadership rating scale has as its focus assessment of the adequacy of leadership activities. It differentiates among the kinds of leadership by a division into three categories: influence in procedure, influence in creative and critical thinking, and influence in interpersonal relations. This scale can be produced for use without permission of the publisher when it is to be used for nonprofit purposes. When used, it must be labeled as shown in Table 11.2 below. Chapter 7 provides suggestions for promoting more effective leadership once difficulties have been identified.

OBSERVING GROUP PROCESSES

The next two information-processing instruments take a broader focus. They are useful for examining the group's effort when the task is decision making. The first allows you to record judgments about the decision-making process and the group's interaction. The decision-making discussion rating sheet is displayed in Table 11.3.

The Brilhart problem-solving process scale is especially useful if your group is following a full agenda that is based on the reflective thinking process. If you were using either the decision-making agenda (based on Dewey's reflective thinking pattern) or the Brilhart-Jochem creative problem-solving sequence, this would be an appropriate rating sheet. The Brilhart problem-solving scale is in Table 11.4.

Sometimes you will want to focus on the individual members' contributions to the group process. This may be the case especially when you believe that there is a wide

Participants' Names

Self-Centered Roles								
1. Blocker								
2. Aggressor								
3. Deserter								
4. Dominator								
5. Recognition seeker								
6. Self-confessor								
7. Playboy/playgirl								
8. Special-interest pleader								

FIGURE 11.4
Self-Centered Roles

Source: Based on Kenneth D. Benne and Paul Sheats, "Functional Roles of Group Members," *Journal of Social Issues* 4 (1948):41–49.

variation in individual participation. You may have as your goal helping members to set their own goals for improvement of their effort. Table 11.5 provides an evaluation form that will focus your attention on some of the key variables in small group member participation.

SELF-REPORT RATING SHEETS

Self-report measures can help you discover what group members are thinking and how they are experiencing the group. But a word of caution is appropriate: Sometimes members will report what they believe the person collecting the data *wants* to hear, rather than what they actually think. This creates a bias in the data. Sometimes you can minimize the bias by asking for anonymous reports.

Three self-report instruments are presented below. The first was designed to be used to collect data about cohesiveness in a work group. The Seashore index of group cohesiveness, Table 11.6, asks three basic questions: How much do you feel you are a part of this group? How willing are you to leave the group? How does your group compare with similar groups with respect to member relations? If the ratings are low, you will want to engage in some of the cohesiveness-building behaviors recommended in Chapter 8.

The postmeeting open-ended reaction sheet, Table 11.7, has a particular advantage. The open-ended nature of the instrument avoids observer bias in collecting data. It does this by allowing the individual group members to identify strengths and weaknesses as they see them. It also asks for member suggestions for improvement and change in the group. These can be valuable kinds of data to collect because group members may point out problems about which the person collecting the data may not have known.

TABLE 11.2   Barnlund-Haiman Leadership Rating Scale

Instructions: This rating scale may be used to evaluate leadership in groups with or without official leaders. In the latter case (the leaderless group) use part A of each item only. When evaluating the actions of an official leader, use parts A and B of each item on the scale.

INFLUENCE IN PROCEDURE
Initiating Discussion

A. 3   2   1   0   1   2   3

Group needed more help   Group got right amount   Group needed less help
in getting started   of help   in getting started

B. The quality of the introductory remarks was:

Excellent   Good   Adequate   Fair   Poor

Organizing Group Thinking

A. 3   2   1   0   1   2   3

Group needed more direc-   Group got right amount   Group needed less direction in thinking   of help   tion in thinking

B. If and when attempts were made to organize group thinking they were:

Excellent   Good   Adequate   Fair   Poor

Clarifying Communication

A. 3   2   1   0   1   2   3

Group needed more   Group got right amount   Group needed less
help in clarifying   of help   help in clarifying
communication   communication

B. If and when attempts were made to clarify communication they were:

Excellent   Good   Adequate   Fair   Poor

Summarizing and Verbalizing Agreements

A. 3   2   1   0   1   2   3

Group needed more   Group got right amount   Group needed less help
help in summarizing and   of help   in summarizing and
verbalizing agreements   verbalizing agreements

TABLE 11.2   Barnlund-Haiman Leadership Rating Scale *(Continued)*

B.   If and when attempts were made to summarize and verbalize agreements they were:

Excellent	Good	Adequate	Fair	Poor

Resolving Conflict

A.   3   2   1   0   1   2   3

Group needed more help in resolving conflict	Group got right amount of help	Group needed less help in resolving conflict

B.   If and when attempts were made to resolve conflict they were:

Excellent	Good	Adequate	Fair	Poor

INFLUENCES IN CREATIVE AND CRITICAL THINKING
Stimulating Critical Thinking

A.   3   2   1   0   1   2   3

Group needed more stim- ulation in creative thinking	Group got right amount of help	Group needed less stim- ulation in creative thinking

B.   If and when attempts were made to stimulate ideas they were:

Excellent	Good	Adequate	Fair	Poor

Encouraging Criticism

A.   3   2   1   0   1   2   3

Group needed more en- couragement to be critical	Group got right amount of help	Group needed less en- couragement to be critical

B.   If and when attempts were made to encourage criticism they were:

Excellent	Good	Adequate	Fair	Poor

Balancing Abstract and Concrete Thought

A.   3   2   1   0   1   2   3

Group needed to be more concrete	Group got right amount of help	Group needed to be more abstract

B.   If and when attempts were made to balance abstract and concrete thought they were:

Excellent	Good	Adequate	Fair	Poor

TABLE 11.2   Barnlund-Haiman Leadership Rating Scale *(Continued)*

INFLUENCE IN INTERPERSONAL RELATIONS
Climate-Making

A. 3   2   1   0   1   2   3

Group needed more help in securing a permissive atmosphere	Group got right amount of help	Group needed less help in securing a permissive atmosphere

B. If and when attempts were made to establish a permissive atmosphere they were:

Excellent	Good	Adequate	Fair	Poor

Regulating Participation

A. 3   2   1   0   1   2   3

Group needed more regulation of participation	Group got right amount of help	Group needed less regulation of participation

B. If and when attempts were made to regulate participation they were:

Excellent	Good	Adequate	Fair	Poor

Overall Leadership

A. 3   2   1   0   1   2   3

Group needed more control	Group got right amount of control	Group needed less control

B. If and when attempts were made to control the group they were:

Excellent	Good	Adequate	Fair	Poor

Source: Dean C. Barnlund and Franklyn S. Haiman, *The Dynamics of Discussion* (Boston: Houghton Mifflin, 1960), 401–404.

A group might use this form to evaluate its performance. If so, the group would set aside a time at the end of a work session to evaluate and decide on alternative ways of working together.

Finally, the Brilhart postmeeting reaction questionnaire, Table 11.8, provides a focused means of collecting self-report data. Asking members to respond to the same ideas has an advantage over the open-ended questionnaire. It allows you to compare answers against the question and discover if members are perceiving the group consistently. Notice that the items correspond to various chapters of this book. We've listed each

TABLE 11.3   Decision-Making Discussion Rating Sheet

Problem: _____ Group: _____

I. Rate the group on the following:

	Poor	Fair	Adequate	Good	Excellent
1. How well did the group understand the problem?	1	2	3	4	5
2. How adequately did the group discuss causes?	1	2	3	4	5
3. Did the group explore an adequate number of solutions?	1	2	3	4	5
4. How consistently did the group apply criteria?	1	2	3	4	5
5. How well did the group interact?	1	2	3	4	5
6. How well did the group handle conflict?	1	2	3	4	5
7. How well did the group involve its members?	1	2	3	4	5
8. How well did the group use available information?	1	2	3	4	5
9. How well does the group solution meet the causes?	1	2	3	4	5

II. Did the group achieve consensus on the decision?   Yes _____   No _____

III. How do you know what you have said is true? Present the evidence and reasoning behind the ratings of the group's performance.

IV. Evaluate this decision-making performance for overall quality.

Poor	Fair	Average	Above Average	Excellent

TABLE 11.4   Brilhart Problem-Solving Process Scale

Instructions: On each scale indicate the degree to which the group accomplished each identified behavior. Use the following scale for your evaluations:

Poor	Fair	Average	Good	Excellent
1	2	3	4	5

Circle the appropriate number in front of each item.

1	2	3	4	5	1. The concern of each member was identified regarding the problem the group attempted to solve.
1	2	3	4	5	2. This concern was identified *before* the problem was analyzed.
1	2	3	4	5	3. In problem analysis, the present condition was carefully compared with the specific condition desired.
1	2	3	4	5	4. The goal was carefully defined and agreed to by all members.
1	2	3	4	5	5. Valid (and relevant) information was secured when needed.
1	2	3	4	5	6. Possible solutions were listed and clarified before they were evaluated.
1	2	3	4	5	7. Criteria for evaluating proposed solutions were clearly identified and accepted by the group.
1	2	3	4	5	8. Predictions were made regarding the probable effectiveness of each proposed solution, using the available information and criteria.
1	2	3	4	5	9. Consensus was achieved on the most desirable solution.
1	2	3	4	5	10. A detailed plan to implement the solution was adopted.
1	2	3	4	5	11. The problem-solving process was systematic and orderly.

TABLE 11.5   Discussion Participant Evaluation

Participant: _____

Poor	Fair	Adequate	Good	Excellent
1	2	3	4	5

Circle the number that describes the participation of the member indicated above.

1	2	3	4	5	1. Prepared to discuss.
1	2	3	4	5	2. Comments were relevant.
1	2	3	4	5	3. Listened to others.
1	2	3	4	5	4. Open-minded.
1	2	3	4	5	5. Argued constructively.
1	2	3	4	5	6. Frequency of participation.
1	2	3	4	5	7. Contribution to analysis.
1	2	3	4	5	8. Contribution to evaluation.
1	2	3	4	5	9. Overall rating of discussant.

How do you know what you have said above is true? Give your specific evidence and reasoning for your ratings.

Evaluator: _____

topic with the chapter or chapters that focus on it in Table 11.9 below, so you can use this book as a reference to help your group improve its performance.

SUMMARY

This chapter has focused on observing and evaluating groups. First, ground rules were established for observing groups. The observer should decide what he or she wants to observe, be careful to distinguish between judgments made on the basis of data and those that go beyond the data, try not to comment on everything that is observed, and balance the positive and the negative.

Instruments for collecting data were presented. They included interaction observation forms, role analysis forms, leadership observation forms, and a variety of decision-making and performance-rating forms.

TABLE 11.6   Seashore Index of Group Cohesiveness

Check one response for each question.

1. Do you feel that you are really a part of your work group?

    _____ Really a part of my work group

    _____ Included in most ways

    _____ Included in some ways, but not in others

    _____ Don't feel I really belong

    _____ Don't work with any one group of people

    _____ Not ascertained

2. If you had a chance to do the same kind of work for the same pay in another work group, how would you feel about moving?

    _____ Would want very much to move

    _____ Would rather move than stay where I am

    _____ Would make no difference to me

    _____ Would want very much to stay where I am

    _____ Not ascertained

3. How does your work group compare with other similar groups on each of the following points?

	Better than most	About the same as most	Not as good as most	Not ascertained
a. The way the members get along together	_____	_____	_____	_____
b. The way the members stick together	_____	_____	_____	_____
c. The way the members help each other on the job	_____	_____	_____	_____

Source: Stanley Seashore, *Group Cohesiveness in the Industrial Work Group* (Ann Arbor: University of Michigan Institute for Social Research, 1954). Used by permission.

TABLE 11.7   Postmeeting Open-Ended Reaction Sheet

1. I would rate today's discussion as:

   _____ Excellent   _____ Very Good   _____ Good   _____ Fair   _____ Poor

2. I would rate the decision we reached as:

   _____ Excellent   _____ Very Good   _____ Good   _____ Fair   _____ Poor

3. The strong points of the group's decision making were:

4. The weak points of the group's decision making were:

5. The group's climate could be described as:

6. I would recommend the following changes for the group:

7. I would set the following goals for this group's future meetings:

Signed (Optional): _____

EXERCISES

1. Provide an overall assessment of your ability to meet the action plans you established at the beginning of this book. (See Chapter 1, Exercise 1.)

2. Diagram the flow of communication in a discussion group for which you serve as observer. You are recording the number of times a person speaks and to whom the person speaks. Which members make the most contributions? To whom do they talk? What conclusions can you draw from these data? Who are the low participators? Were there attempts to include them by addressing comments to them? What would you recommend for this group with respect to low contributors? How often are comments made to the entire group, rather than to specific individuals? How would you describe the communication network of this group? What would you tell members about their network that would help them be a better group? Report your findings orally to the group or submit a critique to your instructor, whichever your instructor assigns.

3. Listen to a tape-recorded discussion. Use Bales's interaction categories to focus on the questions asked and answered. What types of questions were asked? How often were questions asked? Keep track of this by ten-minute intervals. Were more questions asked during a particular interval? What comments can you make about question asking based upon your data? Now focus on answering. What percentage of the questions were answered? Were members being ignored when they asked questions? Write a two-page report critiquing question asking and answering.

4. Choose a decision-making group in your community and observe it for five or six meetings. Each time you observe it focus on a different aspect of the group interaction or dynamics. Use a different data-collecting form each time. You may even be able to get permission for the group to give you some postmeeting reactions on the form provided for that purpose. Submit a report to your instructor that includes a description of the group, a display of the data you collected,

TABLE 11.8   Brilhart Postmeeting Reaction Questionnaire

Instruction: Circle the number that best indicates your reaction to the following questions about the discussion in which you participated.

1. *Adequacy of Communication:* To what extent do you feel members were understanding each other's statements and positions?

0	1	2	3	4	5	6	7	8	9	10

   Much talking past each
   other, misunderstanding

   Communicated directly with
   each other, understanding well

2. *Opportunity To Speak:* To what extent did you feel free to speak?

0	1	2	3	4	5	6	7	8	9	10

   Never had a
   chance to speak

   All the opportunity to
   talk I wanted

3. *Climate of Acceptance:* How well did members support each other, show acceptance of individuals?

0	1	2	3	4	5	6	7	8	9	10

   Highly critical
   and punishing

   Supportive and receptive

4. *Interpersonal Relations:* How pleasant were members, how concerned with interpersonal relations?

0	1	2	3	4	5	6	7	8	9	10

   Quarrelsome, status
   differences emphasized

   Pleasant, empathic,
   concerned with persons

5. *Leadership:* How adequate was the leader (or leadership) of the group?

0	1	2	3	4	5	6	7	8	9	10

   Too weak (   ) or
   dominating (   )

   Shared, group-centered,
   and sufficient

6. *Satisfaction with Role:* How satisfied are you with your personal participation in the discussion?

0	1	2	3	4	5	6	7	8	9	10

   Very dissatisfied

   Very satisfied

7. *Quality of Product:* How satisfied are you with the discussion, solutions, or learnings that came out of this discussion?

0	1	2	3	4	5	6	7	8	9	10

   Very dissatisfied

   Very satisfied

TABLE 11.8   Brilhart Postmeeting Reaction Questionnaire *(Continued)*

8. *Overall:* How do you rate the discussion as a whole apart from any specific aspect of it?

0	1	2	3	4	5	6	7	8	9	10

Awful, waste of time   Superb, time went well

From John K. Brilhart and Gloria J. Galanes, *Effective Group Discussion,* 6th ed. Copyright © 1989 Wm. C. Brown. Publishers, Dubuque, Iowa. All rights reserved. Reprinted by permission.

**TABLE 11.9   Postmeeting Reaction Questionnaire
with Corresponding Chapters**

1. *Adequacy of communication:* To what extent do you feel members were understanding each other's statements and positions?
    Chapter 4, "Understanding Verbal and Nonverbal Messages"
    Chapter 6, "Roles and Role Emergence"

2. *Opportunity to speak:* To what extent did you feel free to speak?
    Chapter 4, "Understanding Verbal and Nonverbal Messages"

3. *Climate of acceptance:* How well did members support each other, show acceptance of individuals?
    Chapter 8, "Promoting Group Cohesiveness"
    Chapter 9, "Managing Relationships in Groups"

4. *Interpersonal relations:* How pleasant were members, how concerned with interpersonal relations?
    Chapter 9, "Managing Relationships in Groups"

5. *Leadership:* How adequate was the leader (or leadership) of the group?
    Chapter 3, "Decision Making in Small Group Meetings"
    Chapter 7, "Leading Group Meetings"

6. *Satisfaction with role:* How satisfied are you with your personal participation in the discussion?
    Chapter 6, "Roles and Role Emergence"

7. *Quality of product:* How satisfied are you with the discussion, solutions, or learnings that came out of this discussion?
    Chapter 3, "Decision Making in Small Group Meetings"
    Chapter 5, "Encouraging Group Development and Evolution"
    Chapter 8, "Promoting Group Cohesiveness"
    Chapter 9, "Managing Relationships in Groups"

8. *Overall:* How do you rate the discussion as a whole apart from any specific aspect of it?

conclusions you have drawn about the group, and an appendix with the completed instruments you used.

5. Tape-record one of your classroom discussions. Listen to the tape and make an analysis of the functional roles members played. You can use the forms for role analysis provided in this chapter. Then consider the adequacy of the roles played for the achievement of the group's goal. Bring your analysis to class and compare your analysis with those of other members of your group.

RECOMMENDED READINGS

John K. Brilhart, "Observing and Evaluating Groups," Robert S. Cathcart and Larry A. Samovar, eds. in *Small Group Communication: A Reader* (Dubuque, Iowa: Wm. C. Brown, 1988), 559–573.

B. Aubrey Fisher, "Communication Research in the Task-Oriented Group," *Journal of Communication* 21 (1971):136–149.

James C. McCroskey and David W. Wright, "The Development of an Instrument for Measuring Interaction Behavior in Small Group Communication," *Speech Monographs* 38 (1971):335–340.

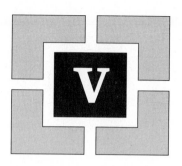

Preparing for and Participating in Public Group Meetings

CHAPTER 12

Groups in Public Settings

OBJECTIVES

After reading this chapter you should be able to:

Specify the chief difference between a public and private group discussion.

Suggest the defining characteristics of a forum, panel, symposium, and colloquium discussion format.

Identify the appropriate discussion format for a particular public group meeting.

Discuss leadership considerations for a public discussion.

Name and explain briefly the steps involved in planning a conference.

Utilize the conference-planning checklist to plan a conference.

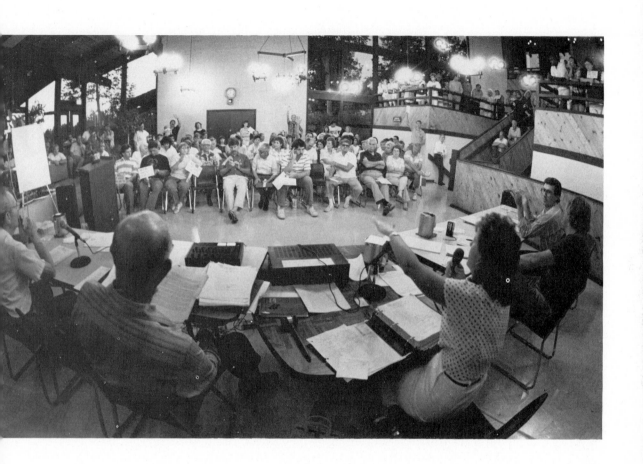

Susan Holbrook works in the engineering department of a power company in the Southeast. One Monday morning she arrived at work to discover a note on her desk:

> Please see me as soon as possible. Management has decided that we should mount a public information campaign on the use of nuclear energy as a power source. I know you have the background to help here. I'd like you to plan a public meeting at which our people can present our position on this issue.
>
> Phil

Susan was surprised at the request for her to participate in this upcoming public information meeting. She was prepared to do so, though she admitted that she was a bit scared.

Organizations that are interested in how they are viewed by the public attempt to provide information about issues. These frequently take the form of some public meeting. Civic organizations and groups that are concerned about community issues do the same. Sometimes classroom teachers ask students to present a discussion for their fellow classmates. Thus you are likely to find yourself in a position to participate in or perhaps organize a public group meeting.

This chapter focuses on the formats and organization of such meetings. We begin by presenting several of the common formats for public discussion. Next we suggest when each format may be appropriate. We conclude with a step-by-step guide for planning and organizing a conference.

FORMATS FOR PUBLIC DISCUSSION

Public discussions usually differ in purpose from private discussions. The principal difference is that public discussion is conducted for the benefit of the audience. Even if a group is engaged in decision making, the fact that an audience is expected means that special attention is being paid to audience needs. For example, in a political group—say a city council meeting—one would sense that members are talking to the audience part of the time, rather than to each other. Thus it seems reasonable to conclude that these discussions are to some extent planned performances. This final section will consider several types of public discussion formats and their uses. These include the forum, panel, colloquium, and symposium.

Forum

A forum is a public discussion that involves full audience participation. Its most familiar form is the New England town meeting. The citizens of the town gather to propose issues, discuss them, and make decisions. Impromptu speeches are made from the floor, members debate each other, questions are asked and responded to, comments are made. The purpose of these meetings is to share information and ideas and to take care of the affairs of the town.

Most of us will not experience the forum in its pure form. Instead, we will experience a forum coupled with some other kind of communication activity. Generally a speech, film, panel discussion, symposium, or interview is presented as a stimulus for the audience discussion. Leading this form of discussion is the responsibility of a chairperson or moderator. This difficult role requires skillful control by the chair. The goals of this leader include:

1. Stimulating the group further by posing provocative ideas and questions.

2. Providing an opportunity for as many people as possible (or practical) to talk. This means urging speakers to keep their comments brief.

3. Recognizing the various viewpoints and trying to give an opportunity for all of them to be heard.

One way to help your audience meet these goals is to suggest some guidelines for participants to follow in their discussion. Here is basic information the chairperson might give the audience:

1. Tell them that there will be a forum after the presentation. Suggest that they write down questions and comments as they are listening so that they are ready to participate fully in the discussion.

2. Ask them to wait to be recognized before they begin to speak.

3. Ask them to hold their comments if they have already spoken, thereby allowing others who have not spoken to have a turn.

4. Suggest a time limit on individual speeches. Suggest some signal you will give when the limit is reached.

5. Have floor microphones available for use.

6. Let them know how much time is allotted for the forum interaction.

7. Call for a different point of view if several persons have presented a similar view.

Panel

A panel discussion is an interaction involving specialists or reasonably well-informed people who share their points of view about a common topic or question. The discussion is carried out for the benefit of the audience, but not with the audience. Panel members generally react to stimulus questions posed by a moderator. A moderator plans such a session by developing five or six primary questions, with several follow-up questions for each. The primary questions are usually given to the participants prior to the discussion so that they can prepare.

A city police department used this format to inform citizens about personal security. They were asked to provide a discussion on self-protection for one of the local high schools. The director of community services for the department gathered a group of experts to discuss the question: What should young people know about self-defense? Subquestions were: What are some common characteristics of attackers? What situations should be avoided if possible? Why? How should you defend yourself against an armed attacker? The panel members discussed each possible subquestion for about ten minutes before an audience of students and faculty.

This kind of public discussion demands special attention to the physical arrangement. The panel members and leader should be seated facing the audience, but in such a way that they can see each other also. A V-shape arrangement is often preferred. Name cards are provided for the participants. The name cards are especially important if the discussion is to be followed by a forum.

The moderator's job includes the following:

1. Preparing the discussion question outline and distributing it to the participants. This includes distribution of the ground rules and stressing the need for fair play and limiting each comment to about a minute.

2. Introducing the topic and the main discussion question or questions.

3. Introducing the panel of participants.

4. Posing questions, maintaining order, and summarizing agreements and differences.

5. Closing the discussion by summarizing, thanking the speakers, and asking the audience for questions.

Symposium

A symposium taken by itself is not a discussion. It is instead a series of brief speeches all related to a central topic, each usually taking a different position on the issue. Its chief purpose in a discussion situation is to provide a stimulus for discussion. It is generally followed by either a discussion among the members of the symposium—a panel discussion—or by audience participation in discussion—a forum. The ideas suggested for forum and panel discussions apply when they are used in connection with a symposium.

Colloquium

A colloquium is a format for public discussion that involves a panel of experts who are asked questions by an audience. The audience knows the general topic of discussion and frequently prepares questions in advance. Often each questioner is given an opportunity to ask a question, and then to ask a follow-up question. The experts generally answer questions but do not ask them. This format seems best suited to enlightenment of the audience, as it does not provide for meaningful two-way communication.

A news conference at which scientists are gathered to announce a medical breakthrough would be an example of a colloquium. Such a colloquium followed the implantation of the first artificial heart. Another example of the colloquium format would be a variation on the police department's panel discussion on personal security described above. If the students and faculty had come prepared to ask questions, instead of the members addressing advance questions, this would have been a colloquium. Also, instead of interacting with one another, the group members would need to interact with the audience.

Larry L. Barker and his colleagues suggest a version of the colloquium that provides two-way communication.[1] Here the panel of experts actually engages in problem solving. Here is how they suggest this process operates:

> When either the chairperson or the panel members determine that some matter is deterring the pursuit of a satisfactory solution to the problem or subproblem, the audience is invited to participate by asking questions or making remarks. For example, as a chairperson you might observe that two panel members disagree on a matter; that a salient issue, subproblem, or solution is being omitted or ignored in the discussion; or that a questionable point is not being challenged. At this point, you would shift from the panel discussion to the forum discussion until the next opportunity occurred for the audience's participation. This process would continue until the discussion was concluded, either by the time limit or by arrival at an agreed-upon solution.[2]

Selecting a Public Discussion Format

Recall that public discussions have as their aim informing the public. This includes programs for segments of the public, such as memberships of clubs and organizations. Regardless of the group, there are some questions that will help you to decide which format you want to use.

Start by asking how informed your audience will be. Then ask what your basic purpose for a public meeting is to be. Table 12.1 is a summary of some of the problems posed by these questions, with the formats that seem most useful for each. Thus, if members of a professional group of speech pathologists in your community want to know about computer applications to speech pathology, they might invite a panel to their meeting. If they knew about some applications, but wanted to be exposed to others, they might choose a symposium-forum. Or, if members are well informed, they might choose to share among themselves in a pure forum format. But if they wish instead to inform the public about the services speech pathologists perform for the community, they might arrange for a colloquium to be videotaped and played over the media. The type of public discussion format you select is related to how informed your membership is and the specific purpose you have in mind for the event. Consider these points with respect to format selection.

TABLE 12.1   Selecting a Public Discussion Format

Situation and/or Problem	*Solution*
1. First exposure of the group to the topic.	1. Group may not be able to generate much dialogue. Invite experts for panel discussion or colloquy.
2. Audience is reasonably well informed but would like to be exposed to different perspectives.	2. A likely format is a symposium-forum.
3. The group is well informed and there are diverse views in the group.	3. A pure forum type of format will allow for an exchange of views.
4. The group wishes to help inform the public on an issue on which the membership is well informed.	4. The format that may best serve this need is a colloquium. Invite a group of experts for several of your quizzes. (This might be videotaped for replay over local media.)

LEADING THE PUBLIC DISCUSSION

The leader of a public discussion will be more successful if he or she keeps several guiding principles in mind. Of course, you will find situations in which one or more of these will not apply, but generally they will.

1. *Limit the number of topics.* A focused discussion will be easier to follow and more meaningful for the listeners. Generally no more than three to four main topics or issues should be addressed within an hour's discussion. Of course, the main issues are generally divided into subtopics. Usually a session should not continue beyond an hour and fifteen minutes.

2. *Plan a series of open-ended questions to guide the discussion.* Open-ended questions call for a general response and allow respondents the freedom to express their views more fully. In contrast, a closed question asks for specific information. An open-ended question might be followed by more specific questions, but open-ended questions are important if you hope to stimulate a lively discussion.

3. *Attempt to keep discussants on the topic.* Of course, you cannot and would not want to try to keep members directly on the topic all the time. Some diversion is likely and not unreasonable. But listeners may soon become bored or perhaps even disappointed if too many long diversions from the issues are permitted. Recall that we presented some specific advice about keeping members on the topic in Chapter 7.

4. *Try to regulate participation so that all members have an opportunity to speak.* There is a good chance that you will discover some members seem to have more to say about the topic of discussion than others. You will not want to be too heavy-handed in regulating, but you also will not want one or two members

to monopolize the discussion. Again, refer to and use suggestions found in Chapter 7 for managing this problem.

5. *Reward group members for their cooperation and participation.* This means that you should compliment both the group and individual members on their good work. You will, of course, want to thank them at the end of the discussion. But you may also find times during the discussion where praise is appropriate. Perhaps at the end of the discussion of one of the main topics you might say, "I appreciate the willingness of each person to speak on this issue. The live discussion of it has been interesting to me and, I suspect, to our listeners, too."

PLANNING THE CONFERENCE

If you are placed in charge of an important meeting, you may hit the panic button, intimidated by the enormous number of details for which you have been made responsible. There are convenient ways to organize your thinking about those details. One way is to think in terms of the two dimensions of group communication, task and social. The task dimension includes the things that must be done if the group is to be productive. The social dimension, equally important, involves the feelings, wants, and images of the people who participate. As we go through each of the steps below, you will see how using the two dimensions can be helpful.

Decide Your Purpose

In the task dimension, deciding your purpose means identifying as clearly as possible the general objectives you wish to accomplish. Consult with your supervisors. Learn from them what they want to accomplish.

Involve top management in the planning as early as feasible. Get their views and take them into account. This will get you around the obstacle of having to make last-minute changes because of their dissatisfaction.

In the social dimension, deciding your purpose means identifying any social concerns that *must* be taken care of. For instance, a company may have a meeting for the purpose of honoring its soon-to-retire employees. The event is almost entirely social. The concerns in the social dimension, then, will center around making people feel very important—like the VIPs they truly are. It may be that on such an occasion management especially wants to honor one individual. You had better know that in advance; it will have a bearing on the seating arrangement. The seating arrangement can be just as important if the issue is task oriented, as we discussed in Chapter 4.

It sometimes happens that many of the arrangements must be made around the requirements of special participants. For instance, a certain speaker may be confined to a wheelchair. Such a person cannot travel up and down staircases unassisted, and should not have to. You should also anticipate that he or she cannot stand at a lectern and may have difficulty with electronic visual aid equipment. Arrangements should be made accordingly.

Sometimes an individual's schedule may require that your meeting be held on a certain date and at a specific time. For example, a U.S. senator from your state will undoubtedly have a full schedule. If you want that individual to appear at your meeting— senators do this as often as they are able—you will have to accommodate that schedule.

Occasionally speakers will provide copies of their address for distribution to participants. Arrangements will have to be made and approved by management in order to accommodate a special speaker.

Plan the Agenda

In the task dimension, planning the agenda involves asking questions like: What topics must be covered to accomplish the purpose? How much time is available? Can we cover everything adequately? Does the agenda need to be focused? Will focusing the agenda mean that a follow-up meeting is necessary? Is that warranted? Is *this* meeting warranted?

In the social dimension, it means taking other people into account. Have you checked with and received input from others? Have you accommodated their suggestions? Their schedules?

Keep in mind that an agenda is a plan of action for a period of time. You would be wise to plan the agenda very carefully. Your success in this task may make all the difference between the success and failure of the entire meeting. Since the things that are most important to all of the members—topics and time—are the substance of an agenda, your care in planning the agenda may have a direct bearing on your personal success in the organization as well.

Identify the Other Participants

In the task dimension, identifying the other participants involves finding out who *must* be at a conference and who *should* be. How many participants are too many? Who can be eliminated?

In the social dimension, that last question is also important. Identifying the participants involves, in part, discovering which people will get along with each other. We suggest, if it is feasible, that you ask the key participants all the task questions above. (Do not ask if you really do not want their advice or if you do not trust them!) Have you accommodated their suggestions? And where have you set limitations? Have you taken care of the social and status problems that might arise from the narrowing process you have applied? (Sometimes it becomes important to invite high-status people for social and not task reasons.)

Select the Setting

In the task dimension, selecting the setting refers to making sure that the meeting place is conducive to the purpose of the conference. It is too large? Too small? Too formal? Too informal? Is it conveniently located? Is it attractive? Will the participants think so? Are the facilities complete? (You would be amazed at the number of conferences that occur in inconvenient places that have no restrooms, no refreshment centers, limited and poor-quality sleeping arrangements, and the like.)

Perhaps you can see that the questions above can be useful in the social dimension, too. Be sure to get some input from the participants and to accommodate that input wherever you can. A key here is the participants' perception that they have influence. To use William Schutz's ideas,[3] individuals are motivated by three things: affection, inclusion, and control. You will instantly see your potential for satisfying participants' needs in each of these areas merely by including them in your planning.

Sometimes participants in a large conference will wish to meet in smaller groups for a variety of purposes. Table 12.2 suggests six different ways to organize physical settings, with reasons why each might be chosen.

Plan for Mechanical Details

Primarily this step has to do with the task dimension. Preparing for audio-visual presentations, food, shipping, hotel procedures, and the like, are all-important in this regard and—as you will see, by implication at least—they are important to the social dimension as well.[4]

Audio-visual If you have elaborate plans for audio or visual support of your meeting, check the facilities before determining where to hold it. It is a good idea, too, to make arrangements for those who will make presentations to rehearse with the equipment if they wish. You may not be able to manage this, but you can try.

If you do not have your own audio-visual equipment and people to run it, then you need to make arrangements for every machine, including operators and spare parts—

TABLE 12.2 A Guide for Planning Group Meetings

Format Called	Arrangement Suggested	Reason for Using	Method
Round table		To promote equality of feelings; maximize participation of all members; ensure as much spontaneity as possible.	Group discussion of problems and solutions for the purpose of making a good decision or sharing information.
Symposium		To present a variety of views in the form of short speeches or reports for the benefit of the audience.	Moderator introduces the panel; provides history of the issues at hand; presents each speaker in turn; monitors time; thanks the participants; ends the meeting with a brief charge to the audience or a summary of the issue.

TABLE 12.2　A Guide for Planning Group Meetings *(Continued)*

Format Called	Arrangement Suggested	Reason for Using	Method
Panel discussion	*[Seating diagram: moderator M at center with panel groups at sides; audience arranged in rows below]*	To conduct a semistructured discussion of issues on a topic for the benefit of an audience.	Moderator introduces the panel and problem and keeps the discussion flowing; restates often; controls (somewhat) equal and fair time allocation. Members are responsible for developing points of view and have some control of agenda.
Forum	*[Seating diagram: speaker and moderator M at front; audience arranged in rows below]*	To encourage audience participation on issues surrounding a topic.	Moderator introduces the program and speaker, who presents a brief statement and interacts with the audience. Moderator participates to encourage audience involvement. A variety of discussion formats can be used.
Colloquy	*[Seating diagram: moderator M with speaker and panel of questioners; audience arranged in rows below]*	To inform an audience through the use of planned questions designed to get unprepared responses from participants for the benefit of the audience.	Moderator introduces the speaker and panel of questioners, then regulates rotation and time. Sometimes summarizing, sometimes clarifying, moderator does not participate as a panelist.
Whole-house decision making	*[Seating diagram: moderator M at front; audience arranged in rows below]*	To debate issues as a body, then decide, using appropriate voting methods.	Moderator regulates the discussion and debate, attempting to get maximum input from both sides in order that members of the house may cast informed votes. Parliamentary procedure is commonly used to govern the event and facilitate orderly progress.

Source: Michael S. Hanna and Gerald L. Wilson, *Communicating in Business and Professional Settings*, 2d ed. (New York: Random House, 1988), 311–312.

even light bulbs! Do this at the time you secure the location. Otherwise you might find out too late that you cannot make such arrangements at the location.

Finally, we suggest that you try everything out before the meeting. By this we mean actually, physically, going to the facility and running through the use of every piece of machinery. Do this in the room where the presentation will be given. Without a doubt, you will find a number of small problems you need to solve.

Food Food can be very important to the success of a meeting. Get copies of all the hotel or meeting place menus. Talk with the catering manager, and ask about what to serve and when. Often the catering manager will be able to give you special prices. For example, in June on the Gulf Coast, shrimp are generally plentiful and therefore relatively inexpensive. You might be able to get a special shrimp meal. Likewise, the house might have other menus that can be made available at reduced prices. Also check on reductions in price for increased numbers. What might cost you so much per plate if you order twenty-five plates might be 20 percent less if you order fifty.

Beware of serving hors d'oeuvres. They're usually expensive, and if they're salty they tend to increase the consumption of expensive beverages. It may be a good idea to limit their use to one occasion at a conference.

One of our reviewers, when responding to this section, offered the following advice. We think it is so appropriate that we have included it here verbatim:

> The standard conference morning fare is coffee and doughnuts. The coffee machine tends to stay set up all day, and often participants drink coffee—and often much more than they normally would—just because it's there. A suggestion for adding variety to conference beverages and also for helping participants keep up their energy is to serve coffee from about eight to ten in the morning. Then take the coffee away. Around eleven make available iced tea, lemonade, soda, or some other refreshing and light drink. These could possibly be served with a light and simple snack. After lunch bring the coffee back for only about an hour. Again, depending on how late the session goes, serve a light beverage in the afternoon. Finishing with a wine and cheese hour to unwind participants also can work well.

Sometimes you will not wish to provide food, but you cannot ignore the appetites of conference goers. Your task in this case is to identify good-quality food at a variety of prices and in places near the meeting site. Participants will eat breakfast, lunch, and dinner—and often in between. They will do so even if your meeting is in progress. So make it easy and pleasant for them. Do not overlook the importance of providing each participant with a sheet of paper showing your suggestions, with maps or descriptions of how to get there.

Hotel The importance of the hotel operation to the success of your conference cannot be overstressed. If the hotel is well run, your meeting is more likely to proceed smoothly. If the hotel is not well run, then no matter how skillfully you arrange your meeting, the chances of its success are at risk. Hotel management, or mismanagement, can make or break your careful planning. Here are some pointers that seem to us worth considering.

First, make arrangements with the hotel management so that whoever you work with in planning the meeting is on hand during the meeting. Sometimes a group will appear for its meeting on a weekend—a common occurrence in professional organizations. While the meeting is on, the hotel staff may well be off. It is possible that without your careful planning, there will be no one on the premises who is aware of or familiar with your arrangements. You need to be sure that a knowledgeable member of the hotel staff is available.

Checking out of a hotel seems simple enough at first glance. But sometimes meetings run beyond the usual hotel check-out times. Be sure to arrange for this variance from usual policy. Set aside an hour or so in the morning, and another at the lunch period, during which members of your group can check out. Incidentally, almost everyone at a meeting will have not only a suitcase but probably a briefcase and perhaps some other luggage as well. Make advance arrangements to store luggage between check-out time and the time the participants actually leave the hotel. No one wants to leave expensive equipment and valuable papers lying around, or to cart them from meeting room to meeting room. The upshot of lack of planning in this regard will be that the participants will take the path of least resistance—they will leave the conference.

It may be a good idea to set up a credit plan with the hotel so that the people who attend the meeting do not have to pay at the time they check out, relieving them of worrying about one more detail.

It is possible to take care of these things in advance, and a hotel manager can help you with this kind of planning. You want the participants' experience to be pleasant and convenient. So does the hotel manager. Incidentally, while no one wants to admit it, some people do not pay their bills. You will wish to discuss this possibility directly with the hotel management to ensure that neither the hotel nor your organization ends up having to pay unexpected expenses.

Finally, the closer you keep advance hotel payments to the beginning of the meeting, the better, since most of these are not refundable and you cannot always predict the future. Over time, you will save your company a good deal of money—and exercise greater influence on arrangements—if you can pattern your payment program carefully. Usually payments to hotels and airlines are not required a long time in advance. Call around. Get an idea of what is standard in the area. Use that information to negotiate for your organization.

Shipping   Shipping is very important, especially if the meeting you call is going to be in another city. A single undelivered package, if the contents are truly important, can make the difference between success and failure of your meeting. Here are some easy-to-follow suggestions:

1. Double-check to be sure that every label is correctly addressed and that the address is legible. We suggest that you include a correct address *inside* every package as well as on the outside.

2. Send a summary of the items you have shipped to the meeting place in advance. Keep a copy of the summary at your office. Include a copy in one of the packages. Request a copy of such a summary from anyone who sends materials to you. Be sure that summaries arrive before the shipments.

3. Make arrangements with your hotel to return materials to their origins following the meeting. Help the hotel to be as thorough as you have been.

4. Determine the best way to ship far in advance. Should materials go by U.S. mail? By express mail? By air? By bus? Should the participants bring the materials? Understand that best is not necessarily cheapest.

Transportation   Typically, the responsibility for transportation lies with the participants. But think about it. If participants take a plane from their home city to Chicago, and a limo from the airport to the hotel, after that they are on foot. If someone has thoughtfully made arrangements, they might be able to take a sightseeing tour. If someone has planned for their needs, they might be able to use the elevated trains for which Chicago is famous. If someone has provided them with bus and train schedules and a list of special bus and limousine services, they could save a bundle by not having to take a taxi or rent a car. All of that kind of planning falls upon you as the one who plans a meeting.

Notice in addition that many companies own private planes. Busy executives will appreciate a list of local airstrips for private planes, or notification if the hotel or resort has an airport.

Miscellaneous   In the final analysis, planning a meeting is an exercise in careful consideration of others. You may wish to accommodate their needs even before the needs occur to them. For instance, you should probably keep a list of the participants, including addresses and phone numbers. There are many possible uses for this list, including having it on hand for Internal Revenue Service agents; responding to requests for information by participants ("What is John Doe's address and phone number? You know, the representative from Du Pont."); returning materials and property lost or misplaced during the meeting; and, perhaps most important, facilitating the all-important follow-through you will do after the meeting.

Your planning should also include securing the necessary materials for each person. Pens, paper, agenda materials, duplicate copies, and the like are necessary and should be available to all. Remember that people are forgetful. Even if you have sent them copies, they might not have them on hand at the meeting. Provide them with another copy if they need it. The success of the meeting is the uppermost concern in their minds. The trick here is to anticipate any possible embarrassment to participants, while at the same time making sure that everyone has everything that you are capable of providing.

Find out about tipping, too. If possible, arrange it so that your participants will not have to tip at airports, at the hotel, at banquets, and the like. Or at least make meeting-related tipping policies available to participants in advance.

The number of miscellaneous details that should be taken care of are myriad. A safety officer related a story that points to how important details can be. He attended an urgent meeting of a government agency in Jackson, Mississippi, held in a hotel in that southern city. He assumed it would be a rather large meeting, but it turned out that he was wrong. The entire conference, which lasted two days, was housed in a couple of meeting rooms on the second floor—one above the mezzanine. When he entered the hotel through the parking lot entrance, he thought he had come to the wrong place. Looking around, he noticed only one person—clearly not a conference participant—in the lobby. There was nothing to indicate that the meeting was to take place in that building. He asked the desk clerk and was told: "That meeting is on the second floor, in the Jackson Room." He went to the Jackson Room. It was empty. He stopped someone walking by—a man who appeared to be a possible participant. He turned out to be the conference director! Our view is that the director could have avoided the safety officer's discomfort by doing two things.

First, he could have provided name badges. They're important, even if the participants are all from the same organization. People are likely to be embarrassed if they have already been introduced but cannot remember a name. The name badges should be distinctive, so that participants recognize their colleagues instantly. They should be large enough so that vain participants who do not wear their glasses can still read them. The large clip-on type is best because it is easiest to handle and does not damage clothing. The sticky-back kind does not stay on long enough, and the pin-on kind can play havoc with good clothing. But anything is better than nothing.

Second, the conference director should have provided directions. Welcome signs and other directional information are a big help. These contribute in at least two ways: They assist in the general sense of welcome that participants should feel, and they help to get the meetings started on time.

Publish the Agenda with the Invitation

In the task dimension, include all the information necessary for participants to prepare well for the meeting. See that it suggests what materials participants should bring and what homework they should do. Be sure that the agenda is couched in moderate language. It is amazing to discover how many times someone runs up a flag with language like "to debate the critical problems of" or "to discover who is responsible for."

In the social dimension, you wish to guarantee that the participants have time to prepare. Remind them once or twice between the initial invitation and the actual conference. You can do this by phone or by note. Or you can arrange to bump into a forgetful individual in the corridor of your building and say, "Sure am looking forward to your part of the meeting Wednesday." Or you might prefer to ask your secretary to confirm the participants' plans to attend. However you do it, remind them gently and skillfully—for obvious reasons. Be sure to encourage and reward inquiry and offers of help or suggestions from participants.

Plan the Arrangement of Participants

In the task dimension, making physical arrangements can be a massive problem or a very minor one. In no case is it something to be left to chance. Seating ought to be arranged with some concern for the effect you wish it to produce. Will seating arrangements maximize participation if that is what you wish? Does the physical arrangement accommodate the camera equipment and the audience's view, when that is necessary?

There are some clear concerns in the social dimension, too. Especially interesting are the implications that an arrangement can have for status consensus, social comparison, interpersonal conflict, and the like. Take a minute to look at the suggestions about space as a message system in Chapter 4.

In both the task and social dimensions, try to anticipate the needs of participants in terms of the arrangement of the meeting by imagining a run-through of the day. To give you a flavor of some of the things that can happen, at a meeting in Denver participants sat at tables arranged in the shape of a large U, illustrated in Figure 12.1. The head table was used by the primary group of speakers. Those of us who were there primarily as listeners but who had some things to contribute were seated around the other tables. Suppose a person was at the position marked X. Do you think that this person would feel somewhat isolated from what was going on?

On another occasion a room was arranged as in Figure 12.2. You might have been amused to watch the squirming among participants who, after about an hour and a half of meeting, had to pass through the doors behind the head table in order to get to the restrooms. Simply turning the arrangement around so that the speakers were at the other end of the room would have solved that embarrassing problem.

If these examples seem a little extreme, it is because they are. Nevertheless, they happened. If you are in charge of a meeting, you need to be concerned about this kind of detail. Someone will surely notice such slip-ups, and you will catch the blame.

Arrange to Meet, Greet, Identify, and Introduce Participants

In the task dimension, greeting and introducing participants means taking care in advance of any protocol requirements, and making sure that each participant can identify every other participant by name and expectation where that is feasible. It also means being sure that each participant who requests or requires it will be picked up and delivered on time or knows how to make such arrangements, and that each has opportunities for last-minute requests.

In the social dimension, this means causing the participants to feel like VIPs. They *are* VIPs, and they should feel that way.

A director of public relations once told a story about a VIP at the airport near Normal, Illinois. He was in charge of meeting and greeting VIPs for his firm. The person he was meeting was obviously tired from a bumpy flight on a commuter aircraft. While

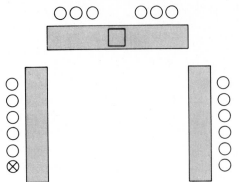

**FIGURE 12.1
A Less than Ideal Set-up**

Source: Michael S. Hanna and Gerald L. Wilson, *Communicating in Business and Professional Settings*, 2d ed. (New York: Random House, 1988), p. 317.

driving to the hotel, he asked the VIP what his favorite drink was, then turned to other topics. When he checked the visitor into the hotel, he made arrangements for that favorite drink to be delivered immediately to the guest's hotel room. Five years later I had occasion to chat with that person myself and asked him if he remembered my friend. "Oh, yes," he said, "I'll never forget him." Then he went on to tell the story of that awful flight and how welcome that drink was. "One of the most welcome surprises in my life," is how he characterized the gesture.

Begin and End on Time

In both dimensions, this means begin and end on time.

Follow Through After the Meeting

In the task dimension, follow-through focuses upon agreements made during the meeting. You and others may commit yourselves to perform certain tasks. Wise leaders will gently remind others, whenever appropriate and in a planned sequence, of these commitments. Mention to the individuals your intention of inquiring and reminding them about the agreed-on pattern; then do it.

In the social dimension, it is worth remembering that participants make a contribution if only in coming to the meeting. They spend a good deal of time, energy, and money to be there, and they want to know and feel that their contribution is valued. Follow through with some old-fashioned stroking where that can be accomplished appropriately.

If the conference goes well, a letter to the conference participant's boss may mean more to him or her than a direct letter. A president of a local firm was a master at this kind of follow-through. Following the meeting of a volunteer group organized to discuss ways of improving the schools, he mailed letters to each person's boss. He commented on the person's fine work and expressed his appreciation to the company. Of course, the participants heard about the compliments through their bosses.

This president's generous remarks to the business leaders were also important to

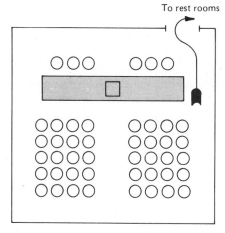

To rest rooms

**FIGURE 12.2
An Inconvenient Way to the
"Conveniences"**

Source: Michael S. Hanna and Gerald L. Wilson, *Communicating in Business and Professional Settings*, 2d ed. (New York: Random House, 1988), p. 318.

him. They worked for *him*, too. Those involved in the project became firm supporters of the man. Do you wonder how much of their faith in him rests on his thoughtful follow-through?

A Conference-Planning Checklist

For your convenience, and as a summary of what's been said so far, Table 12.3 is a checklist that will help you to plan a conference if you are ever called upon to do so. It includes a list of questions that will guide you through the tasks of planning a conference.

SUMMARY

Public discussions are those small group interactions carried on for the benefit of an audience. Forums involve full participation of the audience, either through question-and-answer sessions involving a group of experts or well-informed people, or through actual discussion within the audience. A panel discussion is interaction involving specialists or reasonably well-informed people who share their points of view about a common topic or question. A symposium is a series of brief speeches with an audience present. It is often coupled with a forum or panel discussion. A colloquium is an interaction that involves a group of experts being questioned by the audience. The selection of a format is related to how informed the members of the audience are and the purpose of the meeting.

We suggested that leadership of a public discussion requires limiting the number of topics considered, planning a series of open-ended questions, and keeping the discussants on the topic. Attention should also be devoted to regulating participation and rewarding members for their cooperation and participation.

TABLE 12.3   A Conference-Planning Checklist

1. **Purpose decided?**
   a. Consulted with management?
   b. Special speaker?
      (1) Identified?
      (2) Special arrangements made?

2. **Task and goal thinking complete?**
   a. Homework on subject complete?
   b. Issues identified?
   c. Position on issues clear and supported?
   d. How do issues relate to other participants?

3. **Agenda planned?**
   a. What topics must be covered?
   b. How much time available? Enough?
   c. Who needs to be consulted?
      (1) Have those people been consulted?
      (2) Have their suggestions been accommodated?
      (3) Have their schedules been accommodated?

4. **Other participants identified?**
   a. Who *must* be there?
   b. Who *ought* to be there?
   c. Who *may* be eliminated?
      (1) Implications?
      (2) Actions to smooth ruffled feathers?

5. **Setting and location selected?**
   a. Size appropriate?
   b. Formality/informality appropriate?

6. **Facilities complete?**
   a. Restrooms okay?
   b. Refreshment centers okay?
   c. Acoustics okay?
   d. Seating okay?
   e. Lighting okay?
   f. Public address system okay?
   g. Sleeping arrangements okay?
   h. Food arrangements okay?
      (1) Catering manager: Name? Phone? Office hours? Location?
      (2) Catering specials?
      (3) Snacks and hors d'oeuvres?
      (4) Beverages?
      (5) Restaurants nearby?
         (a) List prepared?
         (b) Maps or location finders available?

TABLE 12.3   A Conference-Planning Checklist *(Continued)*

7. **Hotel procedures checked out?**
   a. Contact person: Name? Phone? Office hours? Location?
   b. Contact person on hand during conference?
   c. Checkout procedure?
   d. Checkout times?
   e. Storage for luggage near checkout desk?
   f. Credit plan available?
   g. Payment schedule and procedures secured?

8. **Audio-visual facilities okay?**
   a. List of equipment needed?
   b. Equipment on hand?
   c. Supplemental parts on hand?
   d. Equipment functioning?
   e. Operator(s) on hand?

9. **Shipping arrangements complete?**
   a. Address labels accurate?
   b. Addresses inside each package?
   c. Summary list of shipping items?
      (1) To hotel?
      (2) From participants?
      (3) Inside one of the packages?
      (4) In file?
   d. Return arrangements made with hotel?
   e. Shipping via . . . ?
   f. Hotel contact person: Name? Phone? Office hours? Location?
   g. Other contact persons?

10. **Transportation arrangements complete?**
    a. Airport location (private and commercial)?
    b. Airport to hotel?
    c. Available tours?
    d. Train, bus, and subway schedules?
    e. Limo service?

11. **Miscellaneous arrangements identified?**
    a. List of participants with addresses and phone numbers complete?
    b. Tipping practices and procedures? No-tip arrangements made?
    c. Welcome posters?
    d. Direction posters?
    e. Name tags and badges?
    f. Meeting and greeting arranged?
       (1) Protocol problems?

Source: Michael S. Hanna and Gerald L. Wilson, *Communicating in Business and Professional Settings*, 2d ed. (New York: Random House, 1988), 320–321.

We presented a checklist that will help you to plan a conference and recommended ten steps to follow in such planning. The discussion focused on the implications of each of the ten steps for both the task and social dimensions of communication.

EXERCISES

1. Record the strengths and weaknesses of your group in its public discussion. What suggestions do you have for improving the effectiveness of your group in this kind of discussion?

2. Write a short paper that distinguishes among the forum, panel, colloquium, and symposium. What are their distinguishing characteristics? How do they differ in degree of formality? How do they differ with respect to audience involvement? How are these formats similar? As examples of each, suggest specific events that seem appropriate for the format.

3. Plan a panel discussion on a topic of interest in your community. Specify who your panel members would be and what you think each person's qualifications for inclusion would be. Plan an agenda for this meeting that includes the questions you would use to carry out the panel discussion. Submit a report that includes a statement of the issue, members, and their qualifications, with the leader's agenda for the discussion.

NOTES

1. Larry L. Barker et al., *Groups in Process: An Introduction to Small Group Communication*, 2d ed. (Englewood Cliffs, NJ: Prentice-Hall, 1983), 221–225.

2. Ibid., 222.

3. William C. Schutz, *FIRO: A Three-Dimensional Theory of Interpersonal Behavior* (New York: Holt, Rinehart and Winston, 1958).

4. Most of these ideas are the good advice of Dennis A. Stone, Director of Public Relations, Manpower, Inc., of Milwaukee, in "We're Having a Meeting and You're in Charge!" *Public Relations Journal* 34 (May 1978):12.

RECOMMENDED READINGS

Ronald L. Applebaum, E. M. Bodaken, K. K. Sereno, and K. W. E. Anatol, *The Process of Group Communication* (Chicago: Science Research Associates, 1974), Chapter 10, "Methods of Discussion."

J. D. Hughey and A. W. Johnson, *Speech Communication: Foundations and Challenges* (New York: Macmillan, 1975), Unit 12, "Public Discussion."

GLOSSARY

abstraction   The process of deriving a general concept from specific details. A partial representation of something whole.

accommodation   Situation in which individuals who are experiencing interpersonal conflict refrain from overt expression of the conflict.

active listening   Process of paraphrasing the other's ideas or statements, including the provision of feedback about nonverbal messages.

affiliation   Attachment or unity on basis or terms of fellowship.

agenda   Agreed-on arrangement of topics for discussion. Sometimes this term is applied to the private issues or problems that individuals bring to a group meeting.

agenda, hidden   A secret plan that a group member has to achieve goals or objectives that are his or her own, rather than those of the group.

agenda setting   Effect of media; focusing attention and discourse on certain issues or problems, usually with the result that the issues or problems are perceived as important. As a group activity, the process of determining and arranging the subject matter for discourse.

anchoring   Point of decision in the process of reach-testing. The cycle that includes an anchoring point follows the sequence: suggestion of an idea, agreement to the idea by others, presentation of examples to clarify the idea, and finally, affirmation, or confirmation, of the idea.

antecedent condition   Any condition that precedes, and thus influences, an event or decision.

approach-approach conflict   Conflict over mutually exclusive but equally attractive outcomes.

approach-avoidance conflict   Conflict resulting when outcomes from an act or decision are perceived as both desirable and undesirable. The actor is attracted by one of the outcomes but put off by another.

arbitration   The process of hearing and determining the outcome of a dispute between factions or persons. A hearing given to disputants by an arbitrator, the aim of which is reaching a settlement.

assembly effect   Ability of a group to be more productive, working together, than the sum total of productivity that individual members can achieve working on their own.

authoritarian leadership   Sometimes called "autocratic leadership." A leadership style in which the leader directs the behavior of others by resort to power and rules.

autocratic leadership   See "*authoritarian leadership.*"

avoidance-avoidance conflict   Conflict that results when avoiding an undesirable outcome will yield a different undesirable outcome.

balance   A sense of psychological well-being in which we perceive the world as harmonious and consistent.

barrier (or) breakdown   Interruption in the flow of communication assigned or attributed to some structural defect in the communication process. This idea is controversial among communication scholars, who perceive it as inconsistent with a "process model" of communication.

brainstorming   Group procedure for generating a large and diverse idea base quickly. Members of a group select a "recorder," then generate as many ideas as may occur. Ground rules prohibit any editorial or judgmental remarks about member contributions. Brainstorming sessions are usually timed, and often a member creates a "group memory" by placing key words or phrases on a chalkboard or flip chart as they are offered by the group.

breakpoint   A transition in the developmental process of a group that is represented by a change in the group activity.

breakpoint, normal   The most common breakpoint by which a group moves from one topic to the next, or from one activity to the next, or moves to plan a task.

centrality   Term used to refer to the location of an individual in a communication network. Centrality is measured by the number of "linkages" required for a position to communicate, through channels, to every other position in the network.

certainty   In logic, the position that what is being observed could not have occurred by chance. 100 percent level of confidence. Certainty also refers to an attitude that is closed-minded, thus not considerate of alternative positions or points of view. The opposite of certainty, from this perspective, is *"provisionalism."*

channel   The means of transmission. The vehicle through which messages are sent.

channel capacity   A measure of the maximum amount of information that a communication channel can handle at any given moment.

coalition   An alliance or agreement between two (or more) individuals. Coalitions are usually temporary, and usually have to do with a controversial position.

code   A system of signs and symbols used to transmit messages between people. Sometimes used to suggest a system of symbols used to translate messages from one form to another.

cognition   The act, power, or faculty of apprehending, knowing, or perceiving.

cohesiveness   A group's sense of unity, or "togetherness." Characterized by mutual attractiveness and willingness to work together. A measure of an individual's commitment to the group.

collective evaluation   A belief shared by members of a group about how members ought or ought not to act.

collective expectation   A standard applied to behavior to discover if it classifies as a norm.

colloquy   A public group meeting format designed to inform an audience through the use of planned questions that produce unprepared responses from a panel of experts.

complementarity   Quality of a relationship. Interaction in which behavior by one individual (stimulus) produces behavior by another (response). Combined, these behaviors produce a complete and coherent unit. In relationship terms, a complementary relationship maximizes individual differences.

compromise   A negotiated conflict settlement in which each party gives up part of what is wanted in order to get the other part. From a game theory perspective, compromise is a lose-lose solution.

conflict, affective   Conflict among people that is generated from differences in emotions or from relational frictions.

conflict, interpersonal   A form of competition. A situation in which one person's behaviors are designed to interfere with or harm another individual (expressed). Disagreement or opposition of ideas or opinions (unexpressed).

conflict, intrapersonal   Condition or status of emotional tension. See *approach-approach, approach-avoidance,* and *avoidance-avoidance conflict.*

conformity   Behaviors produced by an individual that are uniform, or consistent with the expectations of a social system, and least likely to produce negative consequences or influences from the other members of the social system.

confrontation   Conflict management technique in which participants talk directly about the conflict and relationship issues. Sometimes called "confrontation–problem solving method."

connotation   The affective value or meaning of a word. The emotional associations an individual user brings to a word.

consensus   A measure of the extent of agreement or commitment that members feel toward the decisions of a group. Generally, consensus means that the members agree with a decision.

content and relationship dimensions   The notion that language refers to both the world external to a speaker—the objects, phenomena, and events outside of the individual (content dimension)—and to the relationship existing between the speaker and another individual (relationship dimension).

context of communication   The physical, social, psychological, and temporal environment in which a communication event occurs.

contingency model   Fiedler's model of group leadership that predicts leader effectiveness.

cooperation   Process of working together toward a common goal. Sharing effort, expertise, and resources to achieve some mutually desirable outcome.

credibility   Degree to which a receiver believes a source. The believability of an individual.

credibility gap   Tendency of people to disbelieve one another. The difference between the image of integrity an individual attempts to project and the perception of integrity that another holds of that individual.

criteria   Standards of judgment based upon what is valued.

culture (group)   The history, traditions, and rules concerning appropriate and inappropriate behaviors of a group.

decision   A choice among available or imagined alternatives. A group decision is a decision reached by the process of consensus, or by some other decision-making procedure validated by the group.

decision making   The process of choosing among alternatives. The process of arriving at a decision.

decision-making meeting   A group that interacts with its members for the purpose of considering action related to some concern.

decode   The process of taking message value from a code.

delay   A breakpoint that happens when a group moves back to repeat an analysis or activity.

Delphi method   A group decision-making technique in which individuals respond to questionnaires until a final composite list is obtained that represents the opinions of the group. This is *not* a group discussion technique, since the group members do not typically or necessarily meet to talk about their responses to the questionnaires.

democratic leader   A group leader who stimulates the involvement of group members and encourages them to arrive at decisions through the process of consensus.

denotation   The associations usually called up by a word among members of a speech community. The "dictionary definition" of a word. The features of meaning of a word that are usually accepted by native speakers of a language.

designated leader   Any individual who is appointed to a position of leadership, as opposed to an individual who emerges as the result of his or her perceived leadership potential.

deviance   Behavior of a group member that does not conform to the norms or expectations of the group.

disruption   A breakpoint that is represented by either a major disagreement or a conflict.

dyadic communication   Communication between two people. A dyad is not a group, since the minimum number that can be called a group is three.

dysfunctional conflict   Conflict that does not contribute to the group's progress toward its goals, or that is not productive. Not all conflict is dysfunctional, since conflict is inherent in change and in relationship management.

emergence   A gradual process in which groups develop the roles individual members will play, the norms that govern group behavior, and the decisions the group will validate by consensus.

emergence phase   A period in a decision-making discussion in which dissent dissipates as a group comes to agreement on a decision.

emergent leader   The individual who rises to a position of leadership as a result of the group's perception of his or her leadership potential.

empathy   Experiencing what another person experiences, feeling what another person feels.

encoder   The component of the communication process in which information is translated from one form into another. In speech, to encode is to translate ideas into spoken words. A telephone mouthpiece serves as an encoder as it translates spoken sounds into electrical impulses.

equality   The attitude, reflected in communication choices, that each individual is inherently of worth. Equality encourages supportiveness. The behavioral opposite is superiority.

ethics   The branch of philosophy that studies moral value, rightness or wrongness.

ethos   The perception of an individual's character, as, for example, an audience's perception that a speaker is honest, knowledgeable, and of good will and intention.

evaluation   The process of making a value judgment about some person, object, or event.

evolution   The history of an object, idea, or event. The enduring changes.

feedback   Messages sent from a receiver to a source that have the effect of correcting or controlling error. Feedback can take the form of talk, applause, yawning, puzzled looks, questions, letters, increases or decreases in subscription rates, etc. In groups, feedback sometimes is used by members to teach an individual his role, or to extinguish the behavior of a deviant member.

field of experience   The image of the world that an individual holds as a result of interacting and communicating with it. The field of experience is dependent on language (how you talk about the world—the things you say to yourself and others), and on such things as memory and forgetting. Thus an individual field of experience is unique.

FIRO   "Fundamental interpersonal relationship orientation." Analytical system developed by William Schutz for examining and understanding human relationships based upon need for inclusion, control, and affection.

forcing   A method of managing conflict in which the person attempts to gain compliance by applying some sort of pressure.

forgetting curve   A model that traces the amount of material retained or forgotten over time.

forum   Large group meeting designed to encourage audience participation on issues surrounding a topic. Typically, a moderator introduces a speaker and a topic. The speaker presents a brief statement, and then interacts with the audience. The moderator encourages audience participation and involvement.

function   The appropriate activity or action of a person or thing. The purpose for which something is designed or exists. Role.

functional perspective   In group communication theory, the study of the group processes in terms of the functions of a group or its individual members. Applied to leadership of groups, examination of what the individual does, as opposed, for example, to a *trait perspective*, which would study individual features of the leader's character.

game   A simulation, with rules governing the behaviors of the participants. In game theory, games may be played in three forms: win-win, win-lose, and lose-lose.

gatekeeping   The act or process of filtering messages sent. Some messages are allowed to pass intact, others are distorted, still others may be eliminated altogether.

goal conflict   Conflict among group members about what they want to accomplish.

group   Three or more people who perceive themselves as a unit, and who are mutually interdependent, and who interact about some common goal.

group failure   A disruption-type breakpoint that is a result of a group's realizing that its effort is not going to be sufficient to meet the task goals.

group mind   The idea that a group's way of thinking and feeling can exist apart from its individual members. The notion is out of date.

groupthink   A phenomenon that occurs in highly cohesive groups when the members ignore evidence and opinion contrary to their own views, and disregard alternative choices, in order to preserve their feeling of unity. Groupthink often leads to a faulty decision.

hypothesis, motivational-hierarchy   A thesis that Fred Fiedler presented to explain some of his findings about leadership style. It suggests that people are motivated to attain more than one goal at a particular time.

ideational conflict   Disagreements among group members about conceptualizations.

inference   A guess. A judgment, based upon observational data, about the meaning of that data.

information   In information theory, available data. The more the available data, the more the information, and the greater the uncertainty. More commonly used to mean anything that reduces uncertainty.

information overload   Condition in which the amount of information is too great to be processed. Typically, in groups, when the number and complexity of messages is too great to be dealt with.

information processing   Using perceptions to transform data into information, usually followed by action on those perceptions. Can be either an individual or a group process.

information-sharing meeting   A group that interacts for the purpose of enlightenment of its members.

input   In group communication, the contributions of individual members. What the members bring to a group decision-making situation.

interact   Two acts by group members that occur in sequence and are related to each other.

interaction diagrams   Diagrams used to record the flow and number of messages sent in a group.

interaction process analysis (IPA)   A method of content analysis developed by Robert F. Bales that classifies messages into four categories: social-emotional positive, social-emotional negative, questions, and attempted answers.

interdependence   A relationship between elements or people such that each is influenced by the other.

interpersonal communication   Communication between or among people, characterized by give and take. Distinguished from public communication by its more personal nature (as opposed to the impersonal nature of public communication).

interpersonal needs   Motives that produce affiliation. The reasons for establishing a relationship. In William Schutz's system, inclusion, control, and affection.

intrapersonal communication   Communication within oneself.

intrinsic interest   The level of concern and involvement generated by a particular issue or idea.

IPA   See *interaction process analysis.*

issue   A question that is central, or critical, to an argument. Issues may be of fact (something is), value (something is good), or policy (something should be).

jargon   Technical language evolved by specialists so that they can communicate more accurately and efficiently about their interests or concerns.

laissez-faire leadership   A behavioral style employed by some designated leaders in which the leader withdraws from the group process, leaving the group members to their own devices.

leader   One who directs and influences a group to move toward group goal achievement. A leader may be designated, or a leader may emerge.

leader, designated   A person appointed by someone in authority to direct the activities of a group.

leader, emergent   A group member, not appointed to lead by someone in authority, who directs the activities of a group because the majority of group members accept this person's willingness to do so.

leaderless group discussion (LGD)   A task-oriented group that determines its own structures, procedures, and functions.

leadership   In a group, the functional behaviors of a person, usually of high status, that contribute to the group's movements toward its goals.

leadership-structuring style   In a group, the functional behaviors of a person who directs the activities of a group by helping the group plan and organize its activities and set goals, while encouraging relative equality among its members.

leveling   A communication phenomenon in which messages are distorted by reduction of details, intensity, or complexity when they are repeated in a series.

LGD   See *leaderless group discussion.*

linear model   A model of the communication process that describes or implies a line of direction of message flow.

listening   The active process of receiving and processing stimuli.

maintenance   Behaviors by group members that contribute to the cohesiveness of the group.

majority vote   Decision technique sometimes taken by a group to resolve conflict. Not recommended except as a measure of last resort.

mediation   Conflict management technique in which disputing parties agree to negotiate with the help of an arbitrator. Usually understood to be binding.

mental set   Psychological orientation produced by prior events or perceptions that contributes to bias in perception or comprehension.

message   Any sign or symbol, or any combination of signs or symbols, that functions as stimulus for a receiver.

model   A physical representation of an object or process. Models may be visual or verbal, and may be two- or three-dimensional.

modification, nonverbal   A cue or message sent, nonverbally, to modify the meaning of the verbal message.

motivation-hierarchy hypothesis   See *hypothesis, motivation-hierarchy.*

network, communication   In a group, the structure of channel linkages between and among members. A description of who communicates with whom, how often, and through what channels.

neutrality   Impersonal communication response pattern that creates defensiveness. Opposite of empathy.

NGT, (or) NGP   See *nominal group technique.* Sometimes called "nominal group process."

noise   Any source of interference or distortion in message exchange. Noise exists in the process to the extent that message fidelity is damaged. Three broad categories: (1) physical, or channel noise, (2) semantic, or psychological noise, and (3) systemic, or system-centered noise.

nominal group technique   A group procedure for increasing productivity by asking members to follow a five-step sequence: (1) silent listing of ideas, (2) creation of a master list of ideas, (3) clarification of ideas, (4) straw vote for testing acceptance of ideas, (5) follow-through.

norm   A rule that evolves out of a group's interactions to control and govern the behavior of group members.

openness   In language, the phenomenon that allows native speakers to talk about matters that they have not discussed before, and to understand talk they have never heard before. In relationships, the willingness of an individual to receive and consider ideas from another.

operational definition   A definition by example.

opinion leader   A person whose opinion molds public opinion. In a group, an individual whose ideas influence the direction or decision of a group.

organization   A human system designed to achieve some set of specific goals, and characterized by a recurring sequence of events, such as a calendar year.

orientation phase   The initial period in the decision-making process, characterized by the members' establishing goals and getting to know other members.

output   In group communication, the productivity of a group or its individual members. The yield that derives from communication in the task dimension.

participant-analyst   The person in a group who observes and evaluates what is going on and takes action to provide whatever the group needs at that moment.

perception   The process of becoming aware of stimuli that impinge on the five senses.

persuasion   The process of influence. The process of changing attitudes, beliefs, and behaviors.

physical noise   See *noise*.

population familiarity   A feature of a group task having to do with the extent to which a group has had experience with the task.

positive feedback   Feedback that reinforces behaviors for the purpose of increasing the likelihood that the behaviors will recur. For example, nods of agreement, or laughter in response to an anecdote.

positive reinforcement   Increasing the likelihood of a particular response by rewarding it.

power   The perceived influence one person has over another.

primary tension   The experience of tension that individual group members feel during the early stages of group evolution.

problem orientation   Focus upon the components of a problem and its possible solutions, as opposed, for example, to focus upon the group's processes. Encourages supportiveness. Opposite is control.

procedural leadership   Behavior that contributes to group productivity by focusing upon and providing guidance concerning group procedures.

process   Ongoing activity. Continuous changing in the pursuit of a goal.

productivity   The quantity and/or quality of a group's work in the task dimension.

provisionalism   Behavior suggesting an attitude of open-mindedness, tentativeness with respect to a conclusion. Opposite is certainty.

punctuation   In group communication, the arbitrary process of creating the meaning of a sequence of messages by selecting the beginning and ending points of the sequence.

quality circle   A volunteer group of employees that meets to identify work-related problems and propose solutions to them.

question of fact   A discussion issue that does not involve value decisions or policies and that can be resolved by collecting information that addresses the issue.

question of policy   A discussion issue that requires a decision about what should be or ought to be done as a general rule in a particular situation and similar situations.

question of value   A discussion issue that requires a decision about goodness or worth of something.

reach testing   Introduction of a new idea based upon some anchored position in the spiral model. Group members accept, revise, or reject the idea through group discussion.

receiver   A person or thing that takes in messages.

reciprocity   Assumption that people will respond to behaviors with similar behaviors.

redundancy   In information theory, a measure of the predictability of a message. The greater the redundancy the greater the predictability and the less the uncertainty.

referent   The object or event to which a symbol refers.

reflective thinking   A pattern, or sequence, of logical thought that provides a convenient agenda for the tasks of a discussion group: (1) identify the problem, (2) define and delimit the problem, (3) develop evaluative criteria against which to test alternative proposals, (4) seek alternative solutions to propose and test, (5) develop a final solution to advocate.

reflexiveness   A feature of all languages that allows the language to refer to itself. Language for talking about language is said to be self-reflexive.

regulation   In groups, substitution of nonverbal messages for words in order to control the behavior of group members.

reinforcement   Increasing or strengthening the likelihood of a response.

reinforcement phase   A final period in decision making in which members congratulate themselves on completing their task effectively.

reliability   A measure of the extent to which independent observers agree. A measure of the extent to which a measuring instrument will measure the same phenomenon in different cases.

Richards, I. A., triangle of meaning   A theoretical model that shows the relationship among an object, phenomenon, or event, thinking about that object, phenomenon, or event, and the symbolic representations people generate about their observations.

risky shift   The tendency of a group to be less conservative in decision making than an individual. The tendency of a group to take a greater risk than an individual. A group is more likely to gamble—to "go for" the greater payoff, with the less probability of attainment, than is an individual.

role   The part an individual plays in a group. The behaviors evidenced by a group member that have been sanctioned by group approval. The expectations that a group has of an individual's behavior.

role conflict   The result of a person's attempting to play two or more roles that are contradictory in function.

role, self-centered   A role that serves the purpose of personal enhancement of the role player at the expense of progress toward achievement of group goals.

role stability   The point at which a group member performs a particular function in a group and the group reinforces the practice of the function, resulting in general agreement that that member should continue to perform that function.

role strain   The tension that results from a person's trying to perform a role, but being unable to do so.

scapegoating   Blaming others for one's own mistakes.

secondary tension   The discomfort that a group experiences, or that is experienced by individual group members, beyond the *tolerance threshold* for tension. That is, tension experienced by the group or its members that is so great that the group may no longer ignore it.

selective perception   Unconscious process of sorting through available stimuli, and selecting those to be perceived.

self-concept   The image of oneself that has evolved out of interaction with significant others over time.

self-disclosure   Revealing oneself—thinking, feelings, beliefs, and the like—to another.

self-fulfilling prophecy   Process of making a prediction come true. For example, predicting that a group experience will be exciting, then fulfilling the prediction by experiencing the group as exciting.

self-reflexiveness   Ability of something to refer back to itself. Language is self-reflexive. People can be self-reflexive.

self-report rating form   Form used to report self-appraisals of performance in a group context.

semantic noise   Error introduced into a communication event due to peculiarities in the use of language. Sometimes called psychological noise.

scapegoating   Process of placing blame on some outside cause, such as an individual or agency.

situation/context   Terms used interchangeably. The immediate surroundings of an event. The environment in which an event takes place. The presence of variables that may influence a communication event.

situational perspective   A perspective that relies on examination of a situation in order to guide decisions about appropriate leadership.

small group   Three or more individuals, up to about eleven individuals, who perceive themselves as joined to achieve some common goal.

smoothing   A conflict management strategy in which a member attempts to play down or ignore differences in order to keep a disagreement from being addressed by the group.

social dimension   The relationship dimension of group communication, having to do with such relational matters as cohesiveness.

social leadership   Behaviors of individual group members that serve to maintain the group's relationships and cohesiveness.

solution multiplicity   The number of reasonable alternatives to solve a problem.

source   The location of an idea. The originator of a message.

special-events meeting   An unusual, not regular, one-of-a-kind meeting, or an occasional and traditional event meeting, such as the annual sales meeting of a company's marketing division.

spiral model   A model of decision development that encompasses backtracking and reach testing until group consensus is achieved.

spontaneity   Characteristic of interaction in which individuals speak freely and straightforwardly without editing or developing strategies of control. Encourages supportiveness. Opposite is strategy.

stability in perception   Phenomenon of the perceptual process that renders perceptions of people and things relatively constant or consistent with previous conceptualizations of those people and things.

status   Place in a hierarchy. In a group, the social position, either appointed or achieved as the result of interactions.

status, achieved   Position or ranking that a group member gains in a group's hierarchy because of other members' perceptions of the person's contribution and personality.

status, ascribed   Position or ranking that a group member has in a group's hierarchy because of the function that person is assigned to play by the organization of which the group is a part.

status conflict   Conflict over relative, or comparative, status among group members.

status consensus   Agreement among group members that the members place in the status hierarchy is agreeable and appropriate.

stereotype   Application of a fixed set of characteristics about a group or subgroup to an individual member of that group or subgroup in such a way that the uniqueness of the individual is ignored.

stimulus   Data to be perceived. Anything in the experiential field that arouses an individual or impinges upon the perceptual mechanisms of that individual.

strategy   Application of a plan to control another. In interpersonal communication, strategy fosters defensiveness. Opposite is spontaneity.

structure   The arrangement of components of a system at any given moment in time.

style   Having to do with leadership. Style is the general approach that an individual takes while providing leadership to a group.

substantive conflict   Conflict over ideas and issues. In group communication theory, conflict in the task dimension rather than in the social, or relationship, dimension of communication.

substitution   Using nonverbal messages instead of words to regulate another individual during a communication event.

superiority   Attitude or opinion that another individual is not equal to oneself. Opposite is equality.

supportiveness   Category of behavior identified and described by Jack Gibb that implies or suggests an interpersonal attitude characterized by candor, freedom of fear, and a sense of equality. Behaviors that yield a sense of supportiveness are: description, problem orientation, spontaneity, empathy, and equality.

survey interview   A method of collecting data in which a representative group of respondents is asked to answer standardized questions, and the data are tallied and analyzed to make statements about the group, its attitudes, and its opinions.

symbol   Anything that arbitrarily "stands for" something else. Symbols do not usually bear any natural relationship to the things for which they stand. For example, a flag bears no natural relationship to the country for which it stands. A word bears no natural relationship for the thing it represents.

symmetry   In communication, any response that mirrors the antecedent stimulus.

symposium   A form of group meeting used to present a variety of views in the form of short speeches or reports for the benefit of an audience. Moderator introduces a panel, provides history of the issues, presents each speaker, monitors time, and ends the meeting with a brief charge to the audience or a summary of the ideas and issues presented.

system   The sum total of all the components of a thing, plus all the relationships among those components, joined to form a single entity, and interdependent in such a way that any change in the system affects the entire system.

task difficulty   The amount of effort required to complete a task. As a general rule, complex tasks (those which have multiple causes and multiple solutions) are more difficult than simple tasks (those which have few causes and few solutions).

task dimension   The part of a communication event having to do with objects or ideas, as opposed to relationships.

territoriality   The notion of ownership or attitude of possessiveness that individuals develop toward a particular space or to particular objects.

theory   The foundation of an explanation or description of any complex phenomenon. Sometimes described as a complete set of "if-then" statements that serves to allow explanation or prediction.

tolerance threshold   A level of tension experienced by individual or groups such that any tension beyond that threshold must be addressed. The maximum tension that will not debilitate an individual or a group.

trait perspective   Attempt to understand leadership by examining the features of personality and behavior that are evidenced by leaders.

transaction   A pattern of interaction between people.

trust   Confidence in another person. Belief that the behavior of another person can be predicted.

value   The worth of something. The characteristic or quality of a thing that renders it desirable.

variable   Something that can increase or decrease in some dimension, as in the variable worth of the American dollar overseas. Something that can have different values.

withdrawal strategy   A conflict-management strategy in which a disputant leaves the conflict, either physically or psychologically.

TROUBLESHOOTING
THE SMALL GROUP

Many college graduates keep a library of reference works to help them resolve problems in their professional and social life. Sooner or later they encounter communication problems. We want this book to be helpful as a tool for dealing with the common communication problems that occur in small groups.

Many texts written for the college classroom do not lend themselves well to being useful references for solutions to problems. For example, a typical index—like the one at the end of this book—presents a fairly thorough list of key words. But that kind of index is not a very helpful problem-solving reference because it is not problem-specific. Thus you have to read through many sections of a book to find answers to specific questions. Our solution was to develop this troubleshooting guide.

The guide poses over eighty of the most common questions people in groups ask about communication problems. We have indexed these problems in a way that refers you to the locations in the book where solutions are suggested.

How to Use This Problem-Solution Index

1. Verbalize the problem you are experiencing.

2. Look for key words that describe the nature of the problem. Key words are listed alphabetically in the directory that follows.

3. Locate these key words in the problem-solution index.

4. Find a question similar to the one you are asking, and turn to the indicated sections for the answer.

5. If the key words are not listed here, consult the index in the back of the book for the location of information related to your problem.

Directory

Problem Category	Page	Problem Category	Page
Attending	344	Inference problems	348
Climate	344	Interpersonal conflict	348
Cohesiveness	345	Language use	348
Communication effectiveness	345	Leader–member communication	348
Conference planning	345	Leadership	349
Conflict	345	Member development	350
Co-member communication	346	Monthly meeting planning	350
Credibility	346	Nonverbal communication	350
Decision making	346	Perception	350
Dress	346	Primary tension	351
Giving instructions	346	Relationship problems	351
Group	347	Remembering	351
Failure	347	Roles	351
Formation	347	Secondary tension	351
Participation	347	Social dimension	351
Size	347	Task dimension	352
Ideational conflict	347	Tension level	352
Impression management	347	Time analysis	352

PROBLEM CATEGORY AND QUESTION(S)	LOCATION OF SOLUTIONS
A *Attending*	
I find that even though I hear and remember what a group member has said, I have not gotten it straight. What might be the problem?	43–44, 82–87
What can I do to help my group members be more accurate in perceiving what I say?	82–92, 227–228
B *(No Entries)*	
C *Climate*	
Members seem to dread conflict in our group meetings. Why?	238–240, 264–266

PROBLEM CATEGORY AND QUESTION(S)	LOCATION OF SOLUTIONS
There seems to be quite a lot of tension lately in our group. Why might this be the case?	133–137, 150–154 260–264
When I get into an argument, it seems to escalate. Why?	133–137, 255–264

Cohesiveness

Many of our meetings are not very productive. Is there anything I can do?	184–191, 204–212
I've noticed that some groups seem to be too social—they never get much done. Why is this the case? What can be done about the problem?	198–202, 206–214
The members of my group do not seem to enjoy one another; the group does not pull together. What's wrong? What can I do?	150–154, 184–191, 198–212, 262–279

Communication Effectiveness

I know that everything I do as a group member is related to my verbal and nonverbal effectiveness. How can I increase my effectiveness?	90–92, 102–104

Conference Planning

I must plan a conference. What do I do first? Next?	315–327

Conflict

My group has a member who picks fights. Is there something I can do about this?	266–274
My group has a member who is always challenging other people's ideas. Should I put a stop to this? Can I put a stop to it?	262–264, 274–279
I have to work on a committee with a person who does not get along with others. How can I handle this situation?	52–62, 63–65, 240–244, 266–274
There seems to be quite a lot of tension in our group lately. Why might this be the case?	133–137, 150–158, 262–263
When I get into an argument, it seems to escalate. Why?	238–240, 255–260
I've just goofed. If I tell the boss, he'll be angry. If I don't tell the boss, the group project may fail. How can I manage this kind of conflict?	90–92, 238–240, 262–264
Joan and Pete are having trouble getting along. What do I do?	187–191, 238–240, 268–274

PROBLEM CATEGORY AND QUESTION(S)	LOCATION OF SOLUTIONS
Competition is destroying my group. I think it will soon become open warfare. What can I do?	238–240, 263–264, 266–274
I need to manage this conflict successfully. As leader, should I force a decision or should I confront these people and do problem solving?	264–268
Some groups I know about seem to fight all the time. Others seem not to fight at all. Is there some way of knowing what is healthy for a group?	124–130, 255–257

Co-member Communication

I often want reasonable things from my co-members but they do not comply.	83–84, 262–264

Credibility

I am not sure that others will believe me. What can I do?	23–25, 39–45

D
Decision Making

We need to have a meeting to decide _____. What is important to remember about decision-making meetings?	7–8, 51–62, 68–70

Dress

I'm going to attend a meeting of a task force and want to know how I should dress.	98–99

E
(No Entries)

F
(No Entries)

G
Giving Instructions

People don't seem to do what I ask them to. Why? What can I do about this?	79–92, 106–107, 238–240

PROBLEM CATEGORY AND QUESTION(S)	LOCATION OF SOLUTIONS
Group Failure	
When I'm in charge of a group, I want to be sure it is successful. What are some of the common reasons groups fail?	120–141, 150–162, 212–218, 264–266
Group Formation	
I have noticed that I'm nervous when I have to participate in a group. Why is this? Is this normal?	133–135
I have just been given my first big promotion and have been asked to head a special-project group. Are there any special considerations I should give to the makeup of the group?	32–33, 120–124, 204–206
Group Participation	
I have to work on a committee with a person who does not get along with other people. How can I handle this situation?	51–62, 64–65, 240–244, 264–274
The members of my group do not seem to enjoy one another; the group does not pull together. What's wrong? What can I do?	150–154, 184–191, 198–212, 263–264
Many of our meetings are not very productive. Is there anything I can do to change this?	184–191, 204–212
Group Size	
I have just been given my first big promotion and have been asked to lead a special-project group. Are there any special considerations I should give to group size?	32–33, 120–124, 204–206

H
(No Entries)

I
Ideational Conflict

My group has a member who is always challenging other people's ideas. Should I put a stop to this? Can I put a stop to this?	262–264, 274–279
Impression Management	
I am going to start work on a special task force, and I want to make a good impression. What can I do?	34–45, 90–92, 96–104

PROBLEM CATEGORY AND QUESTION(S)	LOCATION OF SOLUTIONS
Inference Problems	
When I am straightforward about the facts of a situation, the other person does not seem to understand these facts. We argue a lot.	79–89
Interpersonal Conflict	
John and Pete are having trouble getting along. What do I do?	187–190, 238–240, 268–274
Competition is destroying my group. I think it will soon become open warfare. What can I do?	238–240, 263–264 266–274
I need to manage this conflict successfully. As leader, should I force a decision or should I confront these people and do problem solving?	264–268

J
(No Entries)

K
(No Entries)

L
Language Use

I often want reasonable things from my co-members but they do not comply.	83–84, 262–264
When I am straightforward about the facts of a situation, the other person does not seem to understand these facts. We argue a lot.	79–89
Leader–Member Communication	
People do not seem to do what I ask them to do. Why? What can I do?	79–92, 106–108, 238–240
I have a member who has a poor self-concept. What can I do to help?	225–236, 238–240
The group leader complains that I do not do things the way I should. (This means the way she wants me to do them.) What are some possible sources of this problem?	79–92, 240–244, 262–264

PROBLEM CATEGORY AND QUESTION(S)	LOCATION OF SOLUTIONS
When I talk to the group leader, I feel tense. What might be wrong? What can I do?	240–244, 262–267

Leadership

I must plan a conference. What do I do?	315–327
I must lead a group. What do I need to consider in my planning?	36–45, 51–70, 184–187
The boss is going on vacation, and I will be in charge of the department's monthly meeting. What do I do first? Next?	7–8, 51–62, 184–187
We need to have a meeting to decide _____. What is important to remember about decision-making meetings?	7–8, 51–62, 68–70
Many of our meetings are not very productive. Is there anything I can do to change the situation?	184–191, 204–212
I've noticed some groups seem to be too social—they never get much done. Why is this the case? What can be done about the problem?	198–202, 206–216
A member won't participate. Why? What can I do?	188–189
A member monopolizes the discussion. What can I do?	188–189
Members are apathetic; they don't seem to care. What are some causes of apathy? What can I do?	188–189
I know that everything I do as a group member, and eventually as a leader, depends on the quality of my thought. What should I know about this?	124–137, 202–212
A member is being disruptive. What's wrong? What can I do?	150–154, 160–162, 262–279
My group has a member who picks fights. Is there something I can do?	266–274
I have to work on a committee with a person who does not get along with others. How can I handle this situation?	51–62, 64–65, 240–244, 264–274
Members of my group do not seem to enjoy one another; the group does not pull together. What's wrong? What can I do?	150–154, 184–191, 198–212, 263–264
There seems to be quite a lot of tension in our group lately. Why might this be the case?	133–137, 150–158, 262–263

PROBLEM CATEGORY AND QUESTION(S)	LOCATION OF SOLUTIONS
Some people seem to want more structure in the group; others seem to want less. What should I do?	36–39
I am anticipating the first meeting of my special-project group next week. I would like to be selected to lead this group. What can I do?	96–101, 171–177, 182–184
Competition is destroying my group. I think it will soon become open warfare. What can I do?	238–240, 263–264, 264–275

M
Member Development

I have group members who have poor self-concept and lack motivation. What can I do to help?	83–84, 262–264

Monthly Meeting Planning

The boss is going on vacation and I am in charge of the department's monthly meeting. What do I do first? Next?	7–8, 51–62, 184–187

N
Nonverbal Communication

I am going to the first meeting of the XYZ committee, and I want to know how I should dress.	98–99
I am going to start work with the special-projects committee, and I want to make a good impression. What can I do?	98–102
I am leading a committee meeting. How should I arrange the room?	96–98
I am anticipating the first meeting of the XYZ group next week. I would like to be selected to lead this group. What can I do to help myself?	96–102

O
(No Entries)

P
Perception

The boss complains that I do not do things the way I should.	79–92, 240–244, 262–264

PROBLEM CATEGORY AND QUESTION(S)	LOCATION OF SOLUTIONS
(This means the way the boss wants me to do them.) What are some possible sources of this problem?	
I find that even though I hear and remember what the boss said, I have not gotten it straight. What might be the problem?	43–44, 83–84
What can I do to help my fellow members to be more accurate in perceiving what I say?	83–86, 227–228

Primary Tension

I have noticed that I am nervous when I have to participate in a group. Why is this? Is this normal?	133–135

Q
(No Entries)

R
Relationship Problems

I have to work on a committee with a person who does not get along with others. How can I handle this situation?	51–62, 63–65, 262–263, 266–274
When I talk to my group leader, I feel tense. What might be wrong? What can I do?	240–244, 262–263
I would like to develop closer relationships with a few of my co-workers. How do I start?	108–112, 225–244

Remembering

When I attend the departmental meeting, I cannot remember what was said. I often need to recall this information. What might I do?	108–112

Roles

My group is having problems completing the task. Might this be a role problem? What are some essential roles?	154–160
How is it that certain people take on certain roles?	149–153

S
Secondary Tension

Some groups seem to fight all the time. Others seem not to fight at all. Is there some way of knowing what is healthy?	133–137

PROBLEM CATEGORY AND QUESTION(S)	LOCATION OF SOLUTIONS
Social Dimension	
I have noticed that some groups seem to be too social—they never get much done. Why is this the case? What can be done about the problem?	198–202, 206–212, 212–217
My group has a member who picks fights. Is there something I can do about this?	266–274
Task Dimension	
My group is having problems completing the task. Might this be a role problem? What are some essential roles?	154–160
Many of our meetings are not very productive. Is there anything I can do?	184–191, 204–212
Tension Level	
The group I am in is often very tense. What can I do to reduce tension?	135–137
I have noticed that I am nervous when I have to participate in a group. Why is this? Is this a normal reaction?	133–135

T
Time Analysis

How can my group manage time better?	37, 51–66

U, V, W, X, Y, Z
(No Entries)

PERMISSIONS
ACKNOWLEDGMENTS

Permission to reprint the following materials is gratefully acknowledged:

Table 3.1: From John K. Brilhart, *Effective Group Discussion*, 4th ed. Copyright © 1982 Wm. C. Brown Publishers, Dubuque, Iowa. All rights reserved. Reprinted by permission.

Figure 4.1: Figure "Thought or Reference" from *The Meaning of Meaning* by C. K. Ogden and I. A. Richards, reprinted by permission of Harcourt Brace Jovanovich, Inc. and Routledge & Kegan Paul Ltd.

Figure 4.4: Adapted from N. F. Russo, "Connotations of Seating Arrangements," *Cornell Journal of Social Relations 2* (1967); 37–44.

Figures 4.5 and 4.6: Adapted from *Use Both Sides of Your Brain*, copyright © 1983 by Tony Buzan. Reproduced by permission of the publisher, E. P. Dutton, Inc., and BBC Publications.

Table 5.1: Table from Marshall Scott Poole, "Decision Development in Small Groups, III: A Multiple Sequence Model of Group Development," *Communication Monographs 50* (1983), p. 327. Reprinted by permission of the Speech Communication Association.

Figure 6.1: Figure from *Discussion and Group Methods: Theory and Practice* by Ernest G. Bormann. Copyright © 1969, 1975 by E. G. Bormann. Reprinted by permission of Harper & Row, Publishers, Inc.

Tables 7.1, 7.2, and 7.3: Leader Adaptability and Style Inventory (LASI). Copyright 1974, *Training and Development Journal*, American Society for Training and Development. Reprinted with permission. All rights reserved.

Table 7.2: Adapted by permission of *Harvard Business Review*. Exhibit from F. E. Fiedler, "Engineer the Job to Fit the Manager," *Harvard Business Review*, September–October 1965, 118. Copyright © by the President and Fellows of Harvard College. All rights reserved.

Figure 7.1: Reprinted with permission from F. E. Fiedler, *A Theory of Leadership Effectiveness* (New York: McGraw-Hill, 1967).

Figure 8.3: Adapted with permission of The Free Press, a Division of Macmillan, Inc., from *Decision Making* by Irving L. Janis and Leon Mann. Copyright © 1977 by The Free Press.

Figure 9.3: Source: Joseph Luft, *Group Processes: An Introduction to Group Dynamics* (Mountain View, Cal., Mayfield, 1984).

Table 9.1: Adapted from Jack R. Gibb, "Defensive Communication," *Journal of Communication* (September 1961), pp. 142–148. Reprinted by permission of the International Communication Association.

Table 11.1: Table 6-1 from *Personality and Interpersonal Behavior* by Robert Freed Bales, copyright © 1970 by Harcourt Brace Jovanovich, Inc., reprinted by permission of the publisher.

Tables 11.4 and 11.8: From John K. Brilhart and Gloria J. Galanes, *Effective Group Discussion*, 6th ed. Copyright © 1989 Wm. C. Brown Publishers, Dubuque, Iowa. All rights reserved. Reprinted by permission.

Table 11.2: Reprinted by permission from Dean C. Barnlund and Franklyn S. Haiman, *The Dynamics of Discussion* (Boston: Houghton Mifflin, 1960), pp. 401–404.

Table 11.6: Reprinted from Stanley Seashore, *Group Cohesiveness in the Industrial Work Group* (Ann Arbor, Michigan: Institute for Social Research, The University of Michigan, 1954). Used by permission.

Tables 12.2 and 12.3 and Figures 12.1 and 12.2: Reprinted by permission of Random House from *Communicating in Business and Professional Settings* by Michael S. Hanna and Gerald L. Wilson.

Chapter Opening Photo Credits

Chapter 1: Susan Lapides/Design Conceptions

Chapter 2: Kathy Sloane

Chapter 3: Ulrike Welsch

Chapter 4: Janice Fullman/The Picture Cube

Chapter 5: David M. Grossman

Chapter 6: Kindra Clineff/The Picture Cube

Chapter 7: Jim Pickerell/Stock, Boston

Chapter 8: Rae Russel

Chapter 9: Steve Payne

Chapter 10: David E. Kennedy/TexaStock

Chapter 11: Richard Kalvar/Magnum

Chapter 12: Spencer Grant/The Picture Cube

NAME INDEX

Alderton, Stephen, 238
Alexander, Elmore R., III, 236

Baird, John E., 99
Bales, Robert, 125, 129, 290–291
Barker, Larry L., 313
Barnlund, Dean C., 263, 277, 278, 297
Becker, S. W., 98
Beisecker, Thomas, 261
Benne, Kenneth D., 154, 157, 160, 291–293
Blanchard, Kenneth H., 174, 193
Bogardus, Emory, 178
Bormann, Ernest G., 133, 150, 151, 162
Brandon, Arlene C., 260
Brilhart, John, 55, 62, 293
Buzan, Tony, 108–111

Campbell, Donald, 107
Canary, Daniel J., 269
Castro, Fidel, 213
Cragan, John, 206
Crowell, Laura, 137–139

Delbecq, Andre, 64, 65
Deutsch, Morton, 236, 255
De Vito, Joseph, 103
Dewey, John, 51, 52
Dobbins, Gregory, 187
Downs, Cal W., 178, 181
Dunphy, D., 202

Ebbinghaus, Herman, 108

Fiedler, Fred E., 179–181, 183
Filley, Alan, 267
Fisher, B. Aubrey, 125, 126, 129, 199, 261, 267, 269
Frey, Lawrence, 238

Gibb, Jack R., 110, 238–241, 244
Gibbs, Jack, 17
Goss, Blaine, 105
Guetzkow, Harold, 259, 277
Guyer, Barbara P., 174
Gyr, John, 259, 277

Haiman, Franklyn S., 263, 277, 278, 297
Hanna, Michael S., 324, 325, 327
Hawes, Leonard C., 257
Hayakawa, S. I., 84
Hearn, G., 97
Hersey, Paul, 174, 193
Heslin, R., 202
Hoffman, L. Richard, 261
Hook, L. H., 97
Howells, L. T., 98

Jago, Arthur G., 50, 51
Janis, Irving L., 212–217
Jochem, Lurene M., 55
Jones, Stanley E., 263, 274, 277, 278

Jourard, Sideny M., 232
Juran, Joseph, 66

Kelly, Charles, 110
Kennedy, John F., 213

Larson, Carl, 57, 58
Leathers, Dale G., 85, 99
Leavitt, Harold J., 255
Likert, Rensis, 268
Lippitt, Ronald, 176
Luft, Joseph, 233

McGrath, Joseph, 153
Mann, L., 216
Mann, R. D., 174
Maslow, Abraham, 96
Miller, George A., 176
Mintz, Norbett, 96
Mortensen, C. David, 178
Murphy, Albert J., 178

Nichols, Ralph, 106, 107

Ogden, C. K., 79
Osborn, Alex, 62

Pax, Timothy B., 176
Phillips, J. Donald, 65
Pickett, Terry, 178, 181

Poole, Marshall S., 128, 130
Powell, Larry, 190

Richards, I. A., 79
Rogers, Carl, 110
Rosenfeld, L. B., 176
Russo, N. F., 97

Sampson, Edward E., 260
Sargent, James F., 176
Scheidel, Thomas M., 137–139
Schlesinger, Arthur M., Jr., 213
Schubert, A., 99
Schultz, Beatrice, 187
Schutz, William, 229–232
Shaw, Marvin E., 178, 199
Sheats, Paul, 154, 158, 160, 291–293
Smith, David H., 257
Steinzor, B., 97
Stevens, L. A., 106
Stogdill, Ralph M., 178
Strodtbeck, F. L., 97

Vroom, Victor H., 50–51

Washington, Grover, 152
Wilson, Gerald L., 324, 325, 327
Wood, Julia, T., 183
Wright, David, 206

Zaccaro, Stephen, 187

SUBJECT INDEX

Abstraction(s):
  defined, 84, 329
  in language use, 84–85
Abstraction ladder, 85
Academy of Management Journal, 42
Achieved status, 262–263, 339
Affective conflict, 259–260, 331
Agenda(s), 329
  adapting to group's needs, 60–61
  for decision making, 51–62
  efficient use of, 61–62
  planning, 316
Agenda items, introducing, 188
Agenda steps, problem characteristics
    matched to, 60
Aggressor role, 160
Ambiguity, defined, 82–83
American Journal of Sociology, 42
American Photography, 42
Appearance, nonverbal codes and, 98–99
Applied Imagination (Osborn), 62
Approach-approach conflict, 256, 329
Approach-avoidance conflict, 256, 329
Arbitration, 70, 276, 279, 329
Ascribed status, 263, 340
Attending, 105, 344
  problems with, 106-107
Attending habits, 106–107
Attraction, 121–123
Audio-visuals, 317, 319
Autocratic leadership style, 175-176, 329

Bales' interaction categories, 290, 291
Barnlund-Haiman leadership rating scale,
    293, 295–297

Basic dynamics of groups, 15–21
Behavior
  basic assumptions of, 225–226
  basic model of, 226–227
Blaming behavior, 265
Blocker role, 160
Bormann's model of role emergence, 150–
    151
Brainstorming, 62–63, 330
Breakpoints, 129, 330
  normal, 129, 330
Brilhart-Jochem ideation criteria, 55–57
Brilhart postmeeting reaction questionnaire,
    297, 303–304
Brilhart problem-solving process scale, 293–
    299
Business Horizons, 42
Buzan curve, 108, 109
Buzz group (Phillips 66), 65–66

Centrality, defined, 245–246, 330
Certainty, defined, 239, 330
Channels, defined, 11, 330
Climate, 89–90, 237–244, 344–345
Closed-mindedness, 108, 215
Code, defined, 9, 330
Code of ethics, personal, in group discus-
    sions, 23–25
Cognition, 228, 330
Cohesiveness, 330, 345
  commitment and, 206–212
  conflict and, 261
  determinants of, 200–202
  effective participation and, 206–209
  group size and, 204–206

Cohesiveness (*Cont.*):
  leadership style and, 204
  productivity and, 198–200
  promoting of group, 196–218
Collective evaluation as group norm, 17–18,
    330
Collective expectation as group norm, 18,
    330
Colloquium, 312–313, 330
Commitment(s):
  cohesiveness and, 206–212
  conflict and, 261
  group goals and, 209–212
Communication:
  basic idea of, 9–15
  group (*see* Group communication)
  nonverbal (*see* Nonverbal communica-
      tion)
  transactional model of, 9–10, 15
  verbal, 82–89
Communication climate:
  creating an effective, 237–244
  defensive, 238–240
  supportive, 240–244
Communication model, 9–15
Communication networks, 244–247
  central positions in, 245–247
Communication process, components of, 9–
    15
Compromise, 68–69, 266, 267, 277–278
  defined, 266, 331
Compromiser role, 158–159
Conference planning, 315–327, 345
Conference-planning checklist, 326–327
Confessor role, 160, 161
Conflict, 345–346
  affective, 259–260, 331
  cohesiveness and, 261
  commitment and, 261
  defined, 255
  dysfunctional, 257, 332
  effect of, in groups, 256–257
  evolution of, 254–255
  functional, 257
  functions of, 260–261
  goal, 263–264, 333
  group productivity and, 261
  hostility and, 260–261

Conflict (*Cont.*):
  ideational, 262, 334
  intergroup, 257–258
  interpersonal, 258, 331, 348
  intrapersonal, 258, 331
  involvement and, 260
  nature of, 255–256
  power, 262–263
  sources of, 262–264
  status, 262–263, 340
  substantive, 259–260, 340
Conflict management, 264–279
  defined, 257
  dysfunctional strategies for, 264–266
  ideational, 274–279
  interpersonal, 268–274
  lose-lose methods for, 267
  strategies for, 266
  win-lose methods for, 267
  win-win methods for, 267–268
Confrontation checklist, 275
Confrontation-problem solving, 266–268,
    274–277
  defined, 266
Connotative meaning, 82, 331
Consensus, 68, 203, 331
Consumer Reports, 42
Content, paraphrasing, 109
Content dimension of group communica-
    tion, 13, 331
Contingency perspective and leader behav-
    ior, 179–182, 331
Control, defined, 238
Cooperation, 265, 331
Cooperation requirements, defined, 39
Coordinator role, 154, 156
Creative problem-solving sequence, 55–57
Creative thinking, stimulating, 190
Creativity, stimulating, 190
Critical thinking, promoting, 191
Culture, defined, 15–17, 331

Data collection, instruments for, 289–304
Decision making, 332, 346
  agendas for, 51–62
  by arbitration, 70
  by compromise, 68–69

Decision making (*Cont.*):
  by consensus, 68
  creative, 55–57
  judgmental, 65
  by the leader, 69–70
  by majority vote, 69
  methods of, 68–70
  in small group meetings, 50–70
Decision Making (Janis and Mann), 216
Decision-making discussion rating sheet, 298
Decision-making group, 5
  goal orientation of, 6
  individual vs., 50–51
  meetings for, 8
  mutual influence in, 6–7
  size of, 6
Decision-making sequences, 51–60
Defensive communication climates, 238–240
Defensiveness:
  categories of behavior and, 241
  conflict strategy for, 264
  defined, 236
Delphi technique, 64, 332
Democratic leadership style, 175–176, 332
Denotative meaning, 82, 332
Description, 241, 242
Descriptive comments, 241
Deserter role, 160
Designated leader, 170, 332, 335
Development, group, 125–133
Diagnostician role, 154–156
Discussion, guiding, 88
Discussion issues:
  focusing, 35–36
  group meetings and, 34–36
  kinds of, 34–35
Discussion participant evaluation, 300
Discussion techniques, 62–68
Discussion topics, research of, 39–45
Dominator role, 160–161
Dynamics of Discussion, The (Barnlund and Haiman), 297

Ebbinghaus curve, 108, 109
Effective Group Discussion (Brilhart), 299
Effective leader, characteristics of, 182–184
Elaborator-clarifier role, 154, 156

Emergent leader, 170, 332, 335
Emotional involvement, 37
Empathize, inability to, 107–108
Empathizing with speaker, 110
Empathy, 235–236, 241, 242, 332
Energizer role, 154, 156
Equality, 241, 243, 332
Ethical responsibilities in group discussion, 23–25
Evaluation, defined, 238, 333
Evaluator-critic role, 154, 157
Experience, different field of, 107
Experience overlap, 81–82

Face and eye behavior, nonverbal codes and, 99–100
Facial expressions in nonverbal communication, 94, 97–98
Fact issues, 34
Fair play, commitment to, 24
Feedback:
  defined, 12, 333
  poor use of, 108
Feeling expresser role, 158, 159
FIRO: A Three-Dimensional Theory of Interpersonal Behavior (Schutz), 229, 330
Follower role, 158, 159
Food, success of meeting and, 319
Forcing, 266–267
  defined, 266, 333
Foreman and QC, The, 66
Forgetting curves, 108, 109, 333
Formal role, 149
Formats for public discussion, 310–314
Forum, 310–311, 333
Frame of reference, 81
Functional perspective and leader behavior, 177, 333
"Functional Roles of Group Members," 292–294

Gatekeeper role, 158, 159
Gestures in nonverbal communication, 94, 99
Goal conflict, 263–264, 333
Goal-oriented, keeping group, 187

Goal setting:
  long-range, 210–212
  short-range, 210–212
Group(s):
  activity, structuring and guiding, 187–191
  basic dynamics of, 15–21
  building and maintenance roles for, 157–160, 292, 293
  cohesiveness of promoting, 196–218
  conflict and productivity of, 261
  in context, 7–8
  decision-making (see Decision-making group)
  defined, 6–7, 334
  dynamics of, 15–21
  evaluation of, 288–305
  goals of:
    commitment and, 209–212
    perceived progress and, 203
  and group processes, 15–23
  and information-processing system, 22–23
  interaction in, 150–151
  needs of, adapting agenda to, 60–61
  observation of, 288–305
    ground rules for, 289
    small group interaction and, 288
  in public settings, 310–327
  reasoning in, 43–44
  size of, 37, 347
    and cohesiveness, 204–206
  structure of, 244–247
Group Cohesiveness in the Industrial Work Group (Seashore), 301
Group communication:
  social-dimension concerns in, 21, 339
  study of, 5–6
  task-dimension concerns in, 21, 341
Group culture, 15–17, 331
Group discussion:
  essential behavior in, determining, 23
  ethical responsibilities in, 23–25
Group meetings:
  discussion issues and, 34–36
  guide for planning, 298–327
  and information sources, 39–43
  kinds of, 7–8
  participant selection and, 32–33
Group norms, 17–19, 336

Group organization:
  amount of order (disorder) in, 36–37
  decisions concerning, 36–39
  efficiency and, 36–37
  group members' feelings and, 37–38
  group size considerations in, 37
  task nature of, 38–39
  time considerations in, 37
Group Processes: An Introduction to Group Dynamics (Luft), 233
Group processes, observation, 293–302
Group task roles, 154–157
Groupthink, 44, 212–217, 334
  antecedent conditions to, 214, 217
Groupthink syndrome:
  consequences of, 215–216
  model of, 217
  symptoms of, 214–215

Harmonizer role, 158
Hostility:
  conflict and, 260–261
  among group members, 37–38
Hotel, success of meeting and, 319–320
How We Think (Dewey), 52

Idea development, 137–141
Ideal solution sequence, 57–58
Ideational conflict, 262, 334, 347
Ideational conflict management, 274–279
Individual filtering system, 226–229
  cognition and, 228
  motivation and, 228–229
  perception and, 227–228
Inferences, 109, 334, 348
Informal role, 150
Information, 334
  adequate, 88–89
  preparing, 44–45
  too little, 87
  too much, 86
Information-giver role, 154, 155
Information overload, 86, 334
Information-seeker role, 154, 155
Information-sharing meeting, 7–8, 334
Information sources and group meetings, 39–43

Initiator-contributor role, 154, 155
Insulation of group, 214
Interaction categories, Bales's, 290, 291
Interaction diagram, 290, 334
Interaction observation forms, 290–291
Intergroup conflict, 257–258
Interpersonal conflict, 258, 331, 348
Interpersonal conflict management, 268–274
Interpersonal Conflict Resolution (Filley), 266
Interpersonal needs, 225–232, 335
Interpersonal needs continua, 230
Interpersonal relationships, 270–274
Intrapersonal conflict, 258, 331
Intrinsic interest, defined, 38, 335
Involvement, conflict and, 260

Johari window, 233–235

"Keep 'em talking" strategy, 266

Labels and language, 85–86
Laissez-faire leadership style, 175
Language use, 348
    abstraction in, 84–85
Leader(s), 169–171
    decision by, 69–70
    defined, 155, 335
    designated, 170, 332, 335
    effective, 182–184
    emergent, 170, 332, 335
Leader Adaptability and Style Inventory
    (LASI), 172–174
Leader behavior:
    contingency perspective and, 179–182,
        331
    functional perspective and, 177, 333
    perspectives on, 171–182
    situational perspective and, 178–179, 339
    style perspective and, 175–177, 340
    trait perspective and, 171, 174–175, 341
Leadership, 169–171, 349–350
    defined, 170, 335
    functions of, 171
    improving skills in, 184–191
    traditional constraints of, 214

Leadership rating form, 293, 295–297
Leadership-structuring style, 176, 335
Leadership style(s), 175
    and cohesiveness, 204
Listener attitudes, 107
Listening problems, 105–108
Listening process, 104–105
    components of, 104–105
Listening skills, developing, 108–112

Majority vote, 69, 276, 278–279, 335
Meaning:
    concept of, 79–81
    connotative, 82, 331
    denotative, 82, 332
Meaning of Meaning, The (Odgen and Richards), 79
Meaningfulness, 84
Mechanix Illustrated, 42
Meeting(s):
    preparing for, 185–186
    routine (information-sharing), 7–8, 334
    special-events, 8, 339
    task (decision-making), 8
Member satisfaction, sources of, 202–204
Memory aid, 110–111
Mental sets, 108, 335
Messages:
    defined, 10
    low intensity of, 107
    nonverbal (*see* Nonverbal messages)
    unaccustomed length of, 107
    verbal, 79–92
Metacommunication, 13
Modification as function of nonverbal messages, 94–95, 336
Morse code, 9
Motivation, 228–229
Motivational-hierarchy hypothesis, 180,
    334, 336

Name-calling, 265
Needs, meeting, 225–232
Network studies, 244–247
Neutrality, defined, 238, 336
Noise, 12–14, 336
    physical, 12, 337

Noise (*Cont.*):
    semantic, 12–13, 339
    systemic, 14
Nominal group technique (NGT), 63–64,
    336
Nonverbal codes, 96–101
    appearance and, 98–99
    face and eye behavior and, 99–100
    gesture, posture, and movement and, 99
    physical environment and, 96–98
    use of time and, 100–101
    vocalics and, 100
Nonverbal communication, 350
    facial expressions in, 94, 97–98
    gestures in, 94, 99
    increasing effectiveness, 102–104
Nonverbal messages, 92–104
    functions of, 94–96
        modification, 94–95, 336
        regulation, 95–96, 338
        reinforcement, 94–95, 338
        substitution, 95–96, 340
    problems with, 101–102
    understanding, 92–96
Norms:
    group, defined, 17–19, 336
    unproductive, 18–19

Observations, 20
Office of Strategic Services (OSS) Assess-
    ment Staff Report (1948), 178
Opinion giver role, 154, 155
Opinion seeker role, 154, 155
Order, need for, 36–37
Orienter-summarizer role, 154, 156
Overestimations of group, 214–215

Panel, 311–312
Paraphrasing, 109
Participant-analyst, 25, 336
Participant selection for group meetings, 32–
    33
Participation:
    cohesiveness and, 206–209
    effective, 206–209
    encouraging, 188
    motivation for, 120–124

Participation (*Cont.*):
    perceived freedom and, 202–203
    regulating, 189
Participative management, 66–67
Perception, 227–228, 350–351
    defined, 82, 336
Perceptual difficulties:
    meaningfulness, 84
    stability, 83–84
    subjectivity, 83
    in verbal communication, 83–84
Personal independence, 18–19
Phases:
    conflict, 126–127, 131
    emergence, 127, 131–132
    orientation, 126, 131
    reinforcement, 127, 131–132
Phillips 66 (buzz group), 65–66
Physical environment and nonverbal codes,
    96–98
Physical noise, 12, 337
Playboy/playgirl–clown role, 160, 161
Policy issues, 34–35
Population familiarity, defined, 39, 337
Postmeeting open-ended reaction sheet,
    294, 302
Posture and movement, nonverbal codes
    and, 99
Power conflict, 262–263
Problem characteristics matched to agenda
    steps, 60
Problem orientation, 241
    defined, 242, 337
Procedural assistant role, 154, 156–157
Procedural leadership functions, 177, 337
Productivity:
    cohesiveness and, 198–200
    defined, 21, 198, 337
Provisionalism, 241, 243, 337
Public discussion formats, 310–314
Public discussions, leading, 314–315
Public settings, groups in, 310–327
Punctuation, 15, 337

Quality circle, 66, 337
Quality Control, 66
Quarterly Journal of Speech, 42

Reaction to behavior as group norm, 18–19
Reasoning in groups, 43–44
Receiver/decoder, defined, 11–12
Recognition seeker role, 160, 161
Reflective thinking, 51–55, 337–338
Regulation as function of nonverbal messages, 95–96, 338
Reinforcement as function of nonverbal messages, 94, 338
Relationship dimension of group communication, 13, 21, 331
Relationships, tasks and, 19–21
Remembering, 105, 109–111, 351
    problems with, 108
Role(s), 351
    analysis of, 291–293
    defined, 149, 338
    formal, 149
    functional, in small groups, 154–157
    group building and maintenance, 157–160, 292, 293
    group task, 154–157
    informal, 150
    self-centered, 160–162, 338
    task, 291–292
Role behaviors:
    identification of, 154–162
    overlapping of, 161–162
Role conflict, 153–154
    defined, 153, 338
Role emergence:
    Bormann's model of, 150–151
    in small groups, 150–153
Role stability, 149, 338
Role strain, 153, 338

Schutz's theory of needs, 229–231
Seashore index of group cohesiveness, 294, 301
Secretary-recorder role, 154, 157
Selecting members, 30–31
Self-centered roles, 160–162, 338
Self-disclosure, 232–235, 339
Self-report rating sheets, 294, 339
Semantic noise, 12–13, 339
Sensing, 104–105
    problems with, 106

Shipping, importance of, 320–321
Single question sequence, 58–60
Situation in communication event, 14–15
Situational-control dimension, 180
Situational perspective and leader behavior, 178–179, 339
Smoothing, defined, 266, 339
Social-dimension concerns in group communication, 21, 339
Social-emotional roles, functional, 292, 293
Social leadership functions, 177, 339
Socioemotional agenda, 263–264
Socioemotional problem, 263–264
Solution multiplicity, defined, 38, 339
Source/encoder, defined, 9–10
Special-events meetings, 8, 339
Special-interest pleader role, 160, 161
Spiral model of idea development, 139–140, 339
Spontaneity, 241, 243–244, 339
Stability, 83–84
Standard setter role, 158, 159
Status, 339
    achieved, 262–263, 339
    ascribed, 262, 340
Status conflict, 262–263, 340
Status consensus, 203–204
    defined, 203, 340
Strategy, defined, 239, 340
Structure, 340
    deciding about, 36–39
Style perspective and leader behavior, 175–177, 340
Subjectivity, 83
Substantive conflict, 259–260, 340
Substitution as function of nonverbal messages, 95, 340
Superiority, defined, 239, 340
Supporter-encourager role, 158
Supportive communication climates, 240–244
Symposium, 312, 340
Systemic noise, 14

Task difficulty, defined, 38, 341
Task-dimension concerns in group communication, 21, 341

Task leadership functions, 177
Task meetings, 8
Task-process activities, 128
Task roles, 291–292
  functional, 292
Tasks and relationships, 19–21
Tension, social, 133–137
Tension levels, reducing, 190, 352
Tension releaser role, 158
Theory of Leadership Effectiveness, A, (Fiedler), 181
Thinking for yourself, 43–44
Thinking tentatively, 44
Thousand Days, A (Schlesinger), 213
Time considerations, 37
Time use, nonverbal codes and, 100–101
Topic activities, 128
Trait perspective and leader behavior, 171, 174–175, 341
Transparent Self (Jourard), 232
Transportation, group meetings and, 321
Triangle of meaning, 79–80

Trust, 236, 341

Understanding, 105
  of nonverbal messages, 92–96
  problems with, 107–108
Uniformity, pressures toward, 215
Use Both Sides of Your Brain (Buzan), 109–111

Value issues, 34, 341
Verbal communication, problems with, 82–89
Verbal effectiveness, increasing, 90–92
Verbal messages, understanding, 79–92
Victims of Groupthink (Janis), 212
Vocalics, nonverbal codes and, 100

Withdrawal, 266, 267
  defined, 266